Getting It Straight: A History of American Orthopaedics

Written by
Henry H. Sherk

Edited by
Robert W. Bucholz, MD
James J. Hamilton, MD

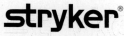

This book was made possible by
an educational grant from Stryker.

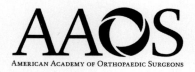

AMERICAN ACADEMY OF ORTHOPAEDIC SURGEONS

Getting It Straight: A History of American Orthopaedics

Published 2008
by the American Academy of Orthopaedic Surgeons
6300 North River Road
Rosemont, IL 60018

The material presented in *Getting It Straight: A History of American Orthopaedics* has been made available by the American Academy of Orthopaedic Surgeons for educational purposes only. This material is not intended to present the only, or necessarily best, methods or procedures for the medical situations discussed, but rather is intended to represent an approach, view, statement, or opinion of the author(s) or producer(s), which may be helpful to others who face similar situations.

Furthermore, any statements about commercial products are solely the opinion(s) of the author(s) and do not represent an Academy endorsement or evaluation of these products. These statements may not be used in advertising or for any commercial purpose.

ISBN 10: 0-89203-419-X
ISBN 13: 978-0-89203-419-2
Printed in the USA

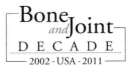

American Academy of Orthopaedic Surgeons

Table of Contents

Foreword

In 2008 the American Academy of Orthopaedic Surgeons celebrates its
75th anniversary. Since its inception in 1933, the exponential growth and
achievements of the Academy have been nothing short of phenomenal.
Few volunteer associations can claim the type of leadership position in a
medical or surgical specialty that the AAOS has assumed in orthopaedic
surgery. Therefore, its 75th anniversary offered an auspicious occasion to
tell its story.

But why write a scholarly book not principally on the history of the
Academy but on the history of orthopaedic surgery over the last century?
A simple answer to this question is that a history of the remarkable
growth of our specialty and the Academy's role in that specialty over the
last century has never been written. A historical text offers a wonderful
perspective on where we have been and even perhaps, where we are headed. Young orthopaedists especially should benefit from reading this history of the changing burdens of different musculoskeletal diseases, the innovations, the occasional technological dead ends, the recurrent socioeco-
nomic challenges, and the creative historical figures of our surgical specialty.

A more practical answer to the question is that while much has been
written on the origins and early years of orthopaedic surgery, little has
been written about the amazing advances of the last century. Such classic
historical texts as Bick's *Source Book of Orthopaedics*, Keith's *Menders
of the Maimed*, Rang's *The Story of Orthopaedics*, and Peltier's
Orthopedics – A History and Iconography provide extensive coverage of
the early founders of the emerging specialty of orthopaedic surgery.
Unfortunately, their coverage abruptly ends with the early twentieth century. None describes the critical role of the Academy during the period
after 1930 when orthopaedic surgery blossomed into the premier surgical
specialty.

The real answer to the question is that the level of historical knowledge possessed by the current generation of orthopaedic surgeons is
abysmal. As lifelong academic orthopaedic educators, we never cease to
be amazed by the rudimentary level of understanding of young
orthopaedic surgeons-in-training of the historical roots of modern
orthopaedic care. Harry Truman purportedly said "nothing is new in this
world but the history that you don't know." The purpose of this textbook
is simply to enhance all of our perspectives on the rich history of
orthopaedic surgery and its impact on our current practices.

Henry Sherk, one of the elder scholars of our specialty, possesses a
keen knowledge and insight into medical history that few orthopaedic surgeons can claim. His credentials as a medical historian are impeccable.
He was an obvious choice to author this textbook. His previous publications in medical history range over such diverse topics as the histories of
medical malpractice, military medicine, prohibition and the roaring twen-
ties, surgical anesthesia, smallpox epidemics, and numerous prominent

medical figures. He served as historian for the Medical Societies of New Jersey, the Camden County Medical Society, and the Somerset County Medical Society. He is currently Professor of Orthopaedic Surgery at Drexel University College of Medicine in Philadelphia.

Despite Dr. Sherk's tireless efforts to be all inclusive in his coverage of Academy and orthopaedic history, a lack of space necessarily curtailed the length of the book. The complexity and details of orthopaedic history preclude coverage of every important and interesting fact and trend in a single text. Consequently, the author had to pass over many of the seminal events in our story. Our specialty's growth over the past 100 years is attributable to the dedication and incremental advances inspired by thousands of practicing orthopaedic surgeons and researchers. Regrettably, not all can be mentioned here.

While drafts of the textbook were vetted by many individuals, historical documents are limited and their accuracy and interpretation are often open to debate. We ask that the readers recognize the problems of verifying many items from the records currently available.

Our Academy and our specialty should be sources of pride and satisfaction to the AAOS fellowship. This authoritative text provides an enjoyable read for all with an interest in our history. If it elevates the awareness of the reader to our origins, the many historical bumps in the road, and the incredible development of our specialty, then it will have met its purpose.

Robert W. Bucholz, MD
James J. Hamilton, MD
The Editors

Preface

One hundred fifty years ago orthopaedics as a surgical discipline hardly existed. A few individuals in New York and Boston and fewer still elsewhere called themselves orthopaedic surgeons, but their impact was minimal. They had little to offer patients suffering with musculoskeletal disease and deformities. They could only prescribe rest and immobilization with braces. In the early 21st century, however, thousands of men and women call themselves orthopaedic surgeons. A vast industry has evolved to support them and their patients with specialized instruments, implants, and medications. The public has instant name recognition for the term "orthopaedic surgeon," and insurers and the government set aside billions of dollars annually to cover the expenses of orthopaedic care.

This book seeks to tell the story of the rise of orthopaedics in America. The specialty originated in Europe and Great Britain in the late 18th and early 19th centuries; American physicians crossed the ocean to study and emulate techniques developing there. They eventually created their own version of musculoskeletal surgery in the United States.

Initially, in the 1850s and 1860s when orthopaedics began to be practiced as such in America, it dealt mostly with the musculoskeletal manifestations of tuberculosis. That disease afflicted large numbers of children during the middle of the 19th century, prompting a demand for physicians to treat them. Later, as the prevalence of tuberculosis declined, the waves of polio epidemics began. This occurred paradoxically because of cleaner water and better sanitation. The enteric poliovirus was present in the drinking water of most Americans until the late 19th century, a fact that conferred a herd immunity to polio. The loss of this immunity allowed polio to infect thousands of children and adults, many of whom required orthopaedic care. After the advent of the polio vaccines, orthopaedics took off in new directions. Total joint replacements and arthroscopic surgery led to a revolution in the specialty in the late 1970s and early 1980s. The stage was set for this revolution, however, by a decision of the Surgeon General of the Army in World War II. He was an orthopaedic surgeon, and ordered that all fractures in the army would be treated or supervised by members of his specialty. Many physicians on active duty during the war years acquired an interest in orthopaedics as a result. They became the men who developed the discipline when the war was over.

This history is a celebration of the 75th Anniversary of the founding of the American Academy of Orthopaedic Surgeons. It has been written by an orthopaedic surgeon for other orthopaedic surgeons to provide insight into the origins of the specialty and how it developed. It is incomplete, of course, because orthopaedics continues to grow and change. The project was made possible with the support of an educational grant from the Stryker Corporation; I am grateful for their interest and help.

Acknowledgments

Dr. Stuart Hirsch, former Chair of the Council on Communications (now the Communications Cabinet), and Dr. Robert Bucholz, then President of the American Academy of Orthopaedic Surgeons, conceived the idea of a book on the history of Orthopaedics in celebration of the 75th anniversary of the Academy. Stryker Inc. provided the AAOS with a grant to fund the publication of the book. Dr. Robert Bucholz and Dr. James Hamilton reviewed and edited the entire text.

Chapter 1. Dr. Zachary Friedenberg provided references and information concerning 18th and early 19th century medicine and surgery in America.

Chapter 2. Dr. John Gartland reviewed and edited this chapter and provided references and information regarding the Philadelphia Orthopaedic Hospital. Dr. David Levine provided information regarding Dr. James Knight and the Hospital for the Ruptured and Crippled (later the Hospital for Special Surgery).

Chapter 3. Dr. Howard Steel provided information regarding the Shriners and the Shriners Hospitals, as did Dr. Peter Armstrong. Dr. Matthew Bueche provided information on the Pediatric Orthopaedic Society of North America. Dr. Dean MacEwen reviewed and edited this chapter.

Chapter 4. Dr. Zachary Friedenberg provided references and information concerning Dr. Norman Kirk and Kirk's role in the growth of Orthopaedics after World War II. Dr. Stuart Green granted an interview concerning his knowledge and experience with Gavriil Ilizarov's system of external fixation. Dr. Jeffrey Anglen provided information on the Orthopaedic Trauma Society, as did OTA Executive Director Nancy Franzon. Dr. Robert Bucholz also reviewed and edited this chapter.

Chapter 5. Dr. Marvin Steinberg and Dr. Richard Brand each reviewed and edited this chapter and made suggestions regarding the history of the total joint revolution. Dr. Henry Bohlman provided information and illustrations regarding the role of his father, Dr. Harold Bohlman, in the development of the Vitallium hip endoprosthesis.

Chapter 6. Dr. Henry Bohlman reviewed this chapter and provided information regarding development of spine surgery in the past 25 years. AAOS General Counsel Richard Peterson provided information on the pedicle screw lawsuits.

Chapter 7. Dr. Robert Leach extensively reviewed and edited this chapter.

Chapter 8. Dr. David Bush and Dr. Charles McDowell provided information and references concerning Sterling Bunnell and the American Society for Surgery of the Hand. Dr. Stuart Green's interview concerning Ilizarov's development of a new system of external fixation included information concerning limb lengthening, correction of deformity, and treatment of chronic infection.

Chapter 9. Ms. Debbie Stallings of Stryker Orthopaedics provided information concerning the manufacture of orthopaedic equipment and the relationship of orthopaedic surgery and industry. She also arranged for many of the illustrations provided by Stryker. Mr. Don Campbell, also of Stryker Orthopaedics, provided illustrations from his personal collection of photographs of orthopaedic devices.

Chapter 11. Mr. Nicholas Cavarocchi granted an interview in which he outlined his role in the opening of the Washington Office of the Academy. AAOS Chief Education Officer Mark Wieting wrote portions of this chapter and reviewed and edited this chapter. AAOS Public Relations Department Director Sandra Gordon wrote a portion of this chapter, as did International Department Director Lynne Dowling.

CHAPTER 1
PROLOGUE

Nicolas Andry and *L'Orthopédie*, 1742

In the late 1730s, the dean of the medical school at the University of Paris lost his job. He had always been arbitrary and opinionated, but now faculty members would openly refer to him as irascible, confused, spiteful, and jealous.[1] The dean had campaigned angrily and relentlessly against would-be surgeons at the University Medical School, even revoking permission—granted by the king himself—from a surgeon who had planned to establish demonstratorships.[2] The faculty and administration could no longer tolerate him; he had to go.

Finding himself suddenly unemployed in his late 70s, the former dean decided to write a book on the care of children with deformities, concentrating mostly on musculoskeletal abnormalities. He may have had trouble coming up with a title, because he had to create an 18th century neologism—orthopédie (French) or orthopaedia (Latin)—to describe his topic. His name was Nicolas Andry.

Priest, physician, professor, dean, and renowned savant, Andry was born in 1658 into middling circumstances during the reign of Louis XIV. Determining that the best way to improve his social standing was to study theology and become a priest, he completed his studies at the College de Grassins in 1685. However, he soon found that ecclesiastical life did not suit him and abruptly changed careers. By 1690, he married an apparently well-connected young woman named Jeanne Larin[3] and enrolled in the medical school at the University of Reims. Reims lost its accreditation through a royal edict, perhaps because the Archbishop at Reims was on the "wrong side" of an ecclesiological dispute; Andry transferred to the University of Paris, where he finished his studies seven years later. He was 39 years old.[1,4-6]

The early years of Andry's practice in Paris did not go well. His theories on the causation of diseases by worms caused people to begin calling him homine verminoso (the man of worms).[7] Even negative publicity, however, introduced him to the public, who then readily recognized his name. He had studied how physicians could interact successfully with patients, writing the thesis for his doctorate on that subject. The title of that work translates as *The Relationship of the Management of Diseases Between the Happiness of the Doctor and the Obedience of the Patient*. He remained unfazed by criticism and adverse remarks, successfully building a large following in Paris. By 1701, he had been promoted to the rank of professor in the medical faculty, and in 1719 he became dean. With the deanship also came the honor of an appointment to the editorial board of *Le Journal des Savants*, the modern world's first scientific journal, predating even the *Transactions of the Royal Society of London*.[8,9]

After he had lost control of the faculty and endured the humiliation of removal from his position as dean of the most prestigious medical school in France, Andry would have faded away into obscurity were it not for his book *L'Orthopédie*. He would have become a very minor figure, unknown and not even contemplated by his contemporaries, let alone their descendants 250 years later. His book, however, captured the attention of the physicians of his era; within several years of its publication in 1741, it was translated into Dutch, English, and German. It was widely read and used extensively as a serious medical text.[10] Andry did not experience *L'Orthopédie's* influence on his profession. He died at the age of 84, soon after he had completed it.

On the first page of the translation as *Orthopaedia*, Andry explains how he derived the term:

> As to the Title, I have formed it of two
> Greek Words, Orthos, which signifies
> straight, free from Deformity, and
> Paidion, a Child. Out of these two Words
> I have compounded that of Orthopaedia,
> to express in one Term the Design I pro-
> pose, which is to teach the different
> Methods of preventing and correcting the
> Deformities of Children.[11]

The frontispiece depicts a seated female figure with several small children beside her (Figure 1). She holds a ruler in her hands, on which the words "Haec est Regula Recti" (This is the rule for straightness) are inscribed. The famous crooked tree symbol for orthopaedics does not appear for more than 200 pages, near the end of the first volume. The symbol of the tree illustrates the text that deals with the correction of the deformed leg in a child:

> If the leg is already crooked you must
> apply as soon as possible a small plate of
> iron upon the hollow side of the leg and
> fasten it about the leg with a linen roller.
> The roller must be made tighter and tighter
> every day till it compresses sufficiently the
> part that buckles out, and that this com-
> pression may not hurt it, you must put a
> large compress under the bandage on that
> part of the leg. In a word, the same method
> must be used for recovering the shape of
> the leg as is used for making straight the
> crooked trunk of the young tree.

Andry's book asserts that preventing deformity in children is better than treating it. He stressed that prevention should entail active, volitional muscle contraction and exercise rather than passive stretching and motion performed by a parent or nurse (Figures 2, 3, and 4). Andry advocated bracing only if exercising and careful attention to posture and proper activities of children failed to prevent crookedness. Much of the first part of the book deals with his assessment of the work of two other authors regarding the treatment of crippled and deformed children. One was Scaevole de Sainte-Marthe,[1,12,13] who in 1584 had written a long poem on the subject of paedotrophia (child nourishment). He had dedicated it to King Henry III who, highly flattered, ordered Sainte-Marthe to translate it from Latin into French so that his subjects would benefit from it. Andry noted, somewhat carpingly, that "the hurry of business hindered him (Sainte-Marthe) to equip himself of this piece of duty to his Majesty." Sainte-Marthe's grandson eventually translated it, however, and it was widely read during Andry's time.

A closer contemporary, Abbé Claude Quillet,[11,14] had entitled his work *Callipaedia* (beautiful child) from the Greek words *kallos* (beautiful) and *paedion* (child). Quillet's book dealt primarily with the correct technique for conceiving a beautiful boy or girl and had relatively little to do with pediatrics per se. Andry noted acidly that Quillet had fallen into disfavor for mentioning royalty critically in his discussion of how to go about conceiving a beautiful child.

In the end, *Orthopaedia* is a minor work that has little relevance to orthopaedic surgery in the 21st century. Indeed, it is ironic that the man who coined the term that describes tens of thousands of physicians and surgeons actually hated surgeons and would rather lose his job than have them on his faculty.

The Enlightenment and John Hunter

Andry published *Orthopaedia* during the roughly 100-year-period known as the Enlightenment. That era spanned most of the 18th century, witnessing the creation of modern science and philosophy. The serious thinkers of the Enlightenment relied on data and experiment, and they based their conclusions on demonstrable facts. Andry was atypical in his reliance on empiricism and his own authority, reputation, and position.

By the end of the 18th century, the mathematicians and scientists of the Enlightenment literally created modern mathematics, chemistry, and physics.[15] Isaac Newton and Gottfried Wilhelm Leibnitz competed in the formulation of calculus, and Newton devised the equations that governed gravity and optics. Galvani, Volta, Ampere, and Benjamin Franklin worked out the nature and behavior of electricity. Names from that era—Bernoulli, Halley, Fourier, and Celsius—are used adjectivally in physics and chemistry. Anton van Leeuwenhoek (born in the 17th century and surviving into the 18th) invented a microscope that could magnify small objects to 200 times their normal size; his work formed the basis for virtually all subsequent medical research involving the study of tissues and microorganisms. Carl Linnaeus of Sweden established the rules of taxonomy in botany, and Joseph Priestley[16] and Antoine Lavoisier[17] were the fathers of modern chemistry. They performed hundreds of experiments proving that air is a mixture of gases and water is a compound of hydrogen and oxygen. Lavoisier established the true nature of combustion and disproved the then-prevalent phlogiston theory. Scientists (including Priestley) held that all flammable materials contained an invisible, weightless substance called phlogiston that combustion would release, leaving an ash that was, itself, the true material. Lavoisier's work on dephlogisticated air led to his discovery and naming of oxygen.

Priestley and Lavoisier paid dearly for their commitment to science. Priestley was a dissenter in the England of King George III. His unpopular opinions and strange experiments inflamed a mob that burned down his house and forced him to flee to America. Lavoisier was seized by the revolutionary tribunal during the Reign of Terror and guillotined on May 8, 1794. When some of Lavoisier's supporters pleaded for his life on the grounds that he was too important to science to face execution, the presiding judge reportedly said, La Republique n'a pas besoins de savants (The Republic has no need for scientists).

The Enlightenment also produced men such as David Hume of Edinburgh, whose philosophic enquiries into morality, religion, and politics contributed to a complete reordering of European and American culture and society. His books and essays (A Treatise of Human Nature, Philosophical Essays Concerning Human Understanding and The Natural History of Religion) established the philosophic basis for the American Revolution and the constitutional form of government that was to follow. Hume's logic refuted the concept of the divine right of kings, and his skepticism concerning the motivations of human beings led to his blueprint for exploiting self-interest for the common good, a concept inherent in the Constitution of the United States. The father of that document was James Madison, educated in the tradition of the Scottish Enlightenment at the College of New Jersey (later Princeton University).[18]

Although the advances in science and philosophy in the 18th century epitomized the Enlightenment, developments in medicine during the period could not be accurately described by that term. For example, Nicolas Andry did not use data obtained from experiments or a critical analysis of clinical results to support his claims and recommendations. He asserted that one or another approach to pediatric deformity would work because he had personally observed it. The conclusion that an outcome follows an intervention because of the intervention, however, does not constitute hard science. Doctors and surgeons of the time had to depend on using whatever seemed to produce a good result without knowing why or how they had achieved a cure, and empiricism was the basis for almost everything they did.

Many modern books on medical history describe the brave and energetic individuals who created the foundation of modern medical science before the arrival of Andry and the Enlightenment. Andreas Vesalius,[19]

William Harvey,[20] and Ambrose Paré[21] deserve honor and respect in this regard, but 18th century physicians could not exploit what their predecessors had begun. Science during the Enlightenment had progressed beyond their reach, and it would take time for doctors to catch up.[22]

Vesalius (1514-1564), for example, defied church doctrine to steal cadavers and conduct dissections in secret by candlelight. After publishing his famous work, *De Humani Corporis Fabrica*, he had to flee from his home in Padua because of the controversy it aroused. Harvey (1578-1657) deduced, after multiple animal experiments, that blood circulates and does not replenish itself day by day or hour by hour; that the heart is a pump that produces circulation of the blood; and that blood flows through arteries, into capillaries, and back to the heart via the veins. These basic concepts were radical ideas when first proposed. Paré (1510–1592) was the military surgeon who stopped the process of searing battle wounds with hot irons or boiling oil to control hemorrhage and reintroduced the idea of tying off bleeding vessels with ligatures. Despite the progress made by these men, the transformation of medical science had to wait for the innovations of anesthesia, x-rays, and a more universal understanding of what true scientists had discovered.

Challenges to the old order of empiricism and unsubstantiated theorizing began to come from some of the schools where medicine was taught in the middle and late 18th century—particularly at the University of Leyden in Holland and at the University of Edinburgh in Scotland. Herman Boerhaave (1618-1738)[23] rejected the hands-off approaches of the earlier medical educators of the day (including Nicolas Andry); he taught his students to examine their patients, consider their problems at the bedside, and to recommend surgery when necessary. His pedagogy contrasted sharply with the airy theorizing of Nicolas Andry and his colleagues at the University of Paris, as well as the philosophies of other elite medical schools of the time. At those institutions, medical students could progress through an entire course of medical study without ever touching a patient. Boerhaave's methods became very popular and were quickly adopted elsewhere, especially in Scotland. There, medical education included anatomy and dissection and exposure to surgical training in the new science, thus blurring the class distinctions between physicians and barber-surgeons. Graduates of the Dutch and Scottish medical schools therefore became more successful in curing disease and repairing the injured. That success translated into more successful practices. Young, aspiring American medical doctors found it mandatory to spend some time polishing their credentials in Edinburgh to build better reputations back home. William Shippen and Benjamin Rush, two of the founders of the first medical school in British North America in 1771 in Philadelphia, attended the University of Edinburgh, as did John Morgan, the one-time Surgeon General of Washington's Continental Army.[24] David Hosack, an eminent New York physician and cofounder of Columbia's College of Physicians and Surgeons, also attended (Hosack was present at the Aaron Burr–Alexander Hamilton duel, and attended Hamilton's wounds until he died 36 hours later).[25]

The Scottish physicians and those they educated established a tradition of succinct, no-frills reporting that persists to this day. Many examples of the Scottish tradition come to mind, but first among them was John Hunter.[26,27] Hunter was born in Scotland, just south of Glasgow, in February 1728. His older brother, William, had a medical degree granted by the University of Glasgow in 1750; William had established himself as a physician and teacher of anatomy in London in 1756. He hired his younger brother, John Hunter, to assist in preparing dissections for the courses he was teaching there. John Hunter did this for 11 years, becoming profoundly knowledgeable about human anatomy as a result. At the end of the 11 years, he decided to study surgery and was trained by William Cheselden at Chelsea Hospital. John Hunter never actually pursued becoming a medical doctor and he never completed a course of study at the university, limiting himself always to the lower ranking of "surgeon." In the 1770s, he began teaching anatomy and surgery on his own. By this time, he had also completed a stint as an army surgeon. With his background in anatomy and practical professional experience, he achieved the ultimate success of being appointed physician extraordinaire to King George III.

John Hunter wrote prodigiously about medicine and surgery. Thousands of pages of his writings survive, but many more have been lost or destroyed. One of the executors of his estate, Sir Everard Home, made off with ten folio volumes of Hunter's manuscripts before they were published. Hunter's biographer, Drewry Ottley, suggested that this accounted for the fact that Sir Everard would in later years contribute more papers to the Royal Society than any other single member. He said that if Hunter's manuscripts could be recovered, they would be found to have furnished the substance of many of Home's numerous papers.[26] Hunter produced papers on the placenta of the monkey, the crop of breeding pigeons, how animals produce heat, hearing in fishes, whale anatomy, the gillaroo trout, bees, and electric eels. Hunter also wrote authoritatively about teeth and, in fact, gave them names still in use, such as incisors, bicuspids, and molars. His book *Principles of Surgery* gave the surgeons of that day logical, concise information that the modern reader can still appreciate. His descriptions of fracture healing, closed versus open fractures, bone growth, wound healing, and especially the classic chapters on inflammation were solidly based on his own observations and experiments.

Hunter died suddenly on October 16, 1793. He had championed the acceptance of two young aspirants for admission to the course of study at St. George's Hospital, but his colleagues and the board determined that they were unqualified and blocked their appointments. Hunter got into a shouting match over the matter and collapsed. He was pronounced dead at the scene.

Despite Hunter's extraordinary productivity, it is chilling to read his descriptions of wounds, infections, fractures, and other injuries and diseases. He continued to practice venisection and treated acutely injured patients by removing more of their blood than they lost from the wound they had sustained. Bullet wounds of the chest and abdomen almost always had fatal outcomes in that era; his patients invariably died despite his ministrations. He almost always autopsied them, detailing the path of the musket ball and describing the damage it had caused. He could not offer them any real treatment, however, and in describing bullet wounds of the limbs, he wrote at length on "the time proper" for removing incurable parts:

> It might appear that the best practice
> would be to amputate at the very first; but
> if the patient is not able to support the
> inflammation arising from the accident, it
> is more than probable that he would not
> be able to support the amputation and its
> consequences. . . The only thing that can
> be said in favor of amputation on the
> field of battle is, that the patient may be
> moved with more ease without a limb
> than a shattered one. . . and it has been
> found, I say, that few did well who had
> their limbs cut off on the field of battle;
> while a much greater proportion have
> done well in similar cases who were
> allowed to go on till the first inflamma-
> tion was over and underwent amputation
> afterwards.[28]

Hunter's complete mastery of human anatomy and his rational theories concerning inflammation, wound healing, and surgical treatment in general did not really help him save lives or limbs. However, his work contributed to orthopaedics by emphasizing the need for better science to be applied to medicine and surgery.

In fairness to the physicians and surgeons of the 18th century, it must be acknowledged that individuals besides Hunter contributed to the art of medicine and the scientific revolution of the Enlightenment. Erasmus Darwin, for example, began formulating the theory of evolution, more fully realized in subsequent generations by his grandson Charles.[29] A physician named Bodo Otto, who had been trained in Germany, came to America in time to apply the techniques of smallpox inoculation to an immunologically naive Continental Army. His successful variolation (as opposed to vaccination) of large numbers of men kept the army in the field.[30] Vaccination (inoculation with cowpox) was developed and popularized by Dr. Edward Jenner, a student of John Hunter. Also during the 18th century, John Lind[31] worked out a controlled experiment that identified the cause and cure of scurvy. Havers developed an understanding of his eponymous haversian canal system; Percival Pott, a competitor of Hunter, described a type of ankle fracture and also gave his name to the spinal infection that later came to be recognized as tuberculosis. During the Enlightenment, Chopart, Scheele, Duhamel, and Haller published papers and books in Europe that still have relevance to modern medicine and orthopaedic surgery in particular. Scheele, Wollaston, and Heberden identified the differences between the various types of arthritis, such as rheumatoid, gouty, and degenerative.[32] Perhaps most important of these was Giovanni Battista Morgagni,[33] who revolutionized medicine with his commonsense analyses of thousands of autopsies. He related a patient's symptoms to specific organic and structural changes, and his writings had a huge effect on the physicians of the 18th century. Among other American physicians, John Morgan did not think his training was complete until he had actually visited Padua and seen Morgagni at work. More ominously, Sir William Blackstone in his 1705 *Commentaries on the Laws of England* discovered mala praxis (malpractice).

The Enlightenment came to an end when Napoleon Bonaparte became First Consul of France in 1799 and the 19th century wars began.

The Ether Dome and Listerism

In the early years of the 19th century, physicians and surgeons had few truly effective therapeutic modalities at their disposal. The short list of drugs that could be used with a clear conscience included laudanum for pain, Jesuit bark (quinine) for malaria, ipecac to induce vomiting, calomel (mercurous chloride) for constipation, and foxglove (digitalis) for dropsy. Jenner and Lind popularized vaccination and lime juice to prevent smallpox and scurvy, respectively, but these two epochal discoveries did not affect doctors' practices in their clinics or at the bedside. At this point, surgical management beyond the use of therapeutics required procedures that doctors could perform only by inflicting nearly unbearable pain. Patients and physicians therefore opted for surgical treatment as infrequently as possible. Amputations of mangled, crushed, or infected limbs; tooth extractions; or lithotomies for bladder stones comprised most of the surgical procedures that patients would accept, but only if the surgeon was known to operate speedily. Clearly, progress in surgery could take place only if it became possible to anesthetize patients during surgical operations. To quell the pain of surgery in previous centuries, physicians had attempted to use alcohol, opium, hashish, *Mandragora* (mandrake), and blows to the head, but these neither singly nor in combination rendered people insensate during surgical procedures; medicine had to wait to catch up to science.

As the philosophers (the label for scientists in the late 18th and early 19th centuries) unraveled the laws of chemistry and physics, physicians who had participated in the development of these disciplines began to recognize their possible applications to medicine. For example, Joseph Priestley discovered nitrous oxide in the 1760s[34] when engaged in the research of "airs," as gases were then called. Thirty years later, Humphrey Davy, while a young medical student, also began work on gases, particularly their therapeutic applications. He worked initially at a private laboratory called the Pneumatic Institution that Thomas Beddoes, with the financial support of Josiah Wedgewood (one of the Lunar Men[29]), organized near

Bristol in the English west country. Beddoes had enlisted Davy to take time off from his medical studies to do research into the possible use of gases for the treatment of tuberculosis. Shortly after he began research at the Pneumatic Institution, Davy investigated nitrous oxide by using himself as a research subject. On April 9, 1799, he recorded in his notes that he had anesthetized himself by inhalation of the gas. Davy soon moved on to bigger and better things. In 1820, he became president of the Royal Society. In the course of his ascendant career, he moved away from investigations of the anesthetic potential of nitrous oxide. He had recognized the potential of nitrous oxide, however, writing that it "seems capable of destroying physical pain, it may probably be used with advantage in surgical operations."[35]

During the early years of the 19th century, physicians, dentists, and thrill seekers experimented with nitrous oxide. They called it "laughing gas."[36] Itinerant lecturers and showmen often used it in demonstrations designed to attract audiences at lyceums and county fairs around the United States. After seeing one of these performances in 1844, Horace Wells of Hartford, Connecticut, made the same connection that Davy had four decades earlier. Wells and his partner, Riggs, used it successfully on a dozen patients for tooth extractions. Wells, buoyed by his success, proposed a public demonstration. He approached John Collins Warren, a surgeon at the Massachusetts General Hospital, requesting an exhibition of his technique there before the staff and students. Unfortunately, Wells did not give his patient enough nitrous oxide. The subsequent screams of pain associated with the unanesthetized tooth extraction elicited a derisive uproar from the spectators, delaying the wider use of nitrous oxide for almost 20 years. In June 1863, Dr. Colton, the itinerant showman who had inspired Wells, once again found himself in Connecticut, this time in New Haven. He attracted the attention of another dentist, Dr. Smith. Together Colton and Smith organized the Colton Dental Association, featuring painless extractions under nitrous oxide anesthesia. In a few weeks they removed 3,000 teeth in New Haven, and then moved on to New York City. Similar success there led to similar ventures in several other cities. Colton stated in his fliers and advertisements, "We have never had a fatal case or a case of serious ill effects from the gas."[36]

When nitrous oxide failed so publicly in 1844, other practitioners naturally wanted to turn to something else. An ancient substance that had been recognized several centuries earlier turned out to be what they were seeking. Valerius Cordus had come upon a new and extremely volatile liquid in 1543 that he called *oleum vitrioli dulce*. He produced it by heating a mixture of alcohol and vitriolic (sulfuric) acid. Others subsequently called it sulfurated ether and later, simply ether.[36] During the late 18th and early 19th centuries, physicians in Great Britain attempted treatment of tuberculosis with it; publications as early as 1818 discussed the anesthetic effect observed during its use for the treatment of consumption.[36] Like nitrous oxide, however, ether first found its widest use as a recreational gas breathed at "ether frolics" to induce drowsiness or sleep for fun. Physicians and dentists probably began to use ether as a serious clinical agent as early as the 1830s. In 1842, William E. Clark of Rochester, New York, had experienced anesthesia himself during one of several ether parties he attended. He subsequently administered ether to a young woman undergoing a tooth extraction. She went into a sleep deep enough to permit removal of the tooth without experiencing any pain. Clark went on to a distinguished medical career but did not report this event until 1881.[36] Crawford Long of Jefferson, Georgia, also used ether in his practice as early as 1842. He performed surgery over a period of 4 years on patients he had anesthetized, but waited until 1849 before reporting this experience in the *Southern Medical and Surgical Journal*.[36]

William G. T. Morton, a Boston dentist with questionable credentials, probably had enjoyed ether frolics in 1838 in the company of Clark, but decided to use nitrous oxide as an anesthetic in his dental practice after hearing about the success of Horace Wells in Hartford. Storing and administering nitrous oxide always presented difficulties, however, so Morton approached the Boston chemist and physician Charles P. Jackson for help. Jackson told Morton to forget about nitrous oxide and use ether instead. Morton then embarked on a series of tests and actively used ether in his dental practice. This culminated in the successful public anesthetizing of a patient undergoing surgery on a mandible by John Collins Warren at the Massachusetts General Hospital on October 16, 1846. More operations under Morton's ether anesthesia followed, and Henry J. Bigelow's "Insensibility During Surgical Operations Produced by Inhalation," was published in the *Boston Medical and Surgical Journal* barely a month later, on November 18, 1846. This publicity enabled the staff at Massachusetts General to lay claim to originality. Morton tried to patent ether anesthesia, but the Boston surgeons brushed aside his claims. Morton spent most of the rest of his life attempting to capitalize on his "discovery." Richard J. Wolfe, Morton's biographer and chronicler of the ether controversies, used words and phrases such as "unsavory," "limited talent," "so many flaws," and "lacking a sense of ethics and decency" in describing Morton, but the myth of his achievement led to the erection of monuments to his memory, and he is still a mainstay of the Massachusetts General Hospital's reputation.[37]

Charles Bullfinch, the New England architect of the early 19th century, designed the surgical amphitheater at Massachusetts General Hospital and supervised its construction from the laying of the cornerstone until he was called away to design the first dome of the U.S. Capitol. Bullfinch's plans for Massachusetts General Hospital called for a copper dome that capped a round tower mounted on a much larger dome-shaped structure. Multiple large windows in the tower let in the daylight necessary to illuminate the surgery below. Prior to October 16, 1846, the screams and pleas of patients undergoing operations reverberated off the walls, but the use of ether brought quiet. Not long after the Morton-Warren collaboration, someone started to call the surgical amphitheater the "Ether Dome" (Figure 5). The structure still stands and recently was completely and accurately restored to its 1846 appearance. The people who pass through there now are primarily tourists. The National Park Service has placed a bronze plaque in the building that reads in part:

> Ether Dome
> Massachusetts General Hospital
> This site possesses exceptional value in
> commemorating and illustrating the history
> of the United States.

Parenthetically, Bullfinch's dome on the U.S. Capitol at one time closely resembled the Ether Dome. Observers complained that the Capitol's dome was too low, too modest, and out of proportion with the rest of the building. During the Civil War, Congress decided to remove it and replace it with the current structure designed by the Philadelphia architect Thomas Ustick Walter.[38]

The discovery of anesthesia revolutionized medicine and surgery, and its use swept the world within a short time after Bigelow's 1846 paper. Two European chemists, Soubeiran in France and von Liebig in Germany, both discovered chloroform in 1831, working independently. Heavier and more difficult to ignite, it had an advantage over sulfurated ether.[36] Surgeons in the United States continued to use primarily ether, despite its volatility and tendency to explode because it seemed safer and less toxic than chloroform. Their counterparts in Great Britain and Europe, however, tended to avoid ether and use the more recently discovered agent chloroform.

Antiseptic Surgery

Anesthesia made modern surgery possible. With its advent, physicians could perform operations carefully, allowing frenetic speed to give way to deliberate and more artful technical undertakings. In the mid-19th century, however, surgery remained prohibitively risky because of the nearly inevitable likelihood of postoperative infection. Physicians could not perform procedures in the chest or abdomen because of the universally septic outcome. Operations on the musculoskeletal system posed such serious risks that patients would rarely accept surgical treatment, even though ether, chloroform, or nitrous oxide could make the actual procedure painless.

John Rhea Barton's case report serves as an example. In 1825, Barton (1794-1871) performed a subtrochanteric osteotomy on the right leg of a young man who had a stiff hip fused in severe flexion and adduction. The patient, 21-year-old John Coyle, had sustained a fracture, dislocation, or both in a fall from a hatchway into the hull of a ship. He received essentially no treatment of the injury and developed stiffness and deformity as a result. When he finally returned home more than a year after his injury, Coyle came under the care of several physicians at Pennsylvania Hospital in Philadelphia. He remained hospitalized there for a year.

Eventually, Barton offered Coyle an osteotomy to correct the deformity and Coyle accepted. Barton has received accolades and virtual academic immortality for his visionary approach to Coyle's problem. In fact, the chairman of the Department of Surgery at the University of Pennsylvania today usually occupies the John Rhea Barton Chair. Barton performed the procedure before the advent of anesthesia, but he did it quickly so that Coyle tolerated it well. Barton expertly exposed the upper femur and sawed through it to facilitate realignment of the leg. The 7-minute operation succeeded admirably in correcting the deformity, and Barton attempted to maintain motion at the joint by moving the leg regularly to prevent bony union at the site of the osteotomy. Subsequent historians have hailed this undertaking as the first arthroplasty done in the United States, if not in the world. A close reading of Barton's report, however, reveals what Coyle went through after the surgery and shows the horror of untreatable sepsis during those times. Barton's postoperative notes read (in part) as follows:

Day 2	Lips of wound much swollen and everted—very painful.
Day 5	Approaching suppuration.
Day 6	Some pus secreted.
Day 8	Wound suppurating.
Day 10	Whole surface of wound covered with granulation.
Day 17	Matter copiously excreted from the cavity of the wound and from under the fascia over the rectus muscle.
Day 30	Pus diminishing in quantity.
Day 61	Considerable fluctuation discoverable along the direction of the rectus femoris.
Day 62	A quantity of fluid escaped by a . . . sinuous opening in the cicatrix.
Day 84	The thigh bore marks of approaching inflammation . . . and erysipelatous blush with tumefaction.
Day 85	Fever much abated . . . erysipelas subsiding.[39]

Through all this, Coyle submitted to frequent, if not daily, passive moving of his leg to prevent union of the osteotomy. All of his systemic symptoms were described by Barton and, as expected, included fevers, nausea, vomiting, and cachexia that gradually subsided. By 3½ months after the surgery, Barton could write that Coyle was "walking about and gaining strength." He could actively move his hip "with perfect ease."

Coyle apparently retained useful motion for about 6 years, but thereafter the hip gradually lost mobility and re-ankylosed, albeit in a position con-

sidered better than his original flexion and adduction. Coyle died of tuberculosis not long thereafter, and Barton performed the autopsy. He found that
the femoral head had fused with the acetabulum as a result of the original
injury and that the osteotomy had solidly united.[39]

Barton had achieved a reasonable result in the treatment of John Coyle's
deformity but at great cost. Coyle's youthful determination and courage
made the good outcome possible; clearly, only young, robust, and extraordinarily well-motivated people could tolerate this surgery even if the operation was performed under anesthesia and painless. There had to be a better way. Surgeons had to find some means of circumventing sepsis and
infection. They found it in the work of Joseph Lister.[40,41]

Joseph Lister (1827–1912) (Figure 6) lived at the same time as Louis
Pasteur (1833–1895). While Pasteur worked as an investigative scientist
and microbiologist, Lister was a surgeon. Lister had achieved academic and
professional success by the middle of the 19th century, but like all of his
surgical predecessors and colleagues he was appalled by the number of
complications that followed his operations. When he reviewed the results of
his own series of amputations done from 1864 through 1866, he found that
45 percent of his patients died from postoperative sepsis. Lister's mentor at
Edinburgh, James Syme, advised careful attention to cleanliness before,
during, and after surgery, but Lister found that his best efforts in this regard
still failed to change the overall results. He observed, however, that closed
fractures, when treated with closed techniques, never got infected, whereas
open fractures almost always did. At about this time, while puzzling over
this phenomenon, he heard about the work of Louis Pasteur in France. A
professor of chemistry at the University of Glasgow, where Lister was
working, had mentioned to him that Pasteur had proved that microorganisms in the air caused fermentation and putrefaction. Lister was ready to
apply Pasteur's conclusions to his own problems. Indeed, in his 1867 article "Observations on the Condition of Suppuration" he noted: "We find that
a flood of light has been turned upon this most important subject by the
philosophic researches of M. Pasteur who has demonstrated by fairly con-
vincing evidence that it is not to its oxygen . . . that air owes this property,
but to minute particles suspended in it, which are the germs of various low
forms of life."[41]

Immediately after hearing of Pasteur's work, Lister began searching for
a chemical agent that would kill the "germs." In short order, he came upon
carbolic acid. He had heard that the town of Carlisle used it to detoxify
sewage, noting that "the admixture of a very small proportion not only prevents all odour from the lands irrigated with the refuse material but, as it
was stated, destroys the entozoa that usually infect the cattle fed upon such
pastures." In his early use of carbolic acid, Lister merely soaked a strip of
calico or lint with it and cleaned out the wound using the cloth as a swab.
He also used dressings that had been soaked in carbolic acid to cover
wounds, placing a strip of tin foil over the dressing to prevent evaporation.
The resultant drop in the number of infections to zero in the first 9 months
of his use of carbolic acid convinced Lister that he had come upon the only

way to control surgical sepsis; he no longer needed to regard erysipelas, pyemia, gangrene, and "laudable pus" as inevitabilities in most of his patients. In Great Britain and the United States, Listerism initially met with indifference, if not hostility, especially after Lister began his attempts to sterilize the air of the operating theater with carbolic acid spray. In fact, it took more than 20 years for Listerism to meet with general acceptance at home and in the United States.

In Europe, however, the discoveries of Robert Koch, Louis Pasteur, and Rudolf Virchow had become widely known; German and French surgeons embraced Listerism almost immediately. The disdainful treatment of Ignaz Semmelweis perhaps lay heavily on the conscience of physicians and surgeons on the continent. Nearly 10 years before Lister's publication, Semmelweis had published his famous paper on the cause of "childbed fever," also known as puerperal sepsis. For 15 years, Semmelweis had studied the problem and had tried to understand why so many women in Vienna hospitals died of this disease. He determined that the contagion was brought to them by carriers who on "the examining finger, the operating hand . . . sponges, the hands of midwives and nurses" transferred organic material to the vulnerable tissues of women in labor.[42] The medical community in Vienna and Budapest scorned Semmelweis, who died insane in 1865, ironically of generalized sepsis resulting from an infected finger.

The bacteriologists of Europe and a surgeon in Scotland had brought surgery to the point at which surgeons could perform operations inside any body cavity (chest, abdomen, cranium, and articulations of the extremities). The elimination of pain during surgery due to the advent of effective anesthesia, along with the conquest of postoperative infection, paved the way for the medical profession to embark on a new era by the 1870s. At that point, the number of surgical procedures began to soar.[43]

References

1. Köhler R, Fischer LP: Nicolas Andry (1658-1742): L'inventeur du mot "orthopédie." *Ann Chir* 1999;53:335-339.

2. DePalma AF: Introduction, in Andry N: *Orthopaedia: or, the Art of Correcting and Preventing Deformities in Children: By such Means as may easily be put in Practice by Parents themselves, and all such as are employed in Educating Children*, ed 4. Philadelphia, PA, JB Lippincott, 1961. [Translated from French]

3. The Gennerat families and their alliances in Champagne (France). Available at http://gennerat.free.fr/english/pafg47.htm#514.

4. Andry de Boisregard N: *L'Orthopédie l'Art de Prevenir et de Corriger dans les Enfans les Difformités du Corps: Le Tout par des Moyens a la Porte'e des Peres et des Meres, et de toues les Personnes qui ont des Enfans à élever.* Paris, France, La Veuve Alix et Lambert et Levand, 1741.

5. Lagard A, Michard L: *The Eighteenth Century.* Paris, France, Bardas, 1961, pp 109, 166.

6. Le Tellier C-M: *The Catholic Encyclopedia.* New York, NY, Robert Appleton, 1910. Available from http://www.newadvent.org/cathen/09200c.htm. (Accessed March 6, 2007)

7. Le Vay D: *The History of Orthopaedics: An Account of the Study and Practice of Orthopaedics from the Earliest Times to the Modern Era.* Park Ridge, NJ, Parthenon Publishing Group, 1990, pp 230-236.

8. Castiglioni A, Krumbhaar EB: *A History of Medicine.* New York, NY, Alfred Knopf, 1941, p 574.

9. Kirkup JR: Nicolas Andry and 250 years of orthopaedy. [editorial] *J Bone Joint Surg Br* 1991;73:361-362.

10. Guthrie D: *A History of Medicine.* Philadelphia, PA, JB Lippincott, 1946, pp 142-149.

11. Andry N: *Orthopaedia: or, the Art of Correcting and Preventing Deformities in Children: By such Means as may easily be put in Practice by Parents themselves, and all such as are employed in Educating Children,* ed 4. Philadelphia, PA, JB Lippincott, 1961. [Translated from French].

12. Gelis J: The child: From anonymity to individuality, in Aries P, Duby G, Chartier R (eds), Goldhammer A (translator): *A History of Private Life:* III. Passions of the Renaissance. Cambridge, MA, Harvard University Press, 1989, pp 313-314.

13. Tallmadge GK: Scaevola of Sainte-Marthe and the Paedotrophia. *Bull Hist Med* 1939;7:279-314.

14. Guillemaine C: Claude Quillet (1607–1661). *Cahiers Lyon Hist Med* 1959;4:3.

15. Hankins RL: *Science and the Enlightenment.* Cambridge, England, Cambridge University Press, 1985.

16. Holt FL: *A Life of Joseph Priestley.* London, England, Oxford University Press, 1931.

17. Holmes FL: *Lavoisier and the Chemistry of Life: An Exploration of Scientific Creativity.* Madison, WI, University of Wisconsin Press, 1985.

18. Herman A: *How the Scots Invented the Modern World.* New York, NY, Crown Publishers, 2001.

19. Saunders JB de CM, O'Malley CD: *The Illustrations from the Works of Andreas Vesalius of Brussels.* New York, NY, The World Publishing Company, 1950.

20. Harrison WC: Dr. *William Harvey and the Discovery of Circulation.* New York, NY, MacMillan Company, 1967.

21. Haas LF: Ambrose Pare, 1510-1590. *J Neurol Neurosurg Psychiatry* 1991;54:1068.

22. Cunningham A, French R: *The Medical Enlightenment of the 18th Century.* Cambridge, England, Cambridge University Press, 2004.

23. Knoeff R: *Herman Boerhaave (1668-1738): Calvinist Chemist and Physician. History of Science and Scholarship in the Netherlands Series.* Amsterdam, The Netherlands, Koninkli, 2002, vol 3.

24. Friedenberg ZB: *The Doctor in Colonial America.* Danbury, CT, Rutledge Books Inc, 1998, pp 160-191.

25. Robins CC: *David Hosack: Citizen of New York.* Philadelphia, PA, American Philosophical Society, 1964.

26. Ottley D: The life of John Hunter, in Palmer JF (ed): *The Works of John Hunter,* London, England, F.R.S. London, 1835, vol 1, pp 1-188.

27. Palmer JF: *The Works of John Hunter*. London, England, F.R.S. London, 1837.

28. Hunter J: *A Treatise on the Blood, Inflammation, and Gun-Shot Wounds.* London, John Richardson, 1794, p 561.

29. Uglow J: *The Lunar Men: Five Friends Whose Curiosity Changed the World*. New York, NY, Farrar, Strauss & Giroux, 2002.

30. Gibson IE: *Dr. Bodo Otto and the Medical Background of the American Revolution.* Springfield, IL, Charles C. Thomas, 1931, p 131.

31. Lind J: *A Treatise of the Scurvy*. Edinburgh, Scotland, Sands, Murray & Cochrane, 1753.

32. Bick EM: *Source Book of Orthopaedics*. New York, NY, Hafner Publishing Company, 1968.

33. Jarcho S: Giovanni Battista Morgagni, his interests, ideas, and achievements. *Bull Hist Med* 1948;22:503-524.

34. Priestley J: *Encyclopaedia Brittanica*, 15th ed, vol 9. Chicago, IL, 1987, p 967.

35. Davy H: *Encyclopaedia Brittanica*, 15th ed, vol 3. Chicago, IL, 1987, p 920.

36. Lyman H: *Artificial Anesthesia and Anaesthetics*. New York, NY, William Wood and Co, 1881, pp 5, 125, 278, 309, 498-450, 509.

37. Wolfe RJ: Tarnished idol, in William GT (ed): *Morton and the Introduction of Surgical Anesthesia*. San Anselmo, CA, Norman Publishing, 2001, p 500.

38. Kirker H: *The Architecture of Charles Bullfinch*. Cambridge, MA, Harvard University Press, 1969.

39. Barton JR: On the treatment of ankylosis by the formation of artificial joints. *North Am Med Surg J* 1827;3:279-400.

40. Lister J: On the antiseptic principle in the practice of surgery. *BMJ* 1867;2:246-248.

41. Lister J: On a new method of treating compound fracture, abscess, etc with observations on the condition of suppuration. *Lancet* 1867;1:326-329.

42. Semmelweis I: *The Aetiology of Childhood Fever*. Orvosi Hetilap (Medical Weekly), Pest, Hungary, 1858, p 33.

43. Pennington TH: Osteotomy as an indicator of antiseptic surgical practice. *Med Hist* 1994;38:178-188.

CHAPTER 2
THE ORIGINS OF AMERICAN ORTHOPAEDICS

Early Nineteenth Century Medicine in America and the Emergence of Orthopaedics

In the early decades of the 19th century, orthopaedics lacked an identity in America. Most people in that era would not have known what Nicolas Andry's invented word really meant. People did not live very long, and their health concerns centered on surviving the epidemics that periodically swept the country. Generally, only those who had orthopaedic conditions focused on orthopaedic problems. Yellow fever killed thousands during hot, mosquito-infested summers in places like New Orleans, Charleston, Baltimore, and Philadelphia. Smallpox and cholera also made dramatic, deadly appearances regularly. Infants and young children faced a multitude of diseases such as diphtheria, dysentery, measles, and tuberculosis, for which no truly effective therapies existed.

Doctors and patients paid little attention to chronic disorders of the musculoskeletal system. These were typically afflictions of older individuals who, in the early and mid-19th century, made up a much smaller percentage of the population than they do today. In 1800, only 18 percent of white men lived beyond 45 years of age, and the median age was 16. In 1998, the average life expectancy for white men at birth was 76.7 years; whoever reached 75 years could expect, actuarially at least, to survive for another 13 years.[1]

The system for educating and certifying physicians in the 19th century could not keep up with the demand. There were not enough men and women educated in the best medical science of the day to care for a population that soared sixfold, from 5.3 million in 1800 to 31.4 million in 1860.[1] The common illnesses (i.e., the infectious diseases) spread doctors too thin for them to develop much interest in the so-called orthopaedic disorders except, of course, for the treatment of musculoskeletal trauma. In addition, the knowledge that physicians possessed in that era did not equip them to deal effectively with many of the conditions they encountered. As a result, numerous diversions developed outside the mainstream of medical progress, such as herbalism, hydropathic therapy, and homeopathy. The top doctors—educated at places like Harvard, Columbia, and the colleges of Pennsylvania, Maryland, South Carolina, and elsewhere—employed useless and often harmful therapeutic measures until midcentury; no one really knew any better. Thus the fear of pain, illness, and even death made people accept almost anything. Doctors administered bleedings, purgings, blisterings, clysters (enemas performed with large volumes of various kinds of liquids), and harsh medications that actually sickened their patients. In a standard medical text published in 1855 that was used by medical students at the University of Pennsylvania, for example, an author recommended for the treatment of typhoid fever "bleeding in the early stages," followed by oral turpentine. If that did not suffice, "in cases of obstinate delirium or coma, great advantage is often derived from shaving the head and applying a blister over the whole scalp."[2] Oliver Wendell Holmes, reacting to the practice of this obviously futile therapy, wrote in 1860: "I firmly believe that if the whole materia medica, as now used, could be sent to the bottom of the sea, it would be all the better for mankind—and all the worse for the fishes."[3]

The public thus often sought out practitioners who would not hurt them, even if they did not help. Hydropathic therapy had considerable appeal for this reason. Hydropathic therapists claimed that patients could expect relief from almost any complaint by immersion in allegedly special waters. These waters came out of the Earth from places like Saratoga Springs in New York, White Sulfur Springs in Virginia, or Warm Springs in Georgia. Because they were bitter, tasted of sulfur, or were warm, the waters were perceived to be curative. Hydropathic therapy proved very profitable for operators of the hotels and spas that developed in such places.[4] Homeopathy, the system of therapeutics devised by Samuel Hahnemann in the early 19th century, also had appeal because it was completely harmless. Hahnemann concocted the theory that "like cures like," that is, a pharmacologic agent that would cause a symptom should be given in a very small dose to counteract that symptom. He held that the homeopathic physician should dilute a given drug serially so that a patient would receive only a minute amount of it. The advantage of this system lay in its failure to harm, thereby allowing the patient to improve on his or her own.[5]

Orthopaedics as practiced in the 1830s and 1840s may have been attractive for the same reasons; it didn't hurt and it might help. In fact, anyone could see that it provided some tangible benefits. Light exercise, rest, massage, and external supports for stiff, painful, and deformed trunks and limbs often did help patients feel better and recover from their illnesses. The practitioners of orthopaedics offered their art without the pompous quackery of the purgers, bleeders, serial diluters, and spa operators, which was also appealing.

For these reasons, the relatively small percentage of the population in the early decades of the 19th century with chronic musculoskeletal diseases sought orthopaedic treatment. The term "orthopaedics" actually appeared in the medical literature in America in the late 1830s, about 100 years after Andry coined it. In Great Britain and in Europe, however, some confusion arose regarding a suitable term to identify the practice of musculoskeletal medicine and surgery. In 1741, Andry's word "L'orthopédie" survived challenges from Scaevole de Sainte-Marthe's "Paedotrophia" and Abbé Claude Quillet's "Callipaedia." In the 19th century, J. M. Delpech used "l'orthomorphie" (1828) and Bricheteau coined "Orthosomatie" (1833) in France, while H. H. Brigg invented "Orthopraxy" (1865) in Great Britain.[6] The people who coined these terms all practiced musculoskeletal medicine and surgery, but none of their designations gained wide use. Curiously, Andry's term won out.

As the efficacy of orthopaedic treatment became more apparent and as Andry's term became more fixed in people's minds, the idea took hold that such treatment could be provided most effectively in one place. This led to the concept of the orthopaedic hospital. Jean André Venel of Geneva opened the first such institution in Orbe, Switzerland, in 1790. He provided manipulation and bracing for clubfeet, recumbency for spinal caries (tuberculosis), calisthenics and bracing for scoliosis, and prolonged treatment with traction for fracture care.[6] In his 1968 book on the history of orthopaedics, Edgar Bick describes the numerous other British, German, French, and Italian orthopaedic hospitals that opened in subsequent decades after Venel's successful venture.[6] The proprietors of these institutions tended to treat their patients with rest or exercise, depending on the modality the institution officially endorsed. Two camps of thought had developed in the profession in Europe in those years: the patients received one or the other (rest versus exercise) based on the prejudices of their orthopaedic (orthopraxic, orthomorphic, or orthosomatic) physician. Venel's hospital in Orbe seemed to offer a rational mixture of therapies.

J. M. Delpech changed the landscape completely in 1828 when he opened his own orthopaedic hospital in Montpellier, France. Delpech had coined the term "l'orthomorphie"; he believed in treating musculoskeletal disorders with exercise and muscle strengthening. He then developed the concept of tenotomy for the rebalancing of the forces across joints caused by "tight muscles." A German surgeon, G. F. Strohmeyer, adopted Delpech's tenotomy operation a few years later, exploiting its dramatic correction of equinus foot deformities at his own Orthopaedic Institute in Hanover in 1831. Done without anesthesia and before Lister's antiseptic surgery, tenotomy carried tremendous risks. Those who have read Gustave Flaubert's *Madame Bovary* will remember how Flaubert described his heroine's feckless husband's attempts to perform this procedure. Dr. Bovary's patient became infected, and his leg had to be amputated. The Bovarys' lives fell apart further as a result. Delpech himself suffered an untimely end as a result of a surgical disaster he inflicted on a patient. Delpech's radical treatment of the man's varicocele ended badly. The patient shot and killed Delpech in revenge.[7]

In the United States, the entrepreneurs, physicians, and concerned citizens who usually joined forces to open hospitals did not begin to show interest in orthopaedics until the 1860s. In 1861, Buckminster Brown opened the House of the Good Samaritan Hospital, a small private hospital in Boston, and Lewis A. Sayre (Figure 7) opened an orthopaedic dispensary at Bellevue Hospital in New York. Brown is regarded as the first physician to devote himself exclusively to orthopaedics during his entire career, and Sayre is known as the first Professor of Orthopaedic Surgery in America at New York University, then called the Bellevue Medical College.[6]

Valentine Mott (1785-1865), a New York surgeon, took six years off in midcareer from his "exhausting labors" to recover his health. During most of those years, he traveled through Europe visiting famous doctors and surgeons. While in Paris, he developed an interest in orthopaedics. In 1841, when he returned home permanently, he wanted to open an orthopaedic hospital in the Bloomingdale section of Manhattan on New York's Upper West Side. His friends dissuaded him, but thanks to Mott, the idea of an orthopaedic hospital had arrived in New York.

Buckminster Brown's father, John Ball Brown, practiced medicine and surgery in Boston during the early decades of the 19th century. He had developed a profound interest in Pott's disease (tuberculous spondylitis) because it caused the death of one of his sons. Buckminster Brown himself contracted the disease but recovered. The elder Dr. Brown had opened an outpatient clinic called the Orthopedique Infirmary in Boston early in his career (1838); Buckminster Brown joined his father's practice there after studying orthopaedics with Strohmeyer, Little, and other leading orthopaedists and tenotomists of the time. Together the Browns opened the House of the Good Samaritan Hospital in 1861 after the younger Dr. Brown returned from abroad. Buckminster Brown donated $40,000 to Harvard in 1883 to establish the John Ball and Buckminster Brown Professorship of Orthopaedics at that institution.

Strohmeyer had two other disciples who came to America during the first half of the 19th century. William Detmold arrived in New York in 1837, performing tenotomies and other orthopaedic procedures at the Bellevue Hospital soon thereafter. He served in the Union army during the Civil War and returned to New York after the war where he died in 1894.

Louis Bauer, who had also studied with Strohmeyer, emigrated to New York in 1853. The following year, he helped found the German General Dispensary in Brooklyn, where he established an orthopaedic hospital based on Strohmeyer's plan (the Dispensary eventually became the Downstate Medical Center of the State University of New York). Bauer, who left Germany to avoid a prison term for unlawful political activities, did not integrate smoothly with his orthopaedic colleagues in New York. In 1869, he left the city and settled in St. Louis, where he remained until he died in 1898. Bauer published a lengthy text on orthopaedics in 1858, revising it in 1864 and 1868. The 1858 book was probably the first orthopaedic text published in the United States.[8]

The Hospital for the Ruptured and Crippled
In 1863, the Society for the Relief of the Ruptured and Crippled opened the first major orthopaedic hospital in the United States (Figure 8).[9] The certificate of incorporation included the following:

> That the particular business and object
> of such a Society shall be to supply
> skillfully constructed surgico-mechanical
> appliances and the treatment of in- and
> out-door patients requiring trusses and
> spring supports, also bandages, laced
> stockings, and other suitable apparatus

> for the relief and cure of cripples, both
> adult and children and, so far as possi-
> ble, to make these benefits available to
> the poorest in the community.

The society, in its original charter of incorporation, thus emphasized bracing and external support of the limbs and trunks of individuals with chronic
musculoskeletal or abdominal wall defects. The original document does not
emphasize the words orthopaedics or orthopaedist, and the men who founded
the Hospital for the Ruptured and Crippled certainly did not intend to make
their institution a center for surgical treatment of musculoskeletal abnormalities. They appointed James Knight to the position of surgeon-in-chief. Knight
had earned his reputation by devising a distinctive truss "for containment of
hernias." He applied his skills and experience to the design of braces and supports for the treatment of congenital and acquired crippling conditions of
bones and joints. Knight held the position for 24 years.

The Hospital for the Ruptured and Crippled opened at 97 Second Avenue,
New York, New York, in Dr. Knight's home. He turned the conservatory of
the house into a workshop where he made braces and other orthopaedic appliances for his patients, converting most of the rest of the building into a hospital for up to 28 inpatients. The society paid him an annual rent of $1,200 for
the first three years and then purchased the building for $15,000. Knight
served as superintendent. Valentine Mott, William Van Buren, Willard Parker,
and John Carnochan, all prominent surgeons, served as consultants. In their
first year together, they treated 828 patients, 50 of whom were pediatric inpatients. They performed no surgery; instead, every patient received some sort
of appliance. The patients included several women with uterine prolapse,
which Knight managed with a brace-like pessary. Very quickly, the institution
outgrew its quarters. Knight and his colleagues tried house calls to ease the
burden, but the board decided to build a new structure at Lexington Avenue
and 42nd Street. Knight designed the facility, making it light, airy, and comfortable, with excellent views of the East River and views to the west extending all the way into New Jersey. He did not provide for an operating room,
however. In 1871, he recruited an assistant, Virgil Gibney, who had received
his medical degree from Bellevue Medical College in New York (Figure 9).
At Bellevue, Gibney came under the influence of Lewis A. Sayre. By
Knight's standards, Sayre improperly inculcated Gibney with the idea that
musculoskeletal conditions might respond more quickly and successfully to
surgery than they would to prolonged rest and bracing. Knight and Sayre thus
drew up the battle lines between conservatism and surgery, with Gibney initially between them. Knight called Sayre mendacious, greedy, and arrogant;
he refused to permit surgical treatment at the Hospital for the Ruptured and
Crippled. He noted in his 1875 report that he had assumed the care of numerous surgical failures, presumably Sayre's, and he would not allow this kind of
thing at his own institution.

The situation changed when Gibney became surgeon-in-chief of the hospital upon Knight's death in 1887. Gibney was forced to resign from the hospital's staff in 1884 over Knight's refusal to permit operations, but with

Knight now gone, Gibney had free rein. During travels abroad after his resignation, Gibney developed an appreciation for the possibilities of antiseptic surgery. This prompted him to recruit William Tillinghast Bull, a surgeon trained in antisepsis and the surgical treatment of hernias. Gibney and Bull developed a productive professional relationship that led to the performance of orthopaedic surgery at the hospital. Gibney acknowledged his lack of surgical training and skill, but with Bull's help he could correct these deficits and change the Hospital for the Ruptured and Crippled (also known as "Dr. Knight's hospital") from a "home for incurables" into an institution where the most up-to-date surgical and rehabilitative techniques could be used to dramatically improve quality of life for its patients. When circumstances warranted, hospital staff would need to be able to perform an operation rather than depend on an "apparatus." In 1894, Gibney expressed this policy as follows:

> The orthopaedic surgeon is prepared to conduct a case from its incipiency to its close; that, if apparatus fails to meet the indications, he is able to conduct an operation, which operation ought to be done as well as any general surgeon can do it, and which operation can be supplemented by the judicious use of mechanical appliances, to bring about the best possible result.
>
> I have no wish whatever to deny to any of my fellows a special predilection for an apparatus alone, or for apparatus combined with minor operations, or for operations alone; but I do feel that if our specialty is to make any advance, and is to maintain its position in the medical and surgical world, an orthopaedic surgeon must be prepared to meet any emergency that may arise.[9]

Under Gibney's direction, the Hospital for the Ruptured and Crippled in 1888 reported 237 operations, 46 of which were for the treatment of abscesses or osteomyelitis. That year, the surgeons there also performed 162 tenotomies, 19 osteotomies, and one hip joint resection. The remaining were miscellaneous procedures such as dressing changes and amputations of supernumerary digits. According to Gibney, the surgeons used nitrous oxide anesthesia and observed the precautions of Listerism, but they still approached surgical treatment with "fear and caution."[9]

After the Civil War, another orthopaedic hospital opened in New York—the New York Orthopaedic Hospital and Dispensary—with Charles Fayette Taylor serving as director. In the mid-1850s, Taylor audited lectures at New

York College and qualified for a medical degree after only a year of study at the University of Vermont. With this relatively brief education behind him, he went to London to study motion and exercise therapy. His faith in these therapeutic modalities did not lead to a successful practice when he returned, so he sought a new way to earn a living. He settled on orthopaedics—designing, fabricating, and fitting braces primarily to patients with spinal deformities. Taylor did well in this endeavor and developed a practice that included such families as Theodore Roosevelt's, fitting a brace for the future president's sister. She recovered with Taylor's treatment, and when Theodore Roosevelt's father participated in the founding of the New York Orthopaedic Hospital, Taylor was put in charge of it. He did not enjoy his position of responsibility, however, and soon resigned. He strongly opposed orthopaedic surgery and did not even use drugs in treatment. Even though he was one of the founders of orthopaedics in America, he really had a limited role in its development.

Taylor had a rancorous relationship with his contemporaries. The Rare Book Library of the New York Academy of Medicine has an extensive collection of material relating to a dispute between Taylor and Sayre. In June 1873, Taylor brought charges of unethical conduct against Sayre, demanding that the academy investigate the matter and censure him.

According to the documents at the Rare Book Library, Dr. Sayre's treatment of a child named Fannie Foote had not proved successful. Fannie had developed hip pain that was so severe, she screamed with apprehension even when she was approached by her parents. At bedtime, she would sit on the side of the bed and refuse to lie down because of the intense pain. After a while, the parents decided to change doctors. They discharged Sayre and asked Taylor to take over the case. Taylor must have had some success with his braces as opposed to Sayre. Fannie began to have less pain, but she developed progressively worse stiffness in the hip.

Sayre stayed in touch with Mrs. Foote, however, writing letters and visiting her and her daughter Fannie. He even suggested to Mrs. Foote that he might bring a patient of his to her residence so that Mrs. Foote could compare Fannie's progress with another child who had a similar problem. When Sayre arrived unannounced with the child and her mother, Mrs. Foote was not at home, but Fannie was there with an aunt who invited him in. Sayre suggested that Fannie should take a look at the other child, and Fannie agreed. Sayre then examined Fannie, lifting up her dress to palpate her hip and check on her range of motion. When Sayre told Fannie that she had no hip motion, Fannie became extremely frightened and could not be consoled. Mrs. Foote arrived home at that point and Sayre departed with the other child, her mother, and his assistant, Dr. Yale. Before he departed, Sayre may have made disparaging remarks about Taylor's course of treatment of Fannie. The next day, Fannie's father went to Sayre's office demanding that Sayre never return to his house unless invited. Foote also informed Sayre that he should not examine Fannie again unless requested by Taylor, and even then only if accompanied by Taylor.

Sayre's actions outraged Taylor, who wrote a multipage complaint to the academy demanding Sayre's formal censure. This could be facilitated only by an investigative hearing. The academy convened a panel of well-known New York physicians to look into the matter. The investigation generated several hundred pages of letters and documents. Later, as the investigation proceeded, Sayre averred that Mrs. Foote had invited him to bring the similarly afflicted child for her examination and that Fannie had asked him to examine her hip while he was in her room. Taylor did not believe it, nor did Mr. Foote, who then wrote a blistering letter to Sayre telling him to stay away. Mrs. Foote, on the other hand, wrote a tender, weepy note to Sayre expressing her devotion and gratitude to him for all that he had done for Fannie.

The panel formally interviewed all of the Footes, Mrs. Birdwell (the aunt), Taylor, Sayre, Sayre's assistant, Dr. Yale, the consultants who had examined Fannie on various occasions, and even the similarly afflicted child (Nellie) and her mother. The panel also dickered with Sayre, Taylor, and the academy about who would pay for the stenographer who took this all down.

In the end, the panel and the academy could not make a judgment. The evidence was contradictory, leading the academy to suggest to Taylor and Sayre that they should let their friends decide the matter.

Philadelphia Orthopaedic Hospital

Orthopaedic hospitals also opened outside of New York and Boston. The fate of an institution that opened in Philadelphia illustrates the way extreme conservatism limited development of the specialty. In 1867, four well-known Philadelphia surgeons collaborated in opening the Philadelphia Orthopaedic Hospital, even though none of them would have identified himself as an orthopaedist. Thomas Eakins, the Philadelphia artist, immortalized two of them in portraits—Samuel D. Gross in "The Gross Clinic" and D. Hayes Agnew in "The Agnew Clinic." The other two men, Thomas Morton and Henry Goodman, did not achieve that level of recognition but were successful and well known in their day. Parenthetically, Agnew served on the medical team that cared for the wounded President James Garfield, but inexplicable rejection of antisepsis and probings for the assassin's bullet led to Garfield's subdiaphragmatic abscess and subsequent death.

None of these four surgeons actually originated the idea of an orthopaedic hospital. At the time, the operations in their surgical clinics gave these well known men and their medical schools strong reputations that attracted medical students and patients. After surgery, however, patients (especially the poor) had to fend for themselves. Many of these patients, often children, needed bracing, physical therapy, and prolonged nursing care to recover, but no one really knew or cared what happened to them. There was one man in Philadelphia, however, who realized the importance of follow-up for these patients.

Mr. Dietrich W. Kolbe had set up shop across the street from the Surgical Clinic of the University of Pennsylvania to serve patients who had undergone surgery there. Frequently, his application of devices he manufactured provided these people with the only aftercare they would receive. Kolbe felt great sympathy for them and mentioned their plight to Dr. Morton, who then discussed it with Gross, Agnew, and Goodman. Eventually, the four surgeons and a lay board of managers they had recruited drew up a charter. They received court approval in October 1867 to establish the hospital and to provide services to patients with musculoskeletal diseases. Their objective was not to perform surgery in the Philadelphia Orthopaedic Hospital, but rather to provide care for those who required nonsurgical treatment of an orthopaedic disorder or who needed postoperative rehabilitation. The casebooks document a list of crippling deformities such as curvature of the spine, joint infections, clubfeet, knock knees, and various other contractures and disorders.

Because most of the clientele had few financial resources, the directors decided to expand their services and enlisted S. Weir Mitchell to establish a neurologic service. They subsequently changed the name from the Philadelphia Orthopaedic Hospital to the Philadelphia Orthopaedic Hospital and Neurologic Infirmary. Mitchell, a wealthy and socially prominent Philadelphia physician, specialized in what today might be called neuropsychiatry. He invented the "rest cure," which he employed in the treatment of depressed affluent women, and spent his summers writing now-forgotten historical novels at his estate near Bar Harbor, Maine. In the winter, at the Philadelphia Orthopaedic Hospital and Neurologic Infirmary, he ran an outstanding service for 40 years and set the standards for the practice of neurology in the United States.

After Mitchell's death, the hospital gradually sank into disrepair and mounting debt. It could no longer maintain itself. In 1937, during the Great Depression, the University of Pennsylvania absorbed its staff and assets. A group of local physicians purchased the building, which they called the "Doctor's Hospital," but this too failed and the structure was torn down. From the beginning, it had been apparent that the "belt-and-bracing" variety of orthopaedics could not sustain an institution. As the experience at the Hospital for the Ruptured and Crippled showed, doctors and patients wanted more; for orthopaedics to survive as a discipline, its practitioners would have to perform operations.

Organized Medicine and the Need For An Orthopaedic Association

Orthopaedics began to coalesce as a recognized medical and surgical specialty as its practitioners increased in number and gave patients more effective care in orthopaedic hospitals. This occurred in a meaningful way in the United States in the 1880s after anesthesia and Listerism were widely accepted and organized treatment centers were established in several major cities. Physicians who called themselves orthopaedists or orthopaedic surgeons lacked a commonality, however, and needed to come together to establish standards, discuss improvements in their treatment techniques, and advance their profession. This happened in 1887 with the founding of the American Orthopaedic Association (AOA).

The AOA, however, did not arise de novo. Rather, it evolved from other medical and surgical organizations that were formed in response to the need of 19th century Americans involved in almost any trade, craft, or profession to meet collegially with their peers.

Physicians' organizations appeared early in the United States. Several local and state societies convened in the 18th century: the Boston Medical Society met in 1735 and a New York society formed in 1749. The first state medical society was established in New Brunswick, New Jersey, in 1766. These and subsequent state and local societies set the standards of medical care by controlling the education and licensing of doctors as well as exposing fraudulent practitioners. (These noble aims often led to the suppression of competition and unfair favoritism, however.) In addition, the societies compared fees for various kinds of patient encounters and distributed lists of charges physicians might submit for their services. Local societies were criticized for pooling information about the reliability of patients in paying their physicians. Although it was obviously useful for doctors to have such a list, this practice gave physicians too much bad publicity for the medical societies to continue it. Lawmakers in various states had difficulty coming to grips with regulating physician licensing and certification, and controlling the profession in general.[10]

A real need for order and organization thus existed in American medicine in the early years of the 19th century. The word "chaotic" does not overstate the atmosphere in which aspirants to a medical career were trained. Medical schools such as those at the University of Pennsylvania, Columbia College of Physicians and Surgeons, Harvard College, the Medical Departments of the College of Maryland in Baltimore, Jefferson Medical College in Philadelphia and the colleges of South Carolina and Georgia offered courses in medicine and awarded degrees, but many students could acquire a medical degree by serving an apprenticeship with a licensed doctor and applying to the state or even the local medical society for the degree. Although the exact mechanism varied from place to place, essentially a committee of censors in the medical society had to approve an aspiring physician before a license would be granted.

Local and state medical societies served regional needs in setting educational and licensing standards as well as developing codes of ethics, but by the 1840s, some physicians felt the need for a national medical organization. In the past, the difficulty of traveling long distances would have precluded any valid effort to set such standards nationally, but an increasingly reliable postal service and better transportation made the concept viable. Railroads between cities and smaller towns first appeared in America in the 1830s. Twenty years later, people could travel much more quickly from city to city than they could have by horseback or stagecoach in earlier decades. The technological and industrial revolution brought people closer together, making person-to-person exchanges of ideas and information possible.

In 1846, the New York State Medical Society confronted a troubling issue. The state legislature had determined that the state society would no longer have the exclusive right to examine and certify applicants for a medical license.[11] The lawmakers had decided that any physician, professor, or college that taught medicine could license the individuals who had taken their courses. Because the students had to pay for the instruction, the teachers and institutions had an incentive to entice as many as possible to their lectures. Simplifying the course material enabled even more students to practice; this meant more money for the instructors, but it produced license holders who were unqualified to practice medicine.

The American Medical Association

The New York State Medical Society could not control this situation. At its request, 28 state societies and several local medical societies sent representatives to the organizational meeting of what became the American Medical Association (AMA) in 1847. Despite the obvious need for concerted group action to correct abusive practices in medical education, the delegates could not agree on a course of action. That first meeting in New York broke up without formally convening an association. The following year, in Philadelphia, the members present found that they could agree on most issues, and founded the AMA.

The AMA initially made little progress in its campaign against dilution of the quality of instruction. Fly-by-night diploma mills proliferated in those decades, cranking out thousands of unqualified, indeed dangerous, practitioners who had merely paid a fee and received a diploma licensing them to practice. Eventually the abuses grew so dangerous to public health that even the state legislators had to recognize the results of their legislation. By the 1880s and 1890s, the states began to establish responsible state boards of medical examiners. By then the AMA had involved itself in writing a code of ethics for physicians and was lobbying for causes such as collection and reporting of vital statistics to study epidemics, causes of death, death rates, and so forth.[12,13]

In those early years, the AMA brought physicians with disparate backgrounds and interests together, but inevitably doctors developed different ways of approaching their disciplines. Those who found surgery more interesting than therapeutics wanted to spend more time debating their own issues. Prior to 1880, the AMA tried to meet the need for surgeons by forming a Surgical Section. In that year, however, Samuel D. Gross convened a rump session of surgeons at an AMA meeting for the purpose of founding the American Surgical Association (ASA). Gross had the idea that a select few of America's best surgeons should form an association "designed to be an elite and exclusive surgical society which would separate the riffraff from its upper crust numbers." The only criterion for membership would be a "name as a surgeon."[14] The leadership of the AMA protested Gross' action, justifiably noting that an ASA would detract from the common effort and siphon the members' prestige and allegiance from its own Surgical Section. Gross addressed this issue in his speech as ASA president at its second meeting in 1881:

> If it be said we are striking a blow at the
> AMA, we deny the soft impeachment. On
> the contrary, we shall strengthen that

body by rousing it from its Rip van
Winkle slumbers, and infusing new light
into it. We can hurt no society now in
existence, nor likely to come into existence. We can hurt only ourselves if we
fail to do our duty . . . and show the
world that we are earnest and zealous
laborers in the interest of human progress
and human suffering.

Gross' lofty remarks set the pattern for the ASA, which remains a small
and quite exclusive organization of surgeons. Mark Ravitch collected and
edited 100 years of the *Transactions of the ASA*[15] and noted that despite its
apparent exclusivity, the Association had a remarkable record of success,
serving as a forum in which America's brightest and best surgeons discussed advances in their profession. The membership of the ASA in 1913
established a new, larger surgical association they called the American
College of Surgeons (ACS). It in turn established the American Board of
Surgery (ABS) in 1937. The ASA and the ACS also sponsored the premiere
surgical journal, the *Annals of Surgery*.

Many of the early papers presented at the ASA meetings concerned
members' experiences and results with musculoskeletal injuries and diseases. They also debated much more general topics, such as Listerism and
the roles of cupping and bleeding. Surgeons in the 1880s still had relatively little experience with abdominal or chest surgery; most of their papers
covered subjects like joint excision for tuberculosis, astragalectomy for
clubfeet, and various maneuvers for the reduction of difficult fractures and
dislocations.[15]

The American Orthopaedic Association

Seven years after Gross convened the ASA, Lewis A. Sayre, an ASA member, permitted the organizational meeting of the American Orthopaedic
Association (AOA) to take place at his office at 285 Fifth Avenue, New
York City, on February 24, 1887.[16] The record shows, after debate and discussion, "Ten votes for the foundation of such an association and two
against it; two gentlemen did not vote on the question."

Sayre, then considered the leading orthopaedic surgeon in the world, did
not believe that there was a need for an orthopaedic association and advised
the members present to join the ASA, of which he was a member.
Presumably, the orthopaedists would form a section on orthopaedics under
the aegis of the ASA, but the record does not state whether Sayre had
cleared this concept with his colleagues in that organization. Sayre would
not join the AOA at the time it was founded, but two years later he accepted active membership and, in 1895, honorary membership.

The AOA conducted its first annual meeting at the New York Academy
of Medicine on June 15 and 16, 1887, about four months after the organizational meeting in Sayre's office. The association conducted its second

annual meeting in Washington, D.C., in September 1888. In the ensuing year, the secretary of the AOA, Robert W. Lovett, compiled the papers that members had presented at the first and second annual meetings, publishing them as volume 1 of the *Transactions of the American Orthopaedic Association*, presumably at least partially at his own expense. A stringency in the money market in 1888 and 1889 resulted in financial stress for the AOA; the published account notes that Drs. John Ridlon and Judson "went after the delinquents (who had not paid their dues) with a bill or a letter every two weeks." The result was "that all arrears and dues were paid," and the debts of the association settled, so that by the fourth annual meeting the treasury contained a balance of $103.70.[16]

In 1896, at the meeting in Buffalo, New York (with Royal Whitman as president and John Ridlon as secretary), the AOA discussed the publication of a journal to replace *Transactions*. Twenty-nine members voted yes and eleven voted no, but most of the no votes were from New Yorkers who were the more prominent members of the association. Without them, the journal would probably not have succeeded. At this time, the attempt to launch a journal was abandoned. Gradually, however, the opposition faded away, and 7 years later, in 1903, the special committee to investigate the possibilities of an orthopaedic journal reported its 16 recommendations. These included a title (the *American Journal of Orthopaedic Surgery*), financial support ($1,000 per year "at the very least"), and sources of papers to be published (original work presented at the annual meeting, British and German contributions, and "odd papers and those of outsiders"). The committee's final recommendation stated, "It is likely that an American orthopaedic journal will, in some form or other, soon be started," suggesting that if the AOA did not publish it, someone else would. The recommendations also noted that subscribing to a journal published outside the AOA would cost members as much or more than if they offered financial support to their own publication and received it free as a benefit of membership.[16]

The minutes of the 1918 meeting recorded a resolution presented by Mark Rodgers, then editor of the *American Journal of Orthopaedic Surgery*. He noted that in Great Britain orthopaedic surgeons had recently convened the British Orthopaedic Association (BOA) and suggested that the membership of the AOA offer the use of the *American Journal of Orthopaedic Surgery* to the BOA as its official organ. The membership approved the action. The *American Journal of Orthopaedic Surgery* would now serve orthopaedists in two countries; thus the AOA would have to change the name it had used for the journal since 1896. Twenty-two years after its launch, the *American Journal of Orthopaedic Surgery* became the *Journal of Orthopaedic Surgery* and later, in 1922, the *Journal of Bone and Joint Surgery* (*JBJS*), its name to this day.[17]

In 1948, the number of articles submitted for publication grew so large and came from so many different countries that the editorial board of the *JBJS* recommended changes to its sponsoring organization. In that year, it appeared as separate British and American issues, "four edited and published in Great

Britain and four edited and published in the United States of America." In 1936, *JBJS* noted on its title page that in addition to the AOA and BOA, it had also become the official publication of the American Academy of Orthopaedic Surgeons (AAOS).

The AOA played a critical role in the development of American orthopaedics, especially through its participation in creating the *JBJS*. For many years, the journal was the only publication in which orthopaedic surgeons could publish their work. These peer-reviewed papers provide a definition of the specialty in the early years of its existence.

The American Board of Orthopaedic Surgery

The two major achievements that placed orthopaedics on its current trajectory, the creation of the American Board of Orthopaedic Surgery (ABOS) and the AAOS, both took place in the early 1930s and appear to have occurred because of initiatives that began with the AMA. In fact, the president of the AOA, Melvin Henderson, of Rochester, Minnesota, acknowledged this at the AOA Annual Meeting in 1932:

> Some twenty odd years ago, when it became apparent that orthopaedic surgery was destined to become a lusty member of the family of medical specialties, the Orthopaedic Section of the American Medical Association was formed. Also in the East, Mid-West and West, orthopaedic clubs and societies were formed to facilitate the gathering together of those who were interested. . . In the Mid-West and West was formed the Central States Orthopaedic Club which soon outgrew its club clothes and was forced to organize into the Clinical Orthopaedic Society. The Pacific Coast gave birth to similar organizations. . .
>
> The last year has seen the launching of the American Academy of Orthopaedic Surgeons, the common system which promises to link these various distinct groups into one . . . society.
>
> The American Medical Association approves this and under the wing of that great organization, much good will be accomplished by this movement. The AOA, not by official action, but through its members and always with the tacit

consent of the Executive Committee, has
fostered these various movements.[18]

Further evidence of the AMA's contribution to the founding of the
ABOS and the AAOS can be found in the minutes of the AMA
Orthopaedic Section of May 1932.[19,20] At this meeting, Henry Meyerding
moved that the AMA Orthopaedic Section appoint a special committee to
consider the plan for establishing the ABOS. The National Board of
Medical Examiners submitted the proposal to the AMA Orthopaedic
Section; Meyerding suggested that the section "heartily approve" their
plan. W. B. Owen of Louisville, chairman of the Orthopaedic Section,
appointed a committee consisting of Meyerding, Philip Lewin of
Chicago, and J. Archer O'Reilly of St. Louis. The ABOS was founded in
1934. Although Dr. Henderson's Presidential Oration and the AMA
Orthopaedic Section minutes offer little evidence of the AOA role in gen-
erating the AAOS and the ABOS, a review of the program at the first
AAOS meeting reveals that virtually all of the papers were presented by
members of the AOA.

Professional Survival
in the Great Depression

The Founding of the American Academy of Orthopaedic Surgeons
AAOS held its first meeting on January 19, 1933, in the auditorium of
Northwestern University Medical School. American orthopaedic surgeons chose a bad year to launch a national professional organization.
The stock market crashed in 1929, about three years before they had
decided to organize, and the national—indeed, the international—economy showed little sign of recovery. President Herbert Hoover tried to protect American businesses by signing the Smoot-Hawley Act, which
placed a tariff on imported goods. He also agreed to support a Federal
Reserve initiative to inject money into the economy with a $500 million
buyback of federal securities. He then attempted to secure the solvency
of the Treasury by enacting a large tax increase, but nothing seemed to
work. Toward the end of 1932, starving World War I veterans rioted in
Washington, D.C., desperate bank managers foreclosed on mortgages,
and people started living in shanty towns called "Hoovervilles." By
November 1932, nearly 1,500 bank failures stripped citizens of their life
savings. To cap it off, Prohibition—based on a 1919 Constitutional
amendment and implemented by the Volstead Act—resulted in
widespread flouting of the law and gangster rule, particularly in the large
cities. Public confidence in the future collapsed, and birth rates fell to the
lowest ever recorded. The 1932 election of a new president, Franklin
Delano Roosevelt, a man paralyzed from the waist down from an episode
of poliomyelitis some years before, must have struck the voters who
were aware of his condition as an ironically fitting selection for a new
national leader (Figure 10).[21]

Despite this dreary outlook, the determined members of the newly formed AAOS convened their first meeting in Chicago in 1933. They had held a preliminary executive committee meeting the day before the formal opening, electing officers and appointing committees. The organization had a distinctly midwestern flavor, holding its first meeting at Northwestern Medical School in conjunction with the Clinical Orthopaedic Society (COS), an amalgam of Midwestern and Western Orthopaedic Clubs.[22]

Edwin W. Ryerson of Chicago served as president at that first meeting, which he called to order on January 12, 1933. Not a single speaker listed in the program came from the East Coast (unless one considers W. E. Gallie of Toronto). Eighteen of the speakers practiced in Chicago; the rest came from Detroit, St. Louis, Memphis, Milwaukee, Minneapolis, Rochester, Minnesota, and Lincoln, Nebraska. One can imagine that a mid-January AAOS meeting in Chicago would have contrasted sharply with the May 1933 AOA meeting in Washington, DC.[23] In Chicago, the weather typically would have featured single-digit temperatures, snow, ice, and high winds, whereas Washington, DC, offered mild days and spring sunshine. Furthermore, a review of the program reveals that 30 of the 45 speakers at the AOA meeting came from East Coast cities such as Boston, New York, Philadelphia, and Baltimore. Only three speakers at the Washington AOA meeting in 1933 came from Chicago. (One of these speakers, Dr. Ryerson, had assumed the presidency of the newly created AAOS nine months earlier.) The format of the meetings also differed. At the AOA meeting, the speakers presented short papers on specific subjects; at the AAOS meeting, the meeting featured five symposia presented by multiple speakers addressing a single topic. This may have conveyed the impression that at the AOA meeting, physicians came to report on their research, whereas at the AAOS meeting they came to learn.

The historical context surrounding the AAOS meeting was significant; events that would have tremendous sociologic and political impact were about to take place. In January 1933, the New Deal had not yet been implemented; Hoover was still in office, and FDR was awaiting inauguration.

Ryerson's presidency at the 1933 AAOS meeting did not come out of the blue. He had worked previously to create a large, inclusive national organization of orthopaedic surgeons, beginning as early as 1912 when, as a founding member, he also helped launch the COS. That organization held regular meetings throughout the Midwest, featuring the live presentation of patients to the members in attendance. It must have appeared to Ryerson that orthopaedics could not satisfactorily serve those suffering with crippling musculoskeletal diseases and conditions unless those who practiced it worked to create a national, inclusive organization. At the October 29, 1931,[24] meeting of the COS, the members discussed this need and appointed Ryerson as chairman of a committee to consider the idea. Willis Campbell, Frank Dickson, Frederick Gaenslen, Ellis Jones, Philip Lewin, E. Bishop Mumford, and H. Winnett Orr served on the committee with Ryerson. The committee came back with a complete report the very next day, recommending that the COS invite practitioners from all over the United States who considered themselves orthopaedic surgeons to attend its 1932 meeting for the purpose of founding a national society. In addition, the committee presented an outline for the organization of such a society. The completeness of the report, ready for presentation only 24 hours after the committee's first meeting, suggests that Ryerson and his committee members had long considered the matter and developed their recommendations. In fact, on October 11, 1931, Campbell initiated discussion of such a national academy of orthopaedists at the Chicago meeting of the AOA. This took place 18 days before the October 29 meeting of the COS. Thus, in 1932, when the COS met again, he was ready to recommend that a much larger organization, a national academy, should convene its own meeting in January 1933 with Ryerson acting as first president.[25-28]

At the 1932 meeting, Willis Campbell was the first president to be elected in an open meeting and would serve until the second annual meeting in December 1934. Campbell deserves special mention as a founder of the AAOS.[29] Energetic and intelligent, he was instrumental in creating a national academy of musculoskeletal surgeons that helped the members realize their best potential in healing the injured and straightening the crippled and lame. Campbell, born in Jackson, Mississippi, in 1880, attended Hampton-Sydney College, Roanoke College, and the medical school of the University of Virginia. He first practiced medicine in Memphis, Tennessee, but early on was determined to pursue orthopaedics. That decision took him to London, Vienna, New York, and Boston over a period of five years. He then returned to Memphis, where he stayed for the rest of his life. Virtually every modern orthopaedist has used *Campbell's Operative Orthopaedics*, which has been revised many times since it was first published in 1939; the 10th edition was published in 2003. Hundreds of practicing orthopaedic surgeons have received their training at the Campbell Clinic in Memphis since 1910, when Campbell organized the Department of Orthopaedic Surgery at the University of Tennessee School of Medicine. He held the position of Professor of Orthopaedics there until his death in 1941.

A 1934 issue of *JBJS* acknowledged the second annual meeting of the AAOS with two brief announcements: one nine lines long on page 214 and the other seven lines long on page 483. The second announcement indicated that "Seminars were held, conducted by men of wide experience." Again, the newly elected officers for the next yearly meeting were from the Midwest, with the notable exception of Philip D. Wilson of Boston and New York, who would serve as the third president at the meeting in New York.

Wilson came from a medical tradition that differed considerably from that which produced Campbell.[30] Born in Columbus, Ohio, Wilson graduated from Harvard College in 1904 and from Harvard Medical School in 1909, cum laude and class president. These achievements led to a surgical internship at Massachusetts General Hospital. This in turn led to a post with the "Harvard Unit" under the famous Harvey Cushing and military service in wartime in 1915 with fellow graduates of the Harvard Medical School, including Marius Smith-Petersen. After the war, Wilson and Smith-Petersen both returned to Harvard. When the position of chief of the orthopaedic service opened up in the early 1930s at Harvard, Smith-Petersen was selected. Wilson, deeply disappointed, accepted the position of surgeon-in-chief of the Hospital for the Ruptured and Crippled in New York in 1934. His legendary achievements there included changing its name to the Hospital for Special Surgery and moving it to its present location on East 70th Street. Wilson's selection as third president of the academy and his willingness to accept the position gave it a heavy coating of East Coast patina. In fact, during Wilson's presidential year, the AAOS met at the Waldorf Astoria Hotel.

JBJS responded to all of this by devoting three pages to the meeting.[31] By 1935, the national character of the academy was emerging, and presenters from Iowa City, Nashville, Seattle, and Pueblo, Colorado, joined those from Chicago, New York, Pittsburgh, and elsewhere. That year the editors of *JBJS* decided to publish DeForest Willard's AOA Presidential Address rather than Wilson's presidential remarks to the AAOS. Willard, however, made respectful reference to the newly formed academy and spoke of the "struggle" of the early years during which the "medical profession and the public were loathe to recognize orthopaedics as a surgical entity." He noted that at the beginning of the 20th century, orthopaedists were only "fitters of apparatus" and "buckle and strap men," not skilled enough to perform operations. World War I, however, produced a great number of youthful, energetic surgeons (such as, Wilson) with experience, interest, and skill in treating musculoskeletal injuries and diseases. Orthopaedics attracted these veterans, and Willard observed that "The number of men who practice [orthopaedics] has grown from a few score to many hundreds." He admitted that the AOA could not cope with these numbers, but he hoped that the "new American Academy of Orthopaedic Surgeons" would provide "an outlet for the clinical and scientific experience of the large number of people coming into the specialty."[32]

The academy met in St. Louis the following year.[33] The brief description of the meeting published in *JBJS* did not impart the energy and intensity the members must have felt. Thirty-two scientific exhibits and thirty-eight technical exhibits were represented. The three best papers received gold, silver, and bronze medals. Four others won honorable mention.

The meeting also featured six "radio talks": (1) *Physically Handicapped Children and Adults*, Dr. J. Archer O'Reilly, St. Louis; (2) *Progress in Orthopaedic Surgery*, Dr. Melvin Henderson, Rochester, Minnesota; (3) *Infantile Paralysis*, Dr. Philip Lewin, Chicago; (4) *Modern Treatment of Bone and Joint Injuries*, Dr. Frank Dickson, Kansas City; (5) *Bone Tumors*, Dr. Henry Meyerding, Rochester, Minnesota; and (6) *Fractures*, Dr. J. Albert Key, St. Louis.

Frank Dickson gave the AAOS Presidential Oration that year, which *JBJS* published in its entirety.[34] Dickson's address proclaimed the academy as one of the preeminent medical societies in America. His 1935 remarks today seem prescient. He showed no self-consciousness in quoting English essayist and poet Joseph Addison: "Knowledge is, indeed, that which, next to virtue, truly and essentially raises one man above the other." He enumerated the aspirations of the organization, among which were "nation-wide representation . . . and influence in establishing orthopaedic surgery, the elevation of the standards of education in orthopaedic surgery, a systematic study of important orthopaedic problems, a freer exchange of information and ideas, and a source of advice and guidance" on public questions.

Dickson described orthopaedics as a "wide field and one that demands the broadest of medical training and deep, if not profound, knowledge," noting as well that "orthopaedic surgery is probably the broadest and most comprehensive of the special branches of medicine." He believed that an orthopaedist should have the knowledge to treat patients medically as well as surgically for musculoskeletal diseases and conditions. His influence on education and certification is still evident today.

In keeping with the times, Dickson also provided commentary on the Great Depression: "In these days of change, social upheaval, and very articulate demands for social security, there seems to be a growing demand for an altered relationship between the medical profession and its patients, the public." His remarks on this subject did not sound as hopeful and optimistic as other parts of his address, but he did accept "the obligation" of the academy to the public in general economic planning. With the AAOS only in its third year, Dickson's remarks sounded ambitious, perhaps even inappropriately so, but his pragmatism, goodwill, and confidence must have set just the right tone for his audience of physicians and surgeons in 1936.

References

1. Grob GN: *The Deadly Truth: A History of Disease in America*. Cambridge, MA, Harvard University Press, 2003, pp 121, 216.

2. Wood GB: *A Treatise on the Practice of Medicine*, ed 4. Philadelphia, PA, Lippincott, Grambo & Co, 1855, p 348.

3. Numb RL: The fall and rise of the American medical profession, in Leavitt JW, Numb RL (eds): *Sickness and Health in America. Readings in the History of Medicine and Public Health*, ed 2. Madison, WI, University of Wisconsin Press, 1985, p 187.

4. Claridge RT: *Every Man His Own Doctor. The Cold Water, Tepid Water and Friction Cure, As Applicable to Any Disease to Which the Human Frame Is Subject, and also the Cure of Diseases in Horses and Cattle*. New York, NY, John Wiley, 1849.

5. Haggard H: *Devils, Drugs and Doctors: The Story of Healing from Medicine Man to Doctor*. New York, NY, Blue Ribbon Books, Inc, 1929, pp 352-353.

6. Bick EM: *Source Book of Orthopaedics*. New York, NY, Hafner Publishing Company, 1968, pp 69, 489, 492.

7. Keith A: Introduction of tenotomy, in *Members of the Maimed: The Anatomical and Physiological Principles Underlying the Treatment of Injuries to Muscles, Nerves, Bones and Joints*. London, England, Henry Frowde, 1919, pp 63-77.

8. Bauer L: Lectures on Orthopaedic Surgery: *Delivered at the Brooklyn Medical and Surgical Institute*, ed 2. New York, NY, William Wood & Co, 1868.

9. Beekman F: *Hospital for the Ruptured and Crippled. A Historical Sketch Written on the Occasion of the Seventy-Fifth Anniversary of the Hospital.* New York, NY, Statistical Press, 1939.

10. Sherk HH: *Colleagues and Competitors: A Sesquicentennial History of the Camden County Medical Society: 1846-1996.* Rochester, MN, Johnson Printing Company, 1996.

11. Shryock RH: *Medical Licensing in America, 1650-1965.* Baltimore, MD, Johns Hopkins Press, 1967, p 34.

12. Bender GA: The founding of the American Medical Association, in *Great Moments in Medicine.* Detroit, MI, Parke-Davis & Co, 1961, pp 226-237.

13. Shryock RH: *The Development of Modern Medicine.* New York, NY, Alfred A. Knopf, 1947, p 110.

14. Rutkow IM: The American Surgical Association. *Arch Surg* 2000;135:872. Medline

15. Ravitch MM: *A Century of Surgery 1880-1980.* Philadelphia, PA, JB Lippincott, 1981.

16. Ridlon J: The Beginnings of the Transactions and Journal of the American Orthopaedic Association. *Am J Orthop Surg* 1918;16:501-512.

17. British Orthopedic Association [editorial]. *Am J Orthop Surg* 1918;16:308.

18. Henderson MS: Leadership in orthopaedic surgery: Presidential address before the American Orthopaedic Association. June 8, 1934. *J Bone Joint Surg* 1934;16:495-498.

19. AMA Section of Orthopedic Surgery. *JAMA* 1932;98:1914.

20. AMA Section of Orthopedic Surgery. *JAMA* 1932;98:1296.

21. McElvaine RS: *The Great Depression: America 1929–1941.* New York, NY, Three Rivers Press, 1993.

22. Organizational meeting of the American Academy of Orthopaedic Surgeons. *J Bone Joint Surg* 1933;15:550.

23. The forty-seventh annual meeting of the American Orthopaedic Association. *J Bone Joint Surg* 1933;15:548.

24. Brackett BE: History Lessons. AAOS Bulletin, July 1997. Available at http://www2.aaos.org/aaos/archives/bulletin/jul97/histor.htm. (Accessed March 7, 2007)

25. A tribute to the first president of the American Academy of Orthopaedic Surgeons: Edwin W. Ryerson (1872-1911). *J Bone Joint Surg Am* 1965;47:1274.

26. Meeting of Orthopaedic Surgeons. *JAMA* 1932;99:2192.

27. Orthopaedic Meeting. *JAMA* 1933;101:2059.

28. Badgley CE: The American Academy of Orthopaedic Surgeons. Orthopaedic Surgery in the United States of America. *J Bone Joint Surg Br* 1950;32:531-533.

29. Willis Cohoon Campbell (1880-1941). *J Bone Joint Surg* 1941;23:716.

30. Philip Duncan Wilson (1886-1969). *J Bone Joint Surg Am* 1969;51:1445.

31. The third annual meeting of the American Academy of Orthopaedic Surgeons. *J Bone Joint Surg* 1935;17:514.

32. Willard DF: Presidential Address, AOA Annual Meeting. *J Bone Joint Surg Am* 1935;17:531.

33. The fourth annual convention of the American Academy of Orthopaedic Surgeons. *J Bone Joint Surg* 1936;18:539.

34. Dickson FD: Presidential address. *J Bone Joint Surg* 1936;18:263.

CHAPTER 3

MUSCULOSKELETAL SURGERY IN CHILDREN: THE SOUL OF ORTHOPAEDICS

Tuberculosis and the Rise of Orthopaedic Surgery

Tuberculosis has virtually disappeared from the United States and Europe during the past 150 years. Although the vast majority of the population in this country remains free of the disease, and orthopaedic surgeons no longer deal with it on a regular basis, tuberculosis triggered the emergence of the new medical and surgical discipline that came to be known as orthopaedic surgery.

In 1900, tuberculosis was the second leading cause of death, killing far more people than heart disease, trauma, and cancer.[1] Children suffered with it in disproportionately large numbers compared to adults. Commonly, in the pediatric population, dissemination of the disease from the lungs produced progressive destructive lesions of the bones and joints (Figure 11). Treatment of the musculoskeletal manifestations of tuberculosis in the late 19th and 20th centuries consisted primarily of immobilization of the involved parts. A few adventurous surgeons, such as Lewis A. Sayre[2] of New York, attempted open drainage or even excision of infected joints, but the results were poor and the morbidity unacceptable. Consequently, orthopaedists at that time placed great importance on the art and science of bracing. Disagreements about the best way to make and apply braces naturally arose, and orthopaedists were not always generous in their public comments about their contemporaries' methods and techniques. Drs. Sayre, Taylor, Davis, and Knight, for example, leveled harsh criticism at each other. Sayre, while on tour in Great Britain, was also particularly harsh about the treatment methods he observed there. It was not surprising that British orthopaedists responded in kind. Hugh Owen Thomas of Liverpool addressed these issues in his 1876 monograph *Diseases of the Hip, Knee, and Ankle Joint with Their Deformities Treated by a New and Efficient Method*. Thomas expressed disapproval of what he considered Americans' misconceptions about how "iron frames" should be designed. Thomas commented as follows:

> Their appliances are variations of one
> type and may be called perineal extension
> instruments illustrating a likely erroneous
> principle which led to the construction of

the original splints of Davis and Sayre, each equally possessing their practical defects. These gentleman had attempted to cure hip disease by relieving pressure, while yet permitting movements of these joints.

I hold that for mechanical reasons, this relief of pressure must be infinitesimal, if at all, and I know, from practical experience that a cure free from defect, is impossible with the use of these appliances.

Since the visit of Dr. Sayre to England in the exposition of his method to the London surgeons, I have seen several instances in which his apparatuses were skillfully applied, and from personal knowledge I am satisfied that in not one of these cases was the disease arrested or even benefited.[3]

Thomas criticized the American designs because they braced the leg only from the ankle to a pelvic band from which perineal slings were usually suspended. Sometimes the Americans also included an ischial support as a sort of chair attached to the upper end of one of the uprights. Thomas held that the painful hip could not be immobilized by these devices, and that trunk support should extend upward to the scapulae, encasing the entire body from the ankle to the axilla.

The belt, strap, and brace school of orthopaedics reached its apogee with Thomas;[3] according to the several accounts of his life and work, he possessed consummate skill in devising and applying these devices. Several interesting aspects of his career deserve mention. His ancestors included a group of Welsh "bone setters," a class of practitioners who in general received little respect from the individuals with medical degrees or formal training in surgery. Despite attending the University of Edinburgh and University College in London, spending a year in Paris, and serving a fellowship at the Royal College of Surgeons, Thomas had virtually no scholarly or collegial interaction with physicians and surgeons, possibly because of his family's practice background. In short, he was a maverick who took no pains to hide or disguise his usually adverse opinions of others. He was a tiny man—very thin, dark, intense, and a heavy smoker. He was almost always pathologically energetic and compulsive. He fabricated and applied his braces himself, and he followed his patients with a smothering intensity, adjusting and continuously modifying the braces for their comfort and improvement. His method of treatment had limited applicability, however. He alone could provide this kind of bracing and external support, and he could handle only a limited number of patients. His importance in the history of orthopaedics rests in part on the fact that he showed how it should be done, but perhaps more significant is that he trained his nephew by marriage in the practice of orthopaedics. His nephew was Robert Jones, who became the putative "father of orthopaedics" in Great Britain.

Gradually, as the art and science of anesthesia improved, coupled with the evolution of asepsis and surgical techniques, surgical treatment of children "crippled" by tuberculosis became more common and efficacious. Hugh Owen Thomas died in 1891 at the age of 57; his publications regarding bracing and immobilizations had a strong influence on American orthopaedics throughout the last years of the 19th century. By 1903, however, when the *American Journal of Orthopaedic Surgery* was first published, American physicians' opinions had begun to shift from bracing to surgery. Augustus Thorndike's experience at Children's Hospital in Boston, described in volume 1 of the journal, serves as an example. He found 55 children younger than the age of 12 years in his survey of patients treated there from 1890 to 1903; Thorndike implied that all had tuberculosis. Some may have had pyogenic infections of the hip or Legg-Calvé-Perthes disease, but Thorndike could not differentiate these conditions at that time. The majority of the children were treated according to Thomas' principles, but Thorndike reported that caregivers' "lack of care in properly applying the apparatus," breakage, poor attendance at clinical follow-up, "ignorance and stupidity," and the "slow course of the disease leading to dissatisfaction" all compromised the ability of bracing to control hip infection. As a result, 21 of the 55 children underwent surgical incision and drainage of their abscesses with curettage of the carious bone in and about the hip. The surgery, however, led to persistent drainage from tuberculous sinuses, which persisted for many months. In the end, almost all of the patients had stiffness and shortening of the hip, but Thorndike did not report any mortalities.

Thorndike discussed the hip resections performed by Franz König at the Royal Berlin Hospital in Germany, maintaining that König did too many of these procedures. Thorndike believed that earlier treatment with more efficient bracing or traction would have cured at least some of these patients, preventing the need for such aggressive surgical intervention.

R. Tunstall Taylor, the surgeon in charge of a hospital for crippled children in Baltimore and clinical professor of orthopaedic surgery at the University of Maryland, also had a paper in volume 1 of the *American Journal of Orthopaedic Surgery*. Taylor appears to have been the first to employ x-ray technology as a means of following the progress of the disease and the efficacy of treatment. Taylor based his decision to supplement traction and bracing with surgery on his analysis of progressive changes seen on the patient's hip radiographs. He reported that he observed "clouding for some distance around the [tuberculous] foci and a worm eaten appearance in the joint." If these appeared to progress despite immobilization and traction, he performed an operation. From his description, his surgery seemed much more aggressive than Thorndike's, but not as aggressive as the joint resections performed by König. "Child was thin, delicate, and ill-looking," "condition very poor," "thigh riddled with sinuses," and "thin, tuberculous looking lad" are descriptions that Taylor used in his case reports. The poor children who underwent these procedures must have suffered terribly.

In all, eight of the articles in volume 1 of the *American Journal of Orthopaedic Surgery* related to tuberculosis. In addition to the articles on hip tuberculosis, Bernard Bartal of the University of Buffalo wrote about tuberculosis of the knee in children. He presented a series of eight patients with tuberculous foci in the femoral condyles that he had treated with early curettage and disinfection of the tuberculous abscesses using zinc chloride, carbolic acid, and iodine in glycerin. If the patient had a contracture of the knee, he also performed hamstring lengthenings and always immobilized the knee in a long leg cast for a prolonged period of time. He claimed that his patients did very well; "before and after" photographs of the actual patients, accompanied by radiographs in some cases, appear to substantiate his claims.

Stuart Leroy McCurdy of Pittsburgh Presbyterian Hospital also had an article in volume 1 of the journal, writing:

> An unusual case of Pott's abscess . . . a young man, age 18, had acute periostitis of anterior surface of maxillary bone, which was followed by infection of orbital cavity with complete destruction of the eyeball. Secondary infections developed, the most important one being destructive disease of the lower dorsal vertebra, which ran an acute course. The destructive process extended over a period of three years. An abscess developed which occupied the left half of the abdominal cavity. A cough had developed, and considerable pus was expectorated. It was not thought that the abdominal abscess had anything to do with this, but it was instead concluded that there has been a secondary deposit in the lungs.
>
> The abscess appeared below Poupart's ligament, and was incised. He was irrigated daily with peroxide of hydrogen. The cough was exaggerated sufficiently to suspect that there might be some connection.
>
> Methylene Blue was added to sterile water, and irrigation of the cavity from below Poupart's ligament is causing the patient to expectorate recoloring matter,

showing conclusively that there was a
continuous passage from the anterior surface of the thigh, through the abdomen,
lungs, air passage, and mouth.

This case is reported for record.

Presented at the 17th Annual Meeting
of the Association, Washington, DC,
May 11-14, 1903.

Rigid bracing, surgical drainage, débridement, and joint excision all had
serious limitations. In the early decades of the 20th century, orthopaedic surgeons began to seek alternatives. Because the goal of treatment was a painless bony ankylosis of an infected joint, it seemed reasonable to achieve this
outcome surgically. Anesthesia and aseptic surgery had made it possible to
open joints safely; several European surgeons had in fact produced fusions
of joints destabilized by paralytic disease such as polio.[4] Russell Hibbs[5] of
New York was the first to report a successful knee fusion in controlling
tuberculosis infection. Hibbs performed a wide resection of all the infected
tissue that he removed, then sculpted the distal end of the femur and upper
end of the tibia to fit well together. He also imbedded the patella into the surgical site and, after closing the incision, immobilized the leg in a long leg
cast. This technique achieved painless stable fusion in most of his patients,
thus avoiding months to years of bracing as well as multiple surgeries to
remove diseased and infected tissues. Hibbs extended his indications for
surgical fusions to the hip,[6] then to virtually any other joint, including the
spine.

Treating tuberculosis operatively seemed to embolden orthopaedic surgeons. In the 1890s, Virgil Gibney referred to approaching a percutaneous
tenotomy with "fear and caution," but by 1911, the year in which Hibbs
began to treat tuberculous joints with fusion, orthopaedists seemed to
believe there was no limit to what they could achieve with surgery.
Orthopaedists in the United States and abroad began to perform resections,
fusions, and osteotomies in large numbers, modifying and improving on
each others' methods. For example, several orthopaedic surgeons who
believed that disturbing an infected joint might disseminate the tubercle
bacilli determined to attempt fusions extra-articularly, and therefore bypass
the infection. Others attempted to hasten fusion using bone grafts; eventually, others tried using internal fixation with metal nails or rods.[7-12]

Until 1945, surgical treatment of musculoskeletal tuberculosis always
carried the serious risk of dissemination of the disease, and the cure of
tuberculosis depended on the patient's ability to fight off the infection.
Thus, the patient's "constitution" (degree of robust health) and nutritional
status were really more important than the finesse with which the surgeon
performed the operation. In the mid-1940s, a soil bacteriologist at the
Agricultural College of Rutgers University in New Jersey, Selman
Waksman,[13] found that tubercle bacilli could not live in cultures on which a

streptomyces fungus had been implanted. Further experiments led to the development of streptomycin, an antibiotic effective against the tubercle bacilli, ushering in a new era for the treatment of tuberculosis. David Bosworth of New York and his associates[14] reported on débridement of tuberculous bone lesions in patients undergoing treatment with the antibiotic, noting that dissemination of the infection did not occur. Since then, the pharmacologic armamentarium has expanded to include rifampin, isoniazid, pyrazinamide, and ethambutol, which are now considered the first-line drugs. Streptomycin is currently one of the second-line drugs used in patients with drug-resistant infections.[15]

Tuberculosis is now a relatively uncommon disease;[16] in 1999, fewer than 10 cases per 100,000 population were reported in the United States. This contrasts starkly with the 300 deaths from tuberculosis per 100,000 population in the mid-19th century. The dramatic decline in the frequency of the disease stems from improved living conditions, better nutrition, more attention to public health, and isolation of the infected. Better treatment with drugs and surgery, while important for a patient with the disease, probably did not cause the decline in the prevalence of tuberculosis. The large numbers of children crippled by the disease forced American physicians and surgeons to devise new techniques, new operations, and new approaches to treat patients with tuberculous infection. The techniques of bracing, physical therapy, surgery, and rehabilitation in the treatment of this disease laid the groundwork for the specialized discipline of orthopaedic surgery.[17,18]

Poliomyelitis

As the incidence of tuberculosis began to decline during the early part of the 20th century, poliomyelitis arose to take its place as a disease that would challenge the inventiveness and skill of the small community of orthopaedists in the United States (Figure 12). Paradoxically, the rising volume of patients with polio and the dwindling numbers of patients with tuberculosis can be attributed to the same causes. Improved public health practices, including better sanitation and clean water, helped decrease the frequency of tuberculosis, but these beneficial measures facilitated outbreaks of polio. The enteric poliovirus had infected nearly everyone who was alive in the mid-19th century. Newborns ingested the virus early in their lives by drinking water contaminated by it, but maternal antibodies protected them from the disease. Thus they acquired immunity during infancy, which made polio a rare disease in those years. When local and state governments provided clean water and efficient sewage disposal, however, the waterborne poliovirus gradually disappeared from the water supply, but the herd immunity of the human population likewise disappeared. The loss of this immunity to polio meant that the immunologically naive general population was now vulnerable to it. Inevitably, in such a population, a carrier who had been infected by the poliovirus would contaminate the water in a swimming pool, well, or even in a glass of water served to another individual, leading to an outbreak of the disease.[19]

Sporadic epidemics of polio occurred in Europe during the second half of the 19th century, particularly in Scandinavia. In the summer of 1894, doctors in Rutland, Vermont, suddenly began to see children with an "acute nervous disease," which almost always left the patient with at least some degree of paralysis. By summer's end and the break in warm weather, the medical community in Rutland had seen 132 cases, the largest epidemic of poliomyelitis reported in the United States to date. Thereafter, multiple epidemics began to occur throughout the United States, with a massive outbreak occurring in 1916. The disease paralyzed (at least partially) 9,000 children in New York City alone that year. Many other cities had similar experiences, coping with large numbers of desperately ill children. The 1916 epidemic overwhelmed the public health bureaucracy in many cities, including New York City. Polio cases eventually subsided spontaneously with the end of the hot weather.[20,21]

Scientists studying the disease realized that poliomyelitis results in the destruction of the anterior horn cells in the spinal cord and the medulla. Karl Landsteiner of Vienna collected fresh specimens of six spinal cords, and under bacteria-free conditions injected them into monkeys. The species of monkeys he used were fortuitously susceptible to the disease; thus, he was able to demonstrate that polio is caused by a transmissible virus actually occurring in three subtypes. Numerous better funded scientists crowded Landsteiner out of polio research, but he redefined himself as an immunologist and went on to identify the human blood groups, a classic work that made blood transfusions possible. Despite this new knowledge, polio epidemics seemed to worsen throughout the decades that followed the 1916 epidemic. They peaked in 1952, the year in which 60,000 Americans contracted the disease and 3,000 died. Overall, some 20 million people worldwide have at least some disability caused by polio. In 1996, the National Center for Health Statistics reported approximately 1 million American polio survivors, 450,000 of whom had endured at least some degree of paralysis.[19]

An acute episode of paralytic polio affects people in unpredictable ways. The death of enough motor neurons in the respiratory centers of the medulla obviously destroys an individual's ability to breathe autonomously. This aspect of polio resulted in rows of children being placed in Drinker respirators, also known as "iron lungs" (Figure 13) during the peak years of the polio epidemics. Many of these acutely suffering children who were afflicted with severe global loss of motor function died.[22]

On the other hand, some patients would experience only a slight residual motor weakness, and after their recovery were normalized with a barely perceptible disability. Many others remained severely disabled, with marked paralysis and deformity. The treatment of the acute stage of paralytic polio had little effect on the eventual outcome of the disease; what really mattered was how many motor cells had survived the infection. An Australian nurse, Sister Elizabeth Kenny, became well known for applying hot packs to painful paralyzed limbs of patients acutely affected by the disease. She lectured to the medical establishment about the benefits of gentle, passive range-of-motion exercises to prevent contractures and maintain mobility.

Sister Kenny received much attention in the lay press during those years. Orthopaedists took exception to Sister Kenny's hot packs, stretching, and manipulations for several reasons. In volume 1 of *Clinical Orthopaedics*, Ned Shutkin of New Haven, later the chief of the division of orthopaedics at Yale, reported on his observations of acute polio in 362 of his patients. The muscle spasm to which Sister Kenny referred never occurred in Shutkin's patients, and hot packs were inconvenient. The paralyzed children hated them; the summertime heat of stifling hospital wards was difficult enough to bear without this added discomfort. In addition, Shutkin felt that rigid adherence to a schedule of ranging, stretching, and manipulating the painful limbs caused more harm than good.[23]

Children in the chronic stage of polio needed more than hot packs and manipulation, and those needs defined the priorities for pediatric orthopaedists for years. Tuberculosis, although universally feared because of the abscesses, caries, and ever-present threat of death, was a familiar opponent. The relatively sudden appearance of polio surprised American society, mandating that the relatively few physicians who called themselves orthopaedic surgeons devise new treatment methods. These would be built on the lessons learned in administering to children with tuberculosis, the gradually disappearing scourge of the previous century.

A child in a chronic stage of polio (two years after acute onset) had two problems: muscle imbalance causing a dynamic deformity, and joint instability caused by paralysis of the muscles controlling a given joint. In the latter case, the orthopaedist could support the limb in a brace. This option for control of the flail joint had the disadvantages of pressure sores, mechanical failure of the brace, the continuous expense of providing new braces as the child grew, and the psychological burden of appearing in public supported by a metal and leather appliance. In the lower limb, ankle, and knee, fusions had the potential to eliminate the need for bracing for many children; however, fusions in the upper limb, shoulder, elbow, and wrist often proved more disabling than helpful. Nevertheless, the textbooks of the day included fusion surgery, and many children underwent these operations.

Dynamic deformities, on the other hand, demanded a more complex approach. Treatment often consisted of combinations of fusions, realigning osteotomies, releases, and tendon transfers, with careful consideration of how the child's growth would impact the deformity. Orthopaedic surgeons in Europe and the United States had performed tenotomies and tendon lengthenings for musculoskeletal deformities for many years. They had considerable experience with outcomes and providing aftercare. Transferring the tendon of a normal muscle to correct loss of function of a paralyzed muscle was a relatively new concept, however. Carl Nicoladoni[24] performed the first such procedure in 1880, but there was scant demand for the operation in America until the rise of polio in the second decade of the 20th century. Thereafter, American orthopaedists responding to the needs of large numbers of polio patients had to learn the principles and methods of tendon transfers. During the period from 1916 to 1961, the orthopaedic community in this country devoted a great deal of attention to the treatment of poliomyelitis. Musculoskeletal surgery for these children became the heart and soul of orthopaedics during those years.

Joel E. Goldthwait of Boston published the first American paper on the treatment of a polio-related musculoskeletal disorder in volume 5 of the *American Journal of Orthopaedic Surgery* in 1908. His paper, "An Operation for the Stiffening of the Ankle Joint in Infantile Paralysis," reviewed his indications for performing an ankle fusion in patients with chronic polio. "The muscles of the lower leg are usually paralyzed, and as a part of the paralysis, the ligaments which support the foot and ankle are usually much weakened, so that when the weight is borne upon the foot, the flattening of the arch with the dropping of the inner side of the foot is marked. The flail foot with a marked toe-drop is the type." Goldthwait described only technique; he did not provide such essential details as number of patients he had treated, their ages and sex, associated deformities, how many achieved a solid ankle fusion, or how the procedure improved gait and function. He did not appear to consider patient satisfaction in the outcome.

In the same 1908 issue of the *American Journal of Orthopaedic Surgery*, Sir Robert Jones of Liverpool described an operation for paralytic calcaneocavus foot deformities, noting that "the literature of flail ankle is copious and conflicting, and that type known as paralytic pes calcaneocavus is, of all others, the most intractable to treat." He referred to the astragalectomy operation of Royal Whitman, but naturally touted his own technique over Whitman's. Jones' operation required a two-stage procedure, the first of which accomplished a wedge-shaped resection of bone from the midfoot. The second operation, done four weeks later, was performed though a direct posterior approach through the heel cord. It included the removal of a wedge of bone from the talus, fusion of the ankle, tightening of the posterior capsule of the ankle, and shortening of the heel cord. Jones did not report outcomes.

After this slow start in reporting their experiences with treating polio-related disorders, American orthopaedic surgeons rapidly developed a profound interest in the disease as the epidemic intensified. The early reports that orthopaedists prepared for their journal reflected the ignorance in the medical community concerning the cause, pathophysiology, and potential interventions for treating these patients. For example, Sir Robert Jones[25] wrote in an invited editorial that the disease follows the distribution of the anterior spinal artery and that the "toxin" responsible for the death of motor cells in the spinal cord spreads from the artery "due to the entrance of some irritant into the vessel walls." He also mentioned the practice of nerve anastomosis, in which a surgeon would transfer part of the healthy nerve into one that was nonfunctional or minimally functional due to the polio. Jones justifiably expressed considerable skepticism about this procedure. He stood on more solid ground when he discussed orthopaedic operations in the treatment of children with paralytic deformities. He reported that he had performed more than 300 tendon transfers in polio patients. From that experience, he learned that a strong muscle transferred under correct tension and solidly secured to its new site would effectively restore useful function to an otherwise paralyzed limb.

Jones expressed less satisfaction with his results in joint fusions, noting that fusions in very young children had the least successful outcomes: "We have not known a case of bony union occurring in a child operated upon under 4, but in children over 10, the fixations rarely failed." The final paragraph of his editorial captured his optimism: "When we look back only a few years to the hopeless state of paralyzed children, we are proud of the advances made by surgery. It is in our power, no matter what the age or condition, to correct deformities . . . we can safely predict that paralytic distortions will cease to exist, and that the hopeless figures seen on crutches will only be known as a parental reproach."

In 1916, the year of the worst polio epidemic to date in the United States, the *American Journal of Orthopaedic Surgery* published an impressive 13 papers related to the disease. By 1916, orthopaedists had treated a much larger volume of patients, providing a wealth of data to support their assertions on treatment more credibly.

After World War I, orthopaedic surgeons codified the treatment of chronic polio. By the late 1940s through the early 1950s, the care of children with polio evolved into a defined specialty. As the number of cases peaked, medical texts, exemplified by *Campbell's Operative Orthopaedics*, devoted hundreds of pages to correction of paralytic spinal deformities, tendon transfers about the major joints, fusion operations, bracing, soft-tissue releases, and follow-up care for these treatments. Several generations of orthopaedic residents-in-training improved their surgical skills by studying the indications for and performing such operations as heel cord lengthening, fascia lata releases for abduction and flexion contractures of the hip, foot-stabilizing operations such as ankle fusions and triple arthrodeses, hamstring transfers for quadriceps paralysis, and tendon transfers in the upper limb to restore elbow flexion or opposition of the thumb. The seemingly endless list of complicated indications and procedures confounded all but the most committed. It grew clear to those who practiced pediatric orthopaedics that they should consider themselves subspecialists within the broader field of orthopaedic surgery.

In reality, what orthopaedic surgeons did during those decades of the polio epidemics mattered relatively little with regard to the impact of poliomyelitis on the public health and psyche. It is hard to conceive of the horror families must have felt when a healthy child suddenly developed a high fever, stiff neck, trouble breathing, and inability to move the arms or legs. People knew what lay ahead for such a child; what the public really wanted was a medical intervention that would eradicate poliomyelitis. Miraculously, this goal was achieved with the advent of mass immunization, thanks to vaccines developed by Jonas Salk and Albert Sabin.

Jonas Salk[19,26] began work on a polio vaccine at the University of Pittsburgh in the late 1940s. His vaccine used an attenuated but live virus. Subsequently, Albert Sabin developed a vaccine using killed poliovirus. A sort of tug-of-war consequently evolved over the relative safety and efficacy of these two types of vaccines. In the United States and most other countries of the world, the live poliomyelitis vaccine has been adopted for general use. In Sweden, possibly because immunization programs are more stringently administered, the killed polio virus vaccines have been selected for general use. Regardless of which vaccine local authorities select, the extraordinary and almost unbelievable success of mass immunizations has resulted in the virtual eradication of poliomyelitis. For a few years after mass immunizations began, children with deformities caused by polio still appeared in clinics and orthopaedic practices, but as polio cases dwindled, so did the need for hospitals and equipage formerly essential for the high volume of epidemic victims.

Nearly 50 years after the discovery of the vaccine, acute poliomyelitis has all but disappeared. The nearly 500,000 individuals still alive who had the disease before the vaccines became available are still impaired by polio's paralyzing effects. In the past 20 years, some of these individuals have shown increasing weakness, fatigue, muscle and joint pain, cold intolerance, and gradually worsening atrophy. Some orthopaedists and physiatrists refer to this as postpolio syndrome. Theories about causation include a gradual, aging-related loss of motor neurons superimposed on an already reduced number from the polio, ongoing denervation of muscles that had been reinnervated following the acute attack, and an as-yet ill-defined immunologic reaction. The therapists and physicians who have described the syndrome do not offer a specific form of treatment. The medical literature suggests swimming exercises, adjustments in lifestyle and activity levels, nonsteroidal anti-inflammatory drugs, and, in one instance, pyridostigmine bromide "for the enhancement of synaptic transmissions."[27-31]

Neurologic Conditions

The conquests of tuberculosis and polio enabled orthopaedic surgeons to focus their attention on diseases and conditions that had not previously involved them. These included cerebral palsy, myelomeningocele, muscular dystrophy, arthrogryposis, spinal muscular atrophy, and other neurologic conditions.

Cerebral Palsy

In the 1830s Dr. William J. Little[32] developed an interest in the condition now called cerebral palsy. Little had a foot deformity, probably caused by polio, which had responded well to percutaneous tenotomy performed by G. F. Strohmeyer, the German surgeon who practiced in Hanover. Little stayed with Strohmeyer for a time after his surgery, learned Strohmeyer's techniques, and returned home filled with enthusiasm for the new specialty called orthopaedics. He founded the Royal Orthopaedic Hospital in London not long thereafter. Little's research into the new specialty of orthopaedics led him into the most complete analysis of birth injury-related deformity of the 19th century. His work culminated in the paper, "On the Influence of Abnormal Parturition, Difficult Labors, Premature Birth, and Asphyxia Neonatorum on the Mental and Physical Condition of the Child, Especially in Relation to Deformities," published in 1861. Little related specific brain injuries to the resultant deformities of the musculoskeletal system; for many years thereafter, cerebral palsy was called "Little's disease."

During the second half of the 19th century and the early years of the 20th century in America, the relatively few physicians who called themselves orthopaedic surgeons showed little interest in cerebral palsy. The first American to address this issue substantively was Winthrop Phelps. In 1932, he presented a paper entitled "Cerebral Birth Injuries: Their Orthopedic Classification and Subsequent Treatment" at the New York Academy of Medicine.[33] Phelps identified five categories of musculoskeletal involvement arising from birth trauma—spasticity, athetosis, synkinesia, ataxia, and tremor—and he correlated these with the kinds of central nervous system injuries his patients had sustained at birth. Phelps took a conservative approach to treating cerebral palsy, and during his career he generally opposed operating on patients with it. His position encountered opposition, however, and by the mid-1950s he apparently felt the need to defend it in a paper published in the *The Journal of Bone and Joint Surgery* (*JBJS*) entitled "Long-term Results of Orthopaedic Surgery in Cerebral Palsy."[34] He personally had examined 200 children on whom orthopaedists from "all parts of the United States had performed nearly 500 operations." He concluded that "tendon transplantation always fails because the injury in cerebral palsy does not involve individual muscles as in polio, but it affects joint position and usage because of the more central cause of the disability." Phelps also concluded that tenotomies and tendon lengthening provided little lasting benefit for most patients with cerebral palsy-related contractures, but he did offer limited endorsement for adductor releases and hamstring lengthenings in a few patients with mild spastic hemiplegia or diplegia. He also concluded that fusions of the hindfoot might be appropriate in some patients, but his basic approach to deformity and cerebral palsy involved only bracing and physical therapy.

Phelps' conservativism has subsequently met with considerable criticism. Even his memorialist in the obituary published in *Developmental Medicine and Child Neurology* in 1972 noted that he did not have "sufficient statistical evidence to support the conclusions to which he had come"; more recently, orthopaedic surgeons have adopted treatment protocols that are more balanced between physical therapy and bracing versus surgery. Since World War II, Samilson, Bleck, Perry, Hoeffer, Sutherland, Renshaw, Waters and others have published numerous papers and monographs on the subject. Their efforts have resulted in a reasonably standardized approach to musculoskeletal conditions associated with brain injury at birth. Most authors now agree that patients with contractures related to spasticity can be improved with surgical lengthening of tight tendons. They also seem to concur that surgery should be done early in the patient's life and that the surgeon should attempt to correct as many things as possible at one sitting instead of subjecting the child to multiple anesthesias and procedures.[35-38]

In the past 30 years, orthopaedic surgeons have developed ways of assessing the effect of surgical releases on cerebral palsy patients preoperatively. At first, this involved performing lidocaine nerve blocks before surgery. However, lidocaine remained effective for too short a time to permit evaluation of the potential effect of the surgical releases of the given muscle, so some surgeons switched to lidocaine and alcohol injections. The discomfort associated with alcohol injections and the limited duration of lidocaine's effectiveness have led to the use of small doses of botulinum toxin for nerve blocks of longer duration.[39] Astereognosis limits the utility of upper limb surgery of cerebral palsy, but tendon transfers and surgical releases can improve the position and appearance of the elbow and wrist. Green and Banks,[40] for example, popularized a procedure that involved transfer of the flexor carpi ulnaris to the dorsum of the hand for the treatment of wrist flexion contractures, and Inglis and Cooper[41] described a release of the wrist flexors from the medial humeral epicondyle for the same kind of deformity. Most orthopaedic surgeons who currently treat cerebral palsy patients, however, publish and present papers on the results of the surgical treatment of lower-limb contractions and deformity, including the problems associated with paralytic hip subluxation and dislocations, foot stabilizations, and the control of pelvic and spinal deformities. Cerebral palsy specialists have also investigated the possibility that dorsal rhyzotomy of lumbar spine nerve roots might decrease lower-limb spasticity in these patients. Despite hopes that this operation would prevent the overcorrection of contractures and deformities that occasionally result from surgical releases of muscles and tendons, dorsal rhyzotomy has been somewhat disappointing to date.[42,43]

Myelomeningocele

Dr. William Sharrard[44,45] in Great Britain popularized a procedure for paralytic hip dislocations in children with myelomeningocele in the 1960s and 1970s (Figure 14). His operation entailed the transfer of the psoas tendon to the greater trochanter through a defect created in the ilium. He postulated that because children with myelomeningocele with an L4 or an L5 paraplegia have no strength in the gluteus medius, transfer of the psoas to the insertion of the gluteus would keep the femoral head in the acetabulum and make the child able to walk more or less normally. Sharrard's book on the orthopaedic aspects of the treatment of patients with myelomeningocele contrasted somewhat with the approach of John Lorber, also in Great Britain. Lorber[46] advocated virtually no treatment of these patients, especially those with severe involvement. His "adverse criteria" included a high level of paraplegia, severe hydrocephalus, and associated malformations, and his concept was that these children should receive no treatment as newborns and be allowed to die in the nursery. For those who did survive, Lorber preferred noninterventional treatment as a management concept, especially for their musculoskeletal problems. The debate apparently caught the attention of American orthopaedic surgeons, and in the early 1970s, Burr Curtis of Hartford and Mark Hoffer and Jacquelin Perry of Rancho Los Amigos in Los Angeles began to present courses and publish papers and monographs on the orthopaedic treatment of patients with myelomeningocele. These children, of course, face a complex array of medical and social issues that necessarily involve several pediatric and surgical subspecialists. These issues include problems with mental deficiency, hydrocephalus and other kinds of brain injury, as well as severe urologic disorders, with atonic bladders, hydroureter, hydronephrosis, bladder and renal calculi, and multiple urinary tract infections. Many die because massive decubiti develop, become infected, and produce uncontrollable sepsis. Many also face very difficult social issues such as abandonment, broken families, and enormous expenses related to their care.

The effort to keep such children ambulatory requires various operations to keep their feet aligned, knees straight, and both hips more or less located and properly aligned with the pelvis and spine. Most children also need at least some bracing to stand upright and walk. If the child has enough strength in the upper limbs, he or she might be able to walk with crutches. Most children and their families give up after years of effort, however, and revert to a wheelchair. Even those with lower-level spinal cord lesions and with quadriceps strong enough to support an upright posture find that skin breakdown on their feet associated with their deformed and insensate limbs make independent ambulation very burdensome. Orthopaedists have concluded that they probably have a limited role in the overall management of children with myelomeningocele. Nevertheless, several orthopaedic surgeons, including, Luciano Diaz, John Banta, Thomas Renshaw, Marc Asher, Malcolm Menelaus, Norris Carroll and others published papers on their treatment outcomes and the results of orthopaedic management. A review of the history of medicine in general and orthopaedics in particular reveals several "blind alleys." Aggressive treatment of foot instability in children with myelomeningocele may be one of these, and prevention and treatment of spinal deformity in such patients may have greater importance for them than multiple operations on the feet, knees, and hips; for many of them, sitting balance is more important than standing upright in a standing brace.[47-50]

Muscular Dystrophy

Guillaime Benjamin Armand Duchenne, a French physician, published his classic article describing pseudohypertrophic muscular dystrophy in 1886.[51] He described the age of onset (2 to 6 years), the hypertrophy of the calves, progressive weakness, and early death in these patients, all of whom were males. Despite the fact that pseudohypertrophic muscular dystrophy would be labeled Duchenne muscular dystrophy, Duchenne had a deeper interest in electrophysiology experiments, and realizing the futility of treating patients with muscular dystrophy, he and others paid little attention to its treatment. British neurologist William Richard Gower, however, discussed Duchenne muscular dystrophy in his 1879 paper, "Pseudohypertrophic Muscular Paralysis." He identified the Gower sign, which describes the peculiar way children with muscular dystrophy stand erect from a sitting or recombinant position. Gower pointed out that they appeared to climb up their own bodies, pushing themselves erect by moving their hands gradually up their knees and thighs. Duchenne, Gower, and others who published papers on this impairment of muscular dystrophy all recognized its progressive behavior and noted that patients afflicted with it all die of respiratory failure in their late teens or early 20s. In the 1960s, P. J. Vignos and K. C. Archibald[52] of the Department of Medicine at Case Western Reserve University published a paper on the maintenance of ambulation in these patients. They hypothesized that the treatment of the contractures of the lower limbs of patients with muscular dystrophy might make it possible for them to remain ambulatory for two years or more beyond what they could expect without treatment. Stretching, bracing, and exercises were the recommended treatment modalities through the 1950s, but in the late 1960s several orthopaedic surgeons began to supplement these measures with tenotomies and surgical releases.[53] More recently, several surgeons have reported on their results in the treatment of scoliotic deformities that muscular dystrophy patients almost invariably developed, particularly in the late phases of the disease. Surgery and anesthesia in these patients, however, carries greater risk than in normal individuals, and surgeons and anesthesiologists have reported an increased incidence of malignant hyperthermia, respiratory complications, and excessive bleeding, especially during scoliosis surgery, in muscular dystrophy patients. The real future of muscular dystrophy treatment most likely lies in developments in molecular biology and gene therapy rather than orthopaedic surgery.

Clubfoot

Lewis A. Sayre published a book on the treatment of talipes equinovarus (clubfoot) in 1869. He advocated aggressive manipulation of the deformity and the use of a specially designed brace to maintain alignment. He also reported that failure of closed treatment could occur, in which case he advocated the use of surgical tenotomy. His book contains an illustration showing how he performed that operation. Surgeons did not wear gowns or gloves at that time, and they operated in their street clothes. Infection complicated many of these procedures.

Papers presented at the early meetings of the American Orthopaedic Association (AOA) in the 1890s detailed techniques for achieving correction with closed methods. Some debate took place regarding the relative merits of the Thomas wrench versus the Bradford tarsoclast. The idea was that the orthopaedist should achieve complete correction of the deformity by a single, very forceful manipulation. Virgil Gibney of the Hospital for the Ruptured and Crippled in New York stated that he preferred the Thomas wrench for this purpose because "the principle of this instrument is so simple that anyone can wrench a club foot into a very good shape." E. M. Phelps reported in 1890 at the AOA meeting that he had invented a machine for forcibly manipulating a clubfoot that could deliver up to one ton of pressure on the foot; he noted that "the operator should not stop operating until the foot is super-corrected." These and other orthopaedists also advocated the liberal use of tenotomies and, for relapsed difficult cases, astragelectomy.

In the first three decades of the 20th century, advocacy for forceful manipulation gradually disappeared from the printed record. By 1920, Frank Ober, Arthur Steindler, Michael Hoke and others described more gentle manipulations; when these failed, they attempted less destructive surgery. Hokes' junior associate, J. Hiram Kite, developed an almost obsessive interest in clubfoot and published numerous papers and a book-length monograph on his ideas regarding etiology, treatment, and outcomes. Kite's basic message was that repeated careful manipulations and serial castings would produce good to excellent outcomes in the overwhelming majority of children without subjecting them to open surgery.[54] Kite succeeded Hoke as director at the Scottish Rite Hospital in Atlanta after Hokes's death in 1944, and Wood Lovell, coauthor of Lovell and Winter's *Pediatric Orthopaedics*, succeeded Kite at that institution. Kite appreciated the nature of the deformity and undertook the gradual correction of each element of it in his patients. This entailed first the gentle manipulation and stretching of the metatarsus adductus, then the correction of the heel inversion, and finally the correction of the equinus. The gradual correction of the deformity required multiple gentle manipulations, repeated cast applications after each one, and patience and determination on the part of all concerned: patient, parents, and physician. Kite usually spent six months or more achieving correction of the deformity, at which point he had the child use a Denis Browne splint for many more months until he felt confident that the clubfoot was well and permanently corrected. Ignacio Ponseti,[55] the academic heir of Arthur Steindler at the University of Iowa, advocated more aggressive manipulation and stretching and usually required less time to achieve correction. Ponseti also had a lower threshold for resorting to Achilles tendon lengthening in his patients; he used that operation frequently to correct the equinus component of the deformity. Like Kite, however, Ponseti maintained contact with his patients for many years, and he required them to use Denis Browne splints, at least part-time, for up to six years after the end of the serial manipulations and casting.

In the late 1960s and early 1970s, several orthopaedists reported that they had moved away from the conservatism of Kite and Ponseti and had determined that early surgical correction of clubfoot deformities would achieve better outcomes in much less time. Much of the current literature on the subject of clubfoot deformity explores how best to do this and how to treat the seemingly inevitable complications. Vincent Turco[56] of Hartford, Connecticut, published a monograph on this subject in 1981. He reported that a seven-year follow-up of patients with clubfoot deformities showed only a 35 percent success rate with nonsurgical management, but he noted that mild deformity was easy to treat and responded well. More severe and more rigid deformities almost always failed conservative treatment and required early surgery if, after a year of manipulation and serial casting, the deformity remained uncorrected or only partly corrected. Turco advocated a one-stage posteromedial release with internal fixation. His procedure involved lengthening of the Achilles tendon and posterior tibial tendon and capsulotomies of the posterior tibiotalar and posterior talocalcaneal ligaments to correct the equinus deformity. The medial part of the release involved dividing the attachment of the plantar fascia and abductor hallucis, the superficial deltoid ligament, the talonavicular capsule, and the spring ligament.

McKay,[57] Simons,[58] and Goldner[59] all published extensively about their own methods of performing this kind of surgery. Alvin Crawford of the University of Cincinnati popularized the "Cincinnati incision"[60] in an article published with Jeffrey Marxen and Diane Osterfeld in *JBJS* in 1982. Crawford reported that Nicholas Giannestras had developed the approach, which according to Crawford had not been described previously. The surgeons who performed and described the tenotomies and releases in young children emphasized the need to accompany these procedures with osteotomies of the os calcis (Dwyer),[61] cuboid (Evans),[62] metatarsal, or distal tibia (Goldner) when soft-tissue surgery alone failed to achieve complete correction. Correction of residual deformity of the foot through a joint instead of through a bone adjacent to a joint would almost inevitably produce fusion of the joint. The resultant disruption of the normal kinematics of the foot would overstress adjacent articulations and result in their deterioration and possibly the early onset of painful osteoarthritis. Children older than ten years of age, however, usually require bony fusion for correction and maintenance of correction of foot deformities[63] Michael Hoke[64] and Edwin Ryerson[65] devised the triple arthrodesis procedure for these situations in 1921 and 1923, respectively. David Grice and William T. Green[66] in 1955 described an extra-articular fusion for use in younger children for whom a surgeon should maintain as much growth potential as possible.

An orthopaedic surgeon whose patient has a relapsed or neglected clubfoot now has the option of using the Ilizarov technique.[67] The Ilizarov frame constructs permit correction with gradual stretching of contracted soft tissues, but any given patient might also require limited soft-tissue releases or bone surgery to gain adequate correction of the deformity. The method carries multiple risks and poses the chance of multiple complications. It is, however, an alternative treatment of a patient with a very difficult deformity.

Pediatric Hip Disorders

Legg-Calvé-Perthes disease, slipped capital femoral epiphysis (SCFE), congenital coxa vara, and developmental dysplasia of the hip (DDH) occupy much of the pediatric orthopaedic surgeon's time and attention. Because developmental dysplasia of the hip occurs more frequently than the others, it will be discussed more thoroughly in a separate section. The history of the other diagnostic entities will be highlighted in this section.

Legg-Calvé-Perthes Disease
Arthur T. Legg of Boston first brought the attention of American orthopaedists to "an obscure affection of the hip joint" subsequently named for him when he presented a paper at the 1909 meeting of the AOA. In 1910, he published a paper in the *Boston Medical and Surgical Journal* (the predecessor of the *New England Journal of Medicine*).[68] Legg had described five children between 5 and 8 years of age who had hip pain and stiffness. Roentgen's discovery of the x-ray enabled Legg to identify flattening of the femoral head and shortening of the femoral neck in these patients with "increased radiability" in the upper part of the head and neck.

One of the children had feverish constitutional symptoms. Legg thought that "deranged circulation" might have caused these changes because he believed that he had ruled out injury, rickets, syphilis, or low-grade infection. He obtained good results treating four of the patients with flannel spica or plaster spica casts. Joel E. Goldthwait, also of Boston, had allowed Legg to mention in the report a similar patient upon whom Goldthwait had operated. Goldthwait had curetted out "necrotic material from the head and neck," although a culture of the necrotic material subsequently showed the presence of staphylococci.

At approximately the same time, Jacques Calvé of France and Georg Perthes of Germany reported their experience with similar kinds of patients. They also used radiographs to differentiate the condition from other diseases such as tuberculosis, which in those years was a common cause of pain and stiffness in children's hip joints. Through the middle years of the 20th century, treatment consisted most often of non-weight bearing. Many children spent months or even years moving about on wheeled stretchers short enough for them to reach the floor and to push themselves wherever they wanted to go. Alternatively, some orthopaedists permitted their patients to walk, but with a sling that held the affected leg in too much flexion to permit weight bearing or with braces that kept the affected leg out of contact with the floor.

Approximately 20 years after Legg, Calvé, and Perthes had identified the "obscure affection," other orthopaedists began to adopt the principles of "containment" of the femoral head in the acetabulum to allow the disrupted physis to heal and remodel while it remained well seated in the spherical socket. Petrie and Bitenc[69] attempted to achieve this with bilateral long leg casts held in 30° of abduction by broomsticks attached to the casts. Walking in this apparatus was difficult, and other orthopaedists attempted to modify it with removable orthoses. Osteotomies on the femoral or acetabular sides of the hip also can improve containment of the head, and in the past 30 years numerous papers have described the indications, techniques, and outcomes of these kinds of procedures. There are, however, few resolved issues regarding Legg-Calvé-Perthes disease, and debate continues over etiology, diagnosis, classification, treatment, and prognosis.[70-73]

Slipped Capital Femoral Epiphysis

Musculoskeletal surgeons have recognized spontaneous displacement of the capital femoral epiphysis since the late 16th century, but accurate diagnosis and effective treatment would not really come about until the advent of x-ray technology. Since then, of course, orthopaedic surgeons usually have been able to make the diagnosis and begin effective treatment early. Several orthopaedic surgeons have investigated the etiology of Slipped Capital Femoral Epiphysis (SCFE). Chung and associates,[74] for example, studied the effect of shear stresses on the physis of children and adolescents in 1976. They reported that the interdigitations of the facing epiphyseal and metaphyseal surfaces could not resist shear forces enough to prevent slips, even in the range of physiologic loads. Their studies show the importance of obesity in adolescence as a causal factor in SCFE. Others have investigated hormonal disorders as causes of physeal failure in adolescents, but these studies have not established any specific endocrinopathy as an etiologic factor.[75-77]

In 1953, David R. Telson[78] of New York reported that he had treated patients with SCFE since 1932 with in situ pinning using threaded stainless steel pins. He documented the importance of early diagnosis to allow fixation before a severe slip developed. He also noted that occasionally he had achieved a closed reduction of a severe slip using the Ledbetter maneuver, making it possible therefore to easily and accurately insert the threaded pins from the lateral approach instead of aiming the pins back into the femoral head from the front of the femoral neck. Telson also reported that using a larger fixation device, such as a Smith-Petersen nail, resulted on several occasions in the displacement of the capital femoral epiphysis; he strongly urged that surgeons use multiple threaded pins instead. Telson and others reported that stabilizing the slipping epiphysis also permits remodeling of the femoral neck, even if a closed reduction of the slip fails to achieve perfect reduction.

Orthopaedic surgeons have reported multiple kinds of operations in patients with severe fixed deformity resulting from the slip. Herndon and associates,[79] for example, claimed that excision of the bony ridge on the anterior surface of the femoral neck would help realign the upper femur and improve motion. If necessary, and if the physis is not completely closed, the surgeon could simultaneously insert multiple short bone grafts from the neck into the head, as described by Beckett Howorth in 1966.[80] For treatment of more severe deformity in skeletally mature patients, many surgeons concluded that only an upper femoral osteotomy could satisfactorily correct deformity. Wayne Southwick[81] popularized a biplane intertrochanteric osteotomy for this purpose, although other surgeons have reported different kinds of osteotomies at different sites.[82-84]

Patients with SCFE face multiple risks (infection, progression of deformity, nonunion of an osteotomy, and late osteoarthritis), but chondrolysis and osteonecrosis relate more specifically to it. In 1930, C. H. Waldenström[85] described chondrolysis, also called acute cartilage necrosis, which consists of attenuation, thinning, and loss of the articular cartilage on both sides of the hip joint, presumably due to an autoimmune process that occurs in some patients with SCFE or due to inadvertent intra-articular placement of fixation pins. Occasionally the process reverses itself, and subsequent radiographs show restoration of the joint space with improved range of motion and decreased hip pain. It can also progress until the joint ankyloses almost completely. Osteonecrosis caused by loss of the blood supply to the femoral head can also occur with or without treatment but is most common in patients with severe acute slips. Osteonecrosis has a poorer prognosis in patients with SCFE than in those with Legg-Calvé-Perthes disease because SCFE occurs in older patients who have less time for their femoral head to remodel.[85,86]

Congenital Coxa Vara
Varus deformity of the upper femur also occurs in patients with congenital coxa vara, a rare developmental condition that causes shortening of the

femoral neck, a decrease in the neck-shaft angle, and relative elongation of the greater trochanter. The condition results from the presence of a cartilaginous defect in the inferior femoral neck just distal to the physis. The loss of mechanical support in this location allows the metaphysis to separate from the epiphysis and migrate upward to produce the coxa vara deformity. European physicians recognized congenital coxa vara as a specific entity of the late 19th century. Reginald Cheyne Elmslie[87] presented a paper at a meeting of the World College of Surgeons on the subject in February 1907. He described "a downward displacement of the head of the femur, carrying with it the adjoining portion of the base of the neck." The fragment of femoral neck that moves with the femoral head has subsequently been called Elmslie epiphysis. With photographs, radiographs, and drawings, Elmslie showed how the abnormality results in the vertical alignment of the physis and progressive deformity. The only treatment is an intertrochanteric osteotomy with the restoration of both the neck-shaft angle and the horizontality of the physis.[87,88]

Developmental Dysplasia of the Hip
Developmental Dysplasia of the Hip (DDH) is an excellent example of how the diagnosis and treatment of a specific abnormality evolves. This single entity illustrates how, over time, orthopaedic surgeons found new ways to modify a disease process of the musculoskeletal system in children.[89]

In the early 20th century, orthopaedic surgeons in the United States did not seem to appreciate the importance of examining newborns for DDH. The literature on the subject ignored the significance of this condition in infants. In fact, to the practitioners of musculoskeletal surgery, congenital hip dislocation was an entity only recognizable well after a child had learned to walk, even into young adulthood. Reduction of the hip in older children who had suffered with a dislocation for many years was obviously a difficult undertaking. One can understand why the members of the AOA were thrilled when Adolph Lorenz, the Viennese surgeon, came to the United States to demonstrate the technique for treatment of congenitally dislocated hips. Many surgeons had discussed how hard it was to reduce and maintain reduction in a femoral head that had been dislocated for 7 to 12 years and noted that open surgery might be a better answer to the problem. Lorenz denounced this approach (not surprisingly, as his allergy to the carbolic acid required for Lister's antiseptic techniques precluded him from performing open surgery). He came upon the idea of "bloodless reduction," a euphemism for the aggressive manipulation of the femoral head into the acetabulum. The charismatic Lorenz conducted a triumphant tour through America, demonstrating his treatment method (principally on patients with congenital hip dislocations) without performing open surgery.[90,91] But by 1903, American orthopaedists began to take a critical look at his results. In that year, H. L. Taylor[92] presented a paper at the annual meeting of the AOA on peripheral palsies following manual replacement of the congenitally dislocated hip. He reported a startling array of complications using the Lorenz technique, including femoral and sciatic nerve ruptures and lumbosacral plexus injuries. Other members present at the meeting corroborated the fact that Lorenz's forceful manipulation could be dangerous. John Ridlon described how Lorenz had performed his manipulation of the hip on Ridlon's patients, producing a femoral shaft fracture in one patient, a fracture of the femoral neck in another, paralysis of the sciatic nerve in another, and a perineal tear in still another. N. M. Shafer reported that when Lorenz manipulated the hip of one of his patients, he tore the soft-tissue envelope about the hip so badly that a massive hematoma developed and the procedure had to be abandoned. B. E. Mackenzie reported that Lorenz claimed to be able to achieve stable reductions in 50% of patients with a unilateral dislocation and in 25 percent of patients with bilateral dislocations. He said that Lorenz's results in his (Mackenzie's) patients were "not that good." He also noted that Lorenz was a man of "Herculean strength and he manifested this while performing his manipulations." Roswell Park of Buffalo opined that "this is not bloodless"; it is not safe to break bones and tear tissue so indiscriminately. DeForest Willard noted, "if the hip is out in a 12 year old, let it be."[92]

Lorenz may have had second thoughts about these aggressive and destructive manipulations; he devised an osteotomy that he claimed would stabilize a dislocated hip, even though the femoral head remained out of and well above the socket.[93,94] He advocated cutting through the femoral shaft just below the level of the acetabulum and angulating the femur medially to provide a kind of prop beneath the socket and along the wing of the pelvis; the patient would bear weight on that part of the femur directly beneath the acetabulum and not on the femoral head, which would be well above the acetabulum up beneath the iliac crest. Viennese surgeons Lorenz, Schanz, and von Baeyer all had basically the same configuration to their various osteotomies, which found a way into American orthopaedic texts well into the 20th century. Arthur Steindler, chairman at the University of Iowa, also from Vienna, included these procedures in his own 1940 book, *Orthopaedic Operations: Indications, Techniques, and End Results*. Steindler called the Lorenz osteotomy "essentially a stabilizing operation because it furnishes a point of support in the unstable hip." None of the modern pediatric orthopaedic texts include descriptions of these osteotomies.

In 1928, Ernest Hey Groves,[95] Professor of Surgery at Bristol University in England and one of the most respected orthopaedic surgeons in that country, was invited to submit a paper for publication in a volume dedicated to a celebration of Sir Robert Jones, the father of British orthopaedics. In writing about congenital dislocation of the hip (now called developmental dysplasia of the hip), Hey Groves noted that "the deformity is very seldom recognized either by parent, nurse, or doctor until the child is between two or three years of age." He recommended that treatment at that stage should consist of closed manipulation under anesthesia and immobilization in a cast with the leg in wide abduction for 6 to 9 months. Such treatment might have a chance to "convert the hip" from a dislocation to a reduced condition. More often, according to Hey Groves, a diagnosis was not made until the patient's waddling gait aroused suspicion. By this time, at 4 to 5 years of age, the ossification centers had appeared and a radiograph of the hip would show the dislocation clearly. Hey Groves noted, however, that because the dislocation did not cause pain at that age, the parents and child did not consider the condition troublesome enough to seek treatment. In the early school years, even if the dislocation had been diagnosed, many physicians felt that it was already too late for treatment and most likely would tell the parents that nothing could be done. Left untreated, by 20 years of age these young adults would experience progressive pain that would eventually be incapacitating.

Hey Groves believed that manipulation and prolonged cast immobilization might work up until 6 years of age. He also postulated that surgical treatment had an excellent chance of preventing late disability and pain, provided the surgeon could operate by the time the child was 12 years old. Hey Groves approached the hip through a long anterior incision and stripped the soft tissue away from the capsule of the hip. The capsule, of course, had stretched to the point that the ball-and-socket joint had migrated up and away from the socket, and it almost always became contracted where the psoas tendon passed over it. This constriction produced an hourglass configuration of the capsule so that the hip could not be reduced unless the psoas tendon was removed and the constriction corrected. Groves advocated cutting across the hip capsule at the level of the constriction, enclosing the head in the upper part of the hourglass, and drawing the capsule over the head with a purse string suture. He then opened the capsule widely about the rim of the acetabulum and placed the head (now covered with the capsule) into it. Several factors could make this difficult. "When after the preliminary steps the acetabulum is found to be so flat that it will not retain the femoral head, the most natural thing is to attempt to hollow out the socket. This is easily done by gouger or reamer, removing the soft cartilage and some of the underlying bone."

When this approach failed, Hey Groves advocated performing a shelving procedure, which is "a way of keeping the head of the femur from slipping out of the socket by making a new rim to the upper part of the acetabulum." He accomplished this part of the operation by driving an osteotome from the outer surface of the pelvic bone across the acetabulum through to the inner cortex. He levered the upper part of the socket down over the femoral head and tried to anchor it with a bone graft or block of ivory wedged into the osteotomy. Part of the graft should extend out to provide more coverage to the head if it remained unstable. Hey Groves' description of this part of the operation and his accompanying drawings resemble the Salter and Pemberton osteotomies popularized by those authors several decades later.

In the paper cited, Hey Groves did not report on the several patients he treated, how they fared, and whether the operation worked over the long term. Nonetheless, his procedure was adopted by several American orthopaedists and became popular as the "Colonna procedure." Paul Colonna, chairman of the Department of Orthopaedics at the University of Pennsylvania, reiterated it in his 1953 paper, "Capsular Arthroplasty for Congenital Dislocation of the Hip."[96] Colonna performed his variation of the procedure in two or three stages. Stage one consisted of the surgical release of tight soft tissues about the hip by appropriate tenotomies, followed by traction to bring down the femoral head to the level of the acetabulum. The second procedure consisted of the capsular arthroplasty as described by Hey Groves, followed by prolonged cast immobilization. Colonna reported that a deformity of the upper femur in which the head and neck projected too anteriorly (anteversion) often made it necessary to perform a supracondylar derotation osteotomy of the femur. Like Hey Groves, Colonna gave no details on number of patients, how long they were followed, or their short-term and long-term results.

Eighteen years later, Stanley Chung, also of the University of Pennsylvania, found all of Colonna's patients who had had this operation. In 56 patients (63 arthroplasties), about half had good to excellent results.[97] Boardman and Moseley[98] of the Los Angeles Shriners Hospital found 17 former patients who had undergone the Colonna procedure 40 years previously. Only four had not yet had a total hip arthroplasty. Boardman and Moseley concluded that the Colonna arthroplasty "apparently plays a very limited role in the management of this relatively common orthopedic childhood disorder."

The remarkable changes that have occurred in the way orthopaedists diagnose and treat DDH have made the statement by Boardman and Moseley possible. There has been, for example, an extraordinary effort on the part of pediatric orthopaedists to diagnose newborns and begin treatment immediately. If the dislocated or unstable hip can be reduced and held in position reliably, the soft cartilaginous structures of the ball and socket can be expected to mold into the normal configuration. Presumably, this would eliminate the need for the much more aggressive, less certain operations that orthopaedic surgeons had devised to treat this problem. In a classic *JBJS* article published in 1976, Paul Ramsey, Steven Lasser, and Dean MacEwen[99] of Wilmington, Delaware, reviewed the issues of early diagnosis and treatment, and reported their results using the techniques first described by Arnold Pavlik. These authors instituted a "routine nursery examination of all newborn babies" in which experienced examiners would evaluate each newborn's hips with the Barlow and Ortolani maneuvers. If the examiner does, in fact, elicit instability, treatment can begin at once using the soft Pavlik harness with front and back straps that hold the hips in flexion and slight abduction, the position of stability. The authors reported that they used the Pavlik harness on 23 infants younger than 6 months of age with 27 dislocations and that all but three were successfully reduced. Furthermore, all of the hips that were reduced developed normally. As a result of this study and others like it, the benefits of early diagnosis and early effective treatment could now be realized with elimination, or at least a sharp reduction in the prevalence of, a major cause of disability in young adults.

Despite the optimism stimulated by such reports, DDH has not been eradicated. Regardless of early diagnosis and treatment, it remains the subject of many reports in recent years. Screening neonates for hip instability in the nursery, however, has at least reduced the number of older children presenting with dislocated or unstable hips.

After walking age, children with DDH usually have more obvious physical signs such as shortening of one leg, change in the distribution of thigh creases, a Galeazzi sign (apparent shortening of the thigh), and easily observable changes on radiographs. At that point in their lives, the tenotomies, traction, manipulative closed reduction, and immobilization techniques used by Hey Groves and Colonna might still be employed. If the diagnosis is made even later, open reduction and an osteotomy of the pelvis and femur might be required to maintain reduction.[100] In younger children, up to 8 years of age, a single osteotomy (Salter[101] or Pemberton[102]) may suffice to rotate the socket over the femoral head to achieve coverage, but as a child gets older these operations do not mobilize the acetabulum sufficiently. The Chiari osteotomy[103] can produce good coverage of the femoral head, but coverage is achieved at the cost of considerable distortion of the pelvis. It produces coverage of the femoral head with capsule interposed between the femoral head and the ilium instead of coverage of the femoral head with the articular cartilage of the acetabulum. Double or triple osteotomies of the pelvis (Sutherland and Greenfield,[104] Steel[105]) mobilized the socket more completely; in adolescents or young adults in whom there is persistent acetabular obliquity, incomplete coverage of the femoral head presages early osteoarthritis. Periacetabular osteotomy (Ganz and associates[106]) permits rotation of the acetabulum into a position covering the head without significantly distorting the pelvis.

Using clinical examination and ultrasound, pediatric orthopaedists have lowered the age at which DDH can be diagnosed. As a result, treatment begins earlier and is easier on the child and the parents. Research on DDH, however, is ongoing, and inquiry into improving detection and treatment outcomes persists at a high level.

The Crippled Children's Hospitals

In 1953, Alfred Shands, Jr.,[107] addressed the annual meeting of the AOA on "the care and treatment of crippled children." That year, representing the peak of the polio epidemics and just before the polio vaccines from Jonas Salk's laboratory came into general use, marked the high point of the need for crippled children's hospitals. Shands enumerated many of the physicians, philanthropists, and organizations involved in the crippled children's crusades during the late 19th and early 20th centuries. Indeed, many thousands of physicians, nurses, administrators, therapists, brace makers, and patients had passed through the wards of these institutions. Most have either closed or dramatically changed to remain open.

In his address, Shands cited one hospital in particular, the Gillette Children's Hospital in St. Paul, Minnesota. In 1998, a former resident physician there, Steven Koop, wrote a history of the hospital.[108] Koop's book captured the poignancy of such an institution during the decades of tuberculosis and polio. It details how orthopaedic surgeons practiced, how young patients were hospitalized for years at a time, and how parents and children coped with their separations. Koop's book also describes how Gillette Children's Hospital has tried to redefine itself since the annihilation of polio, which removed the patient base and eliminated the hospital's reason for existence. Koop writes:

> The first 25 years of the hospital were dominated by infections of bones and joints, especially tuberculosis. The next 40 years were dominated by poliomyelitis . . . Gillette has clearly moved into a third phase of its existence. The conditions that bring children to a hospital like Gillette are uncommon, but together they comprise a group far larger than those of polio during the epidemic years. Between two and four of every 1,000 children will be found to have cerebral palsy; spina bifida, muscular dystrophy, and childhood brain and spinal cord injury are less common. Perhaps one child in a thousand is born with a clubfoot or a dislocated hip . . . one child in a thousand develops a serious spinal curvature.[108]

Although the patients with these diseases may number more than the total of polio patients, only a few children need to be hospitalized at any given time. The need for the hospital came into question. As Koop stated, "The hospital . . . is much smaller and less obvious in the community."

The events that overtook Gillette Children's Hospital (shifting patient base, changes in practice from prolonged hospitalization to outpatient surgery and brief courses of hospital care, and emphasis on cost-cutting) have affected all but a few such institutions. Even Shands' well-funded institution, the A. I. duPont Institute, has had to become a more general purpose pediatric hospital to survive. State and local hospitals for crippled children all over the country have either closed or changed into general pediatric or rehabilitation facilities, and the specialized pediatric orthopaedic institute has essentially disappeared. The irony of this fact is that bracing, exercises, physical therapy, and rehabilitation used to be part of orthopaedics; the rehabilitation hospital has to some degree assumed the role that these orthopaedic children's hospitals used to play.

The one system of orthopaedic children's hospitals that has persevered is both operated and supported by the Shriners of North America. Shriners Hospitals for Children is a network of 22 pediatric specialty hospitals dedicated to providing specialized pediatric care, innovative research, and outstanding teaching programs. Children up to age 18 with orthopaedic conditions, burn injuries of all degrees, spinal cord injuries, and cleft lip and palate are eligible for admission and receive all care at no charge—regardless of financial need or relationship to a Shriner.

The impetus for the hospital system came from Freeland Kendrick, who visited the Scottish Rite Hospital for Crippled Children in Atlanta in 1919 and became aware of the overwhelming need for orthopaedic care for children in North America, largely because of polio epidemics. As Imperial Potentate (leader of the Shriners, elected annually), he worked hard to have the Shriners establish an official philanthropy to address this problem, which they did at the 1920 Imperial Council Session (national convention). Each Shriner would help support the hospital through a $2 annual assessment. Today that fee is $5.

In the beginning, Shriners Hospitals served only those unable to afford care and treatment. Today, Shriners Hospitals provide state-of-the-art, expert treatment to any patient, who, in the opinion of a hospital's chief of staff, can be helped. Ability to pay is not a consideration. In fact, Shriners Hospitals do not accept payment for services provided in their facilities, even if it is offered. Clearly, the $5 assessment cannot possibly finance this undertaking; the hospital system relies on the generosity of others, including bequests and donations from Shriners, their families, and the general public.

The first Shriners Hospital opened in Shreveport, Louisiana, in 1922. Since then the network of pediatric orthopaedic hospitals has expanded to 18 additional hospitals in these locations opened in this order: Honolulu; Minneapolis; San Francisco (later relocated to Sacramento, California); Portland, Oregon; St. Louis; Spokane, Washington; Salt Lake City; Montreal; Springfield, Massachusetts; Chicago; Philadelphia; Lexington, Kentucky; Greenville, South Carolina; Mexico City; Houston; Los Angeles; Erie, Pennsylvania; and Tampa, Florida.

In the 1960s, Shriners Hospitals expanded their mission to include treatment of pediatric burns of all degrees, and opened hospitals specifically for burn care in Galveston, Texas; Cincinnati; and Boston. The relocated hospital in Sacramento, California, which opened in 1997, provides pediatric orthopaedic, burn, and spinal cord injury care. In addition, in 1980, Shriners Hospitals opened the first pediatric spinal cord injury unit in the country within the Philadelphia hospital, and in 1984 added a similar program at the Chicago hospital.

In the 1980s, Shriners Hospitals began an aggressive rebuilding and renovation program. Since 1981, 21 hospitals have either been rebuilt or totally renovated. These efforts continue today, with the recent groundbreaking ceremony for a new facility in Honolulu. When possible, new hospitals were located near or adjacent to university hospitals, giving Shriners patients immediate access to services such as intensive care, specialized imaging, and specialists usually available only in university hospitals. In addition, many partnerships have been formed with the universities allowing academic opportunities for Shriners physicians and collaborative research efforts.

Although known by many primarily for marching in parades while wearing odd hats and costumes, the Shriners actually are profoundly serious in their support and management of their philanthropy, Shriners Hospitals for Children.

Since 1922, Shriners Hospitals have spent about $8.2 billion to operate the 22-hospital system, and $1.76 billion on hospital construction and renovations (as of the end of 2006). The operating budget for 2007 is $655 million, including $37 million for research; the capital expenditures budget for 2007 is $66 million.

In addition, the Shriners provide transportation assistance to and from the hospitals for countless patients, and many Shriners also routinely volunteer for a wide variety of tasks at the hospitals. Shriners of North America support the ultimate worthy cause.

The Evolution of Fracture Care in Children

Classification of Pediatric Fractures
The skeleton of the child differs from an adult's most obviously because it grows; those who treat children have been preoccupied by injuries to children's growth plates since these anatomic structures were known to exist. John Poland[109] of Guy's Hospital in London published one of the most complete pre-Roentgen monographs on this subject in 1898; in it, he summarized virtually everything written about physeal injuries from the time of Hippocrates. Because he published his monograph 3 years after Roentgen's discovery of the x-ray, Poland based his analysis of physeal injuries on autopsy and amputation specimens instead of radiographs. Nevertheless, his classification of physeal injuries has served as the basis for most subsequent classification schemes. He identified four types of injuries (Figure 15): separation of the epiphysis from the metaphysis through the growth plate, epiphyseal separations with an attached metaphyseal fragment, a fracture through the epiphysis with separation of one epiphyseal fragment, and a double fracture through the epiphysis with separation of both fragments. Poland cited many publications as well as his own experience in attempting to predict the effect that a given physeal injury could have on growth (Figures 16 and 17). Since his classic work was published, many authors have addressed the same issues. E. Bergenfeldt[110] of Stockholm modified Poland's system in 1933 by adding two additional types of physeal injury, and Alexander Aitken[111] of Winchester, Massachusetts, modified Poland's classification in 1936 by reducing the number of physeal injury types to three. Both Bergenfeldt and Aitken, however, included a type of injury that involved a fracture through both the epiphysis and metaphysis. Both authors' studies were significant because they successfully identified ways to prognosticate how physeal injury would affect growth, and they related the effects of the injury to the histology and physiology of the growth plate.

In 1963, Robert Salter and W. R. Harris[112] of Toronto published their fracture classification system in *JBJS*. It included the same type of injuries described by Poland, Bergenfeldt, and Aitken, and added the following: a crushing injury of the physis due to axial compression, with no radiographic changes. Salter and Harris firmly based their prognosis for fracture healing and alignment with or without growth arrest on their classification system, but subsequently many observers have challenged their assertions. John Ogden, Frederic Shapiro, and Hamlet Peterson have all modified the Salter-Harris system to include virtually any kind of complex injury of the meta-

65

physis, physis, and epiphysis. Peterson and others challenged the existence of the Salter-Harris type VI injury, and Ogden was apparently unable to produce a Salter-Harris type V in the laboratory.[113-117]

In 1967, A. Langenskiöld[118] published a paper that raised awareness about physeal injuries in which all or part of the growth plate stops growing prematurely, resulting in deformity of the limb. Langenskiöld demonstrated that an osseous bridge from the epiphysis to the metaphysis across the growth plate could be resected and filled with fat to permit the resumption of growth, thus preventing a deformity. Others have obtained the same results using a silicone rubber implant or methylmethacrylate.

Fracture care in children has changed considerably over the past 50 years. Orthopaedic surgeons previously depended almost exclusively on closed reduction and immobilization in casts or with traction. Today the principles of open or closed reduction with internal fixation, commonly accepted for the treatment of adults, have increasingly been applied to the treatment of injuries in children. In the late 1950s and early 1960s, Walter Blount considered only fractures of the lateral humeral condyle and fractures of the upper femur to be suitable injuries for open reduction and internal fixation.[119] Increasingly, however, orthopaedic surgeons use internal fixation for skeletal injuries much as they would use it in adults. In the past, fractures of the femur in older children were almost always treated with skeletal or skin traction, but reports of successful intramedullary or plate fixation now appear in the orthopaedic literature. For infants and very young children, immediate fixation in a cast remains the best option for treatment of femoral shaft fractures; however, children as young as 7 years of age can now be successfully treated with internal fixation techniques, thus eliminating the 6 to 8 weeks in a spica cast previously thought necessary to treat these injuries. Bryant's traction for infants and Russell's traction for older children are no longer regarded as necessary or safe. Both led to skin problems or serious vascular compromise in the lower limbs when weights were applied to the legs of infants and young children after injuries severe enough to fracture a femur. Despite the attention given to these methods in fracture texts in the 1950s and 1960s, they have been abandoned.[120,121]

Supracondylar Fractures in Children

The treatment of fractures in children has undergone a critical reappraisal in recent papers and editorials in the *Journal of Pediatric Orthopaedics*. Robert Hensinger,[122] with coeditor Lynn Staheli, wrote a 2002 editorial about the effects of that reappraisal on his practice. In "Changing Expectations" Hensinger mildly lamented the fact that "anatomic reduction has become an important goal in our management of childhood trauma." He noted that in the past, nonsurgical intervention and apposition, rather than surgical reduction, was the treatment of choice, and outcomes were acceptable. Now, parents and referring physicians tend to demand perfection, which often mandates an operation that may not be necessary for a growing child. Hensinger concluded that "guidelines that define current acceptable standards seem to be a moving target."

The routine use of fluoroscopy with image intensification has changed the way orthopaedists care for children with fractures and dislocations. The image intensifier has changed orthopaedics dramatically; comparing the current management of supracondylar fractures of the humerus with past treatment modalities makes this clear.

Walter Blount, chairman of the orthopaedic section of Milwaukee Children's Hospital and professor at Marquette University (now the Milwaukee Medical College) published *Fractures in Children* in 1955. This text was the standard reference for a generation of orthopaedic residents and greatly influenced the way fracture surgeons practiced. Blount devoted 17 pages to the subject of supracondylar fractures of the humerus. He recommended that the fracture be manipulated and reduced immediately if the child was seen before swelling became severe. Reduction, according to Blount, was achieved by applying traction to the axilla, hyperextending the fracture, correcting malrotation by twisting the arm in whichever direction seemed necessary, pushing the distal fragment medially or laterally (depending on the way in which the distal fragment was displaced), and finally manipulating the distal fragment into the reduced position relative to the humeral shaft. He maintained that the elbow should then be flexed until the radial pulse began to disappear, and that a splint should be applied with the elbow in that position. If radiographs obtained immediately thereafter did not reveal adequate alignment, the process should be repeated. If the second attempt failed, Blount suggested "Dunlop's traction."[123] Dunlop's traction required an adhesive strip applied to the forearm containing a few pounds of weights attached via a sash cord that had been run over a pulley; the fracture and the elbow were kept in 60° of flexion, and a counterweight was suspended over the arm just above the fracture. The child had to remain in this position for up to 2 weeks, until the swelling began to subside, at which time reduction was to be attempted again.

The grave concern in treating this fracture, as every orthopaedist knows, is Volkmann's ischemic contracture, usually the end result of a compartment syndrome, with death of the forearm muscles and their subsequent scarring caused by too much pressure in the compartment. Damage to the brachial artery, in Blount's opinion, seemed to be the main reason for Volkmann's contracture; he did not actually refer to the ischemic death of forearm muscles resulting from a compartment syndrome. Compartment syndromes were not recognized as such by Blount and his contemporaries. He did note, however, "if there is evidence of circulatory embarrassment . . . no time should be lost before exploring the cubital fossa and volar aspect of the forearm." He also suggested "blocking the appropriate sympathetic ganglia," and/or the injection of 300 to 500 turbidity-reducing units of hyaluronidase into the hematoma of a badly swollen elbow to "hasten the restoration of the tissues to normal." However, he did not define his exact indications for either of these methods.

Blount condemned internal fixation, stating that "permanent limitation of motion is all too frequent. This method cannot be justified . . . Blind pinning with protruding pins is always undesirable in children whose urge to wiggle and scratch cannot be controlled."

To Blount, more than 50 years ago, safe preservation of the circulation in the arm and avoiding a Volkmann's contracture were the central issues. In his writing on prognosis and outcome, he discussed fracture malunion with considerable equanimity, noting that a gunstock deformity, that is, a reversal of the carrying angle, might follow a perfect reduction and probably would be due to overgrowth of the lateral condylar epiphysis. When manipulation and traction left the fracture "grossly malunited," one might consider an open reduction two months later or even "a year or more after the injury."

Blount's dependence on closed manipulation, splinting, and/or traction for the treatment of supracondylar fractures in children was not shared by all. Alvin L. Swenson[124] of Phoenix, Arizona, described his method of closed reduction and percutaneous pinning in ten patients in *JBJS* in 1948. He noted the difficulty of inserting pins through the medial and lateral humeral condyles, but reported that radiographs confirmed good position of the pins and good alignment of the fracture in all ten patients. Dr. Swenson published his report seven years before Blount's book, but Swenson's technique apparently failed to capture the imagination of the orthopaedic community for several years. Edgar Ralston,[125] for example, professor and chairman of orthopaedics at the University of Pennsylvania, published his *Handbook of Fractures* in collaboration with Alfred Shands, Jr., Herndon Lentz, and Frederick Fitts in 1967, 12 years after Blount's book and 19 years after Swenson's paper. In the section on supracondylar fractures in children, Ralston essentially reiterated Blount's recommendations. He did not condemn open or closed pinning—he ignored it. Andrew G. Pollen,[126] a British orthopaedic surgeon at the Bedford General Hospital, also produced a book on fractures and dislocations in children in 1973, 6 years after Ralston's book. He used the same formulaic approach described by Blount: reduction, possibly repeated two or three times, followed by Dunlop's traction if needed.

In 1964, Martin Gruber and Otto Hudson[127] reported their experience with 145 supracondylar fractures in children over a six-year period. In their introduction, they noted that "success with open reduction has been reported by Scandinavian authors, but it has not been accepted by Americans." They cited several publications by Scandinavian and American physicians, including the book by Walter Blount. Gruber and Hudson, however, performed open reductions in children with displaced fractures, and they secured fixation with two crossed K-wires. They had wide exposure and full visualization of the fracture because they split the triceps tendon and reflected the ulnar nerve. In other words, they exposed virtually everything from the back of the arm, making reduction and internal fixation fairly easy. Postoperatively, they immobilized the fracture in a shoulder spica cast for eight weeks. They performed this operation in 31 patients with severely displaced fractures.

In their follow-up one to five years later, the results were good. Some patients had some limitation of motion, but no patients had malunions and none had infection or Volkmann's contractures. Gruber and Hudson's report, along with that of the Scandinavian authors, must have stimulated others to do the same, because several more papers soon followed on the same subject. In 1974, 19 years after the publication of Blount's book, Joseph C. Flynn, Joseph Matthews, and Roger Benoit[128] from Orlando, Florida, reported their technique for reduction and percutaneous pinning of these injuries. They reduced the fracture first, but in describing this part of the procedure they glossed over a key point—the positioning of the forearm when the distal fragment was medially or laterally displaced. Pronation will secure the position when the fragment lies medially and supination when it is laterally displaced. Their paper was published at a time when numerous others were challenging the orthodoxy of closed techniques. In fact, Ramsey and Griz[129] began their article by challenging Blount: "The objection that permanently restricted motion is all too frequent is not supported by this study or the literature."

The detailed analysis of this important work and surgeons' willingness to challenge existing standards led to a profound change in the way in which this particular fracture is treated.

Mercer Rang's 1980 text established the protocol for the now widely accepted way to treat this injury.[130] Rang's book was written in a casual, jocular style, starkly different from Blount's dour prose. Rang supplemented his text with drawings and cartoons that instructed in a positive way. This was quite a change from Blount's representation of the orthopaedic surgeon with the head of a jackass, congratulating himself on the good reduction seen on a radiograph while the child was suffering with "pain, pallor and paralysis." Rang also published photographs of the sections of the distal humerus, which emphasized the point that Flynn and associates made about the position of the forearm, that is, pronation versus supination in maintaining reduction of the fracture while the surgeon performed the fixation to maintain reduction. Those who had courageously tried something new had established a new standard of care for a difficult and dangerous injury.

Pinning of supracondylar fractures has now become standard. The methods rejected or ignored by Blount, Ralston, or Pollen 50 years ago get a full history and description in the following texts: the fifth edition of Lovell and Winter's *Pediatric Orthopaedics*, edited by Raymond Morrissy and Stuart Weinstein; a discussion by Neil Green[131] in Green and Swiontkowski's *Skeletal Trauma in Children*; and the chapter "Elbow Injuries and Fractures in Children," in the fifth edition of Rockwood and Wilkins' *Fractures in Children*, edited by James Beaty and James Kasser. In Beaty and Kasser's book, the authors of the chapter on elbow injuries (Kaye Wilkins, James Beaty, Henry Chambers, and Renato Maria Tonalo) devoted 269 pages to the subject of elbow fractures, referencing 226 articles on the subject of supracondylar fractures alone. They describe reduction techniques in meticulous detail and show how the child should be positioned, how to place the pins and/or wires, and how one should use the power equipment. In a modern American hospital with trained pediatric orthopaedic surgeons, these injuries now have far less potential for producing deformities, loss of function, and lifelong disability.

A badly displaced supracondylar humerus fracture is still a terrible injury for a child; the orthopaedic surgeon should always be acutely sensitive to the severe physiologic and psychologic trauma of this injury for the young patient. However, now that the surgeon has image intensification for fluoroscopic guidance, elegant power tools, and a well-run operating room, at least an injured child does not suffer very long.

The evolution of treatment of supracondylar fractures of the humerus is but one subject in the vastly broader field of pediatric orthopaedics. The clinicians of this subspecialty within the larger discipline of orthopaedic surgery must deal with a daunting array of disorders. Some of these are minor, such as intoeing and out-toeing, mild bowlegs or knock-knees, and lumps and bruises. All these problems require sensitivity in dealing with the patients and their family members. Others are much more serious: clubfoot, DDH, spinal deformity, limb-length discrepancies, dwarfism, various syndromic malformations, osteomyelitis, septic arthritis, tumors, and many others.

History of the Pediatric Orthopaedic Society of North America

The Pediatric Orthopaedic Society

The origins of a group dedicated to pediatric orthopaedics can be traced to 1969 when Douglas McKay, Paul Griffin, and Mihran Tachdjian envisioned an organization where those few practitioners devoted to the musculoskeletal care of children could discuss problems and techniques. These three met in a hotel room at the American Academy of Orthopaedic Surgeons (AAOS) meeting in San Francisco along with William Green, Burr Curtis, and Frank Stelling. They compiled a list of twelve physicians who devoted the majority of their practices to the care of children.

In 1971, Tachdjian hosted a meeting in Chicago with both clinical and organizational components. In attendance were those mentioned above as well as Anthony Bianco, Dean MacEwen, and Robert Samilson. While some concern was voiced regarding the separation of children's care from the body of general orthopaedics, the separatist mood prevailed and the Pediatric Orthopaedic Society (POS) was born. Officers were elected and an official meeting was planned for later that year, to follow the Scoliosis Research Society meeting.

That first meeting, in September 1971, was held at the Newington Children's Hospital and featured 12 surgeons, adding Sherman Coleman, Charles Ryder, and Wood Lovell to the group. It was agreed at that meeting to invite nine others to join. Membership continued to be by invitation only, a principal at odds with the inclusivity espoused by the AAOS. For this reason, the POS did not affiliate with the academy. The decision in 1972 to limit membership to 35 and in 1973 to allow the roster to increase by no more than five members a year resulted in the exclusion of a growing number of surgeons interested in the care of children.

70

The Pediatric Orthopaedic Study Group
In 1974, in a hotel room in Dallas during the AAOS annual meeting, Hamlet Peterson and Henry Cowell discussed the need for a forum for young pediatric orthopaedists. A letter was drafted announcing a meeting to be held at the Mayo Clinic in November of that year. Included in the mailing list were Walter Bobechko, Stanley Chung, Liebe Diamond, James Drennan, Robert Eilert, Robert Fisher, Roger Gallien, Robert Hensinger, Rudolph Klassen, Stephen Kopits, Dennis Lyne, Maureen Malloy, E. William Schmitt, George Simons, and Lynn Staheli. Originally called the Pediatric Orthopaedic Travel Group, by the time of their second meeting the name had been changed to the Pediatric Orthopaedic Study Group (POSG). The spirit of the POSG meetings was informality and egalitarianism, with brief paper presentations followed by lengthy open discussion.

Like the POS, interest in membership was considerable, and by 1976 there was discussion of limiting membership. While an inclusive policy was generally followed, it was decided that membership requirements would include fellowship in the AAOS and a practice profile devoted at least 75 percent to the care of children.

The Move Toward Unification
Over time, several members of the POSG were invited to join the POS, and the duplication of effort of the two separate societies, both devoted to a single specialty, became evident. There remained, however, some differences in approach and outlook. Several years of effort by multiple individuals resulted in a combined annual meeting in Charlottesville, North Carolina in 1984. There the POS and POSG agreed to formal unification in 1984 under the name Pediatric Orthopaedic Society of North America.

Pediatric Orthopaedic Society of North America (POSNA)
Since the amalgamation of its two precursor societies, POSNA has undergone remarkable growth. Membership now numbers over 900. Additional membership categories added over the years include candidate membership for those not yet board certified, associate membership for non-physician medical personnel devoted to care and research of pediatric orthopaedic conditions, and corresponding membership for pediatric orthopaedic surgeons who practice in countries other than the United States and Canada. Numerous alliance societies increase communication between POSNA members and their colleagues around the world.

The annual meeting continues to emphasize short papers followed by lengthy discussion. Additional afternoon sessions devoted to subspecialty concerns including spinal deformity, trauma, gait, sports medicine, and orthopaedics in underserved areas have proven popular. The meeting is preceded by a one-day course devoted to a single topic of interest.

POSNA supports research grants through generous grants from the St. Giles Foundation and the Angela Kuo Foundation. The Steel Foundation funds a lecture at the annual meeting, always devoted to a subject other than orthopaedics.

POSNA members have always been leaders in academia, despite the relatively modest numbers of orthopaedists enrolled in pediatric fellowships. Numerous POSNA members are or have been department chairs. POSNA past-presidents Newton McCollough, Robert Hensinger, S. Terry Canale, Vernon Tolo, Stuart Weinstein, and James Beaty have all served as president of the AAOS.

References

1. Grob GN: *The Deadly Truth: A History of Disease in America.* Cambridge, MA, Harvard University Press, 2002, p 90.

2. Sayre LA: *Lectures on Orthopedic Surgery and Diseases of the Joints, Delivered at Bellevue Hospital Medical College during the winter session of 1874-1895.* New York, NY, D Appleton & Co, 1876.

3. Le Vay D: *The Life of Hugh Owen Thomas.* Edinburgh, Scotland, Livingstone, 1956.

4. Ollier L: Des opérations conservatives dans la tuberculose articulaire. *Neu de Chir* 1885:3.

5. Hibbs RA: An operation for stiffening the knee joint. *Ann Surg* 1911;53:404-407.

6. Hibbs RA: A preliminary report of twenty cases of hip joint tuberculosis tested by an operation devised to eliminate motion by fusing the joint. *J Bone Joint Surg* 1926;8:522-533.

7. Henderson MS: Resection of the knee joint for tuberculosis. *Trans Orthop Sec AMA* 1914:150.

8. Albee FH: Extraarticular arthrodesis of the hip for tuberculosis. *Ann Surg* 1929;89:404.

9. Wilson JC: Extraarticular fusion of the tuberculous hip joint. *Calif West Med* 1927;27:774.

10. Schum HC: Extraarticular immobilization of the hip joint. *Surg Gynecol Obstet* 1929;48:112.

11. Freiberg JA: Experiences with the Brittain ischiofemoral arthrodesis. *J Bone Joint Surg Br* 1946;28:501-512.

12. Gibney VP: The part arthrotomy plays in the treatment of tuberculous joints: More particularly the knee joint. *Am J Orthop Surg* 1909;7:22-30.

13. Ryan F: *The Forgotten Plague: How the Battle Against Tuberculosis Was Won and Lost.* Boston, MA, Little, Brown & Company, 1993, p 209.

14. Bosworth DM, Pietra AD, Farrell RF: Streptomycin in tuberculous bone and joint lesions with mixed infection and sinuses. *J Bone Joint Surg Am* 1950;32:103-108.

15. Dye C, Watt CS, Bleed DM, Hosseini SM, Raviglione MC: Evolution of tuberculosis control and prospects for reducing tuberculosis incidence, prevalence, and deaths globally. *JAMA* 2005;293:2767-2775.

16. Dye C, Scheele S, Dolin P, Pathania V, Raviglione MC: Global burden of tuberculosis: Estimated incidence, prevalence, and mortality by country. *JAMA* 1999;282:677-686.

17. Somerville EW, Wilkinson MC: *Girdlestone's Tuberculosis of Bone and Joint*, ed 3. London, England, Oxford University Press, 1965, p 25.

18. Blumberg HM, Leonard MK Jr, Jasmer RM: Update on the treatment of tuberculosis and latent tuberculosis infection. *JAMA* 2005;293:2776-2784.

19. Paul JR: *A History of Poliomyelitis*. New Haven, CT, Yale University Press, 1971.

20. Vermont State Department of Public Health: *Infantile Paralysis in Vermont*. Brattleboro, VT, 1924.

21. Medin O: An epidemic of infantile paralysis (presented to the pediatric section at the International Congress in Berlin, August 7, 1890). Reprinted in *Clin Orthop Relat Res* 1966;45:5-11.

22. Drinker PA, McKhann CF: The use of a new apparatus for the prolonged administration of artificial respiration: 1. A fatal case of poliomyelitis. *JAMA* 1929;92:1658-1660.

23. Shutkin NM: Treatment of poliomyelitis based on pathophysiology. *Clin Orthop* 1953;1:178-186.

24. Gurunluoglu R, Shafigli M, Huemer GM, Gurunluoglu A, Piza-Katzer H: Carl Nicoladoni (1847-1902): Professor of surgery. *Ann Surg* 2004;239:281-292.

25. Jones RW: Editorial. *Am J Orthop Surg* 1908;6:312-338.

26. Marchant CD, Kumar ML: Immunization, in Jenson HB, Baltimore RS (eds): *Pediatric Infectious Diseases*, ed 2. Philadelphia, PA, WB Saunders, 2002, p 256.

27. Silver JK, Gawne AC: Postpolio Syndrome. Philadelphia, PA, Hanley and Belfus, 2004, p 6.

28. Raymond CA: Decades after polio epidemics, survivors report new symptoms. *JAMA* 1986;255:1397-1399.

29. Rothschild H, Cohen JC: *Virology in Medicine*. New York, NY, Oxford University Press, 1986, p 304.

30. Melnisk JL: Enteroviruses, in Evans AS (ed): *Viral Infections of Humans: Epidemiology and Control*, ed 3. New York, NY, Plenum Medical Book Company, 1989, p 191.

31. Modlin JF: Poliomyelitis in the United States: The final chapter? *JAMA* 2004;292:1749-1751.

32. Little WJ: On the influence of abnormal parturition, difficult labors, premature birth, and asphyxia neonatorum on the mental and physical condition of the child, especially in relation to deformities. *Trans Obstet Soc London* 1861;3:293.

33. Phelps WM: Cerebral birth injuries: Their orthopedic classification and subsequent treatment. *J Bone Joint Surg* 1932;14:773-782.

34. Phelps WM: Long-term results of orthopaedic surgery in cerebral palsy. *J Bone Joint Surg Am* 1957;39:53-59.

35. Obituary: Dr. Winthrop M. Phelps. *Dev Med Child Neurol* 1972;14:265.

36. Bleck EE: *Orthopedic Management of Cerebral Palsy*. Philadelphia, PA, WB Saunders Company, 1979.

37. Samilson RL: *Orthopedic Aspects of Cerebral Palsy*. Philadelphia, PA, JB Lippincott Company, 1975.

38. Saraph V, Zwick EB, Zwick G, Steinwender C, Steinwender G, Linhart W: Multilevel surgery in spastic diplegia: Evaluation by physical examination and gait analysis in 25 children. *J Pediatr Orthop* 2002;22:150-157.

39. Delgado MR: Botulinam neurotoxin type A. *J Am Acad Orthop Surg* 2003;11:291-294.

40. Green WT, Banks HH: Flexor carpi ulnaris transplant and its use in cerebral palsy. *J Bone Joint Surg Am* 1962;44:1343-1352.

41. Inglis AE, Cooper W: Release of the flexor-pronator origin for flexion deformities of the hand and wrist in spastic paralysis: A study of eighteen cases. *J Bone Joint Surg Am* 1966;48:847-857.

42. Peacock WJ, Staudt LA: Spasticity in cerebral palsy and the selective posterior rhizotomy procedure. *J Child Neurol* 1990;5:179-185.

43. Carroll KL, Moore KR, Stevens PM: Orthopedic procedures after rhizotomy. *J Pediatr Orthop* 1998;18:69-74.

44. Sharrard WJW: Posterior iliopsoas transplantation in the treatment of paralytic dislocation of the hip. *J Bone Joint Surg Br* 1964;46:426-444.

45. Sharrard WJW: *Pediatric Orthopedics and Fractures*, ed 2. Oxford, England, Blackwell Scientific Publications, 1979, p 1139.

46. Lorber J: Results of treatment of myelomeningocele: An analysis of 524 unselected cases, with special reference to possible selection for treatment. *Dev Med Child Neurol* 1971;13:279-303.

47. Mackenzie WG, Bowen JR: Muscle and nerve disorders in children, in Chapman MW (ed): *Chapman's Orthopaedic Surgery*, ed 3. Philadelphia, PA, Lippincott Williams & Wilkins, 2001, p 4505.

48. Hobbins JC: Diagnosis and management of neural-tube defects today. *N Engl J Med* 1991;324:690-691.

49. Mazur JM, Shurtleff D, Menelaus M, Colliver J: Orthopaedic management of high-level spina bifida: Early walking compared with early use of a wheelchair. *J Bone Joint Surg Am* 1989;71:56-61.

50. Asher M, Olson J: Factors affecting the ambulatory status of patients with spina bifida cystica. *J Bone Joint Surg Am* 1983;65:350-356.

51. Duchenne GBA de Boulogne: Recérches, sur la paralysie musculaire pseudo-hypértrophique, ou paralysie myosclosique. *Arch Gen Med* 1886;11:5.

52. Vignos PJ, Archibald KC: Maintenance of ambulation in childhood muscular dystrophy. *J Chronic Dis* 1960;12:273-290.

53. Miller J: Management of muscular dystrophy. *J Bone Joint Surg Am* 1967;49:1205-1211.

54. Kite JH: *The Clubfoot*. New York, NY, Grune & Stratton, 1964, p 15.

55. Ponseti I, Smoley E: Congenital club foot: The results of treatment. *J Bone Joint Surg Am* 1963;45:261-275.

56. Turco V: *Clubfoot*. New York, NY, Churchill Livingstone, 1981.

57. McKay DW: New concept and approach to clubfoot treatment: Section II. Correction of the clubfoot. *J Pediatr Orthop* 1983;3:10-21.

58. Simons GW: Complete subtalar release in club foot: Part II. Comparison with less extensive procedures. *J Bone Joint Surg Am* 1985;67:1056-1065.

59. Goldner JL, Fitch RD: Classification and evaluation of congenital talipes equinovarus, in Simons GW (ed): *The Clubfoot*. New York, NY, Springer-Verlag, 1993.

60. Crawford AH, Marxen JL, Osterfeld DL: The Cincinnati incision: A comprehensive approach for surgical procedures on the foot and ankle in childhood. *J Bone Joint Surg Am* 1982;64:1355-1358.

61. Dwyer FC: Causes, significance and treatment of stiffness of the subtaloid joint. *Proc R Soc Med* 1976;69:97-102.

62. Evans D: Relapsed club foot. *J Bone Joint Surg Br* 1961;43:722-733.

63. Herring JA: Congenital talipes equinovarus (clubfoot), in Herring JA (ed): *Tachdjian's Pediatric Orthopaedics*, ed 3. Philadelphia, PA, WB Saunders, 2002, vol 2, p 922.

64. Hoke M: An operation for stabilizing paralytic feet. *J Orthop Surg* (Hong Kong) 1921;3:494.

65. Ryerson EW: Arthrodesing operations on the feet. *J Bone Joint Surg* 1923;5:453-471.

66. Grice DS: Further experience with extra-articular arthrodesis of the subtalar joint. *J Bone Joint Surg Am* 1955;37:246-259.

67. de la Huerta F: Correction of the neglected clubfoot by the Ilizarov method. *Clin Orthop Relat Res* 1994;301:89-93.

68. Legg AT: An obscure affection of the hip-joint. *Boston Med Surg J* 1910;162:202-204.

69. Petrie JG, Bitenc I: The abduction weight-bearing treatment in Legg-Perthes' disease. *J Bone Joint Surg Br* 1971;53:54-62.

70. Herring JA: Legg Calve Perthes disease, in Herring JA (ed): *Tachdjian's Pediatric Orthopaedics*, ed 3. Philadelphia, PA, WB Saunders, 2002, p 655.

71. Mose K, Hjorth L, Ulfeldt M, Christensen ER, Jensen A: Legg Calve Perthes disease: The late occurrence of coxarthrosis. *Acta Orthop Scand Suppl* 1977;169:1-39.

72. Catterall A: The natural history of Perthes' disease. *J Bone Joint Surg Br* 1971;53:37-53.

73. Herring JA, Neustadt JB, Williams JJ, Early JS, Browne RH: The lateral pillar classification of Legg-Calve-Perthes disease. *J Pediatr Orthop* 1992;12:143.

74. Chung SM, Batterman SC, Brighton CT: Shear strength of the human femoral capital epiphyseal plate. *J Bone Joint Surg Am* 1976;58:94-103.

75. Dulligan PJ: The etiology of slipping of the capital femoral epiphysis. *NY J Med* 1953;53:2643-2646.

76. Ferguson LB, Howorth B: Slipping of the upper femoral epiphysis. *JAMA* 1931;97:1867.

77. Howorth MB: Slipping of the upper femoral epiphysis. *J Bone Joint Surg Am* 1949;31:734-747.

78. Telson DR: Reduction and pinning of slipped femoral epiphyses. *NY J Med* 1953;53:2047.

79. Herndon CH, Heyman CH, Bell DM: Treatment of slipped capital femoral epiphysis by epiphyseodesis and osteoplasty of the femoral head: A report of further experiences. *J Bone Joint Surg Am* 1963;45:999-1012.

80. Howorth B: The bone-pegging operation for slipping of the capital femoral epiphysis. *Clin Orthop Relat Res* 1966;48:79-87.

81. Southwick WO: Compression fixation after biplane trochanteric osteotomy for slipped capital femoral epiphysis: A technical improvement. *J Bone Joint Surg Am* 1973;55:1218-1224.

82. Pauwels F: *Biomechanics of the Normal and Diseased Hip*. New York, NY, Springer-Verlag, 1976.

83. Kramer WG, Craig WA, Noel S: Compensating osteotomy of the femoral neck for slipped capital femoral epiphysis. *J Bone Joint Surg Am* 1976;58:796-800.

84. Dunn DM, Angel JC: Replacement of the femoral head by open operation in severe adolescent slipping of the upper femoral epiphysis. *J Bone Joint Surg Br* 1978;60:394-403.

85. Waldenström CH: On necrosis of the joint cartilage by epiphyseolysis capitis femoris. *Acta Chir Scand* 1930;67:936.

86. Moore R: Aseptic necrosis of the capital femoral epiphysis following adolescent epiphysiolysis. *Surg Gynecol Obstet* 1945;80:199.

87. Elmslie RC: Injury and deformity of the epiphysis of the head of the femur: Coxa vara. *Lancet* 1907;1:410.

88. Weighill FJ: The treatment of developmental coxa vara by abduction subtrochanteric and intertrochanteric femoral osteotomy with special reference to the role of adductor tenotomy. *Clin Orthop Relat Res* 1976;116:116-124.

89. Chung SMK: *Hip Disorders in Infants and Children*. Philadelphia, PA, Lea & Febiger, 1981, p 105.

90. Lorenz A: The operative treatment of congenital hip dislocation. *Trans Am Orthop A* 1895;7:99.

91. Lorenz A: Cure of congenital luxation of the hip by bloodless reduction and weighting. *Trans Am Orthop A* 1896;9:254.

92. Taylor HL: Peripheral palsies following manual replacement of the congenitally dislocated hip. *Am J Orthop Surg* 1903;1:273.

93. Lorenz A: Uber die behandlung der irreponiblen angeborenen hüftluxationen und der schenkelhalspseudarthosen mittels gobelung (bifurkation des oberen femurendes). *Wien Klin Uchnschr* 1919;32:997.

94. Haas J: *Congenital Dislocations of the Hip*. Springfield, IL, Charles C. Thomas, 1951, p 292.

95. Hey Groves EW: *The Treatment of Congenital Dislocation of the Hip Joint*. London, England, Oxford University Press, 1928.

96. Colonna PC: Capsular arthroplasty for congenital dislocation of the hip: A two-stage procedure. *J Bone Joint Surg Am* 1953;35:179-197.

97. Chung SM, Scholl HW Jr, Ralston EL, Pendergrass EP: The Colonna capsular arthroplasty: A long-term follow-up study of fifty-six patients. *J Bone Joint Surg Am* 1971;53:1511-1527.

98. Boardman DL, Moseley CF: Finding patients after 40 years: A very long term follow-up study of the Colonna arthroplasty. *J Pediatr Orthop* 1999;19:169-176.

99. Ramsey PL, Lasser S, MacEwen GD: Congenital dislocation of the hip: Use of the Pavlik harness in the child during the first six months of life. *J Bone Joint Surg Am* 1976;58:1000-1004.

100. Galpin RD, Roach JW, Wenger DR, Herring JA, Birch JG: One-stage treatment of congenital dislocation of the hip, including femoral shortening. *J Bone Joint Surg Am* 1989;71:734-741.

101. Salter RB: Innominate osteotomy in the treatment of congenital dislocation and subluxation of the hip. *J Bone Joint Surg Br* 1961;43:518-539.

102. Pemberton PA: Pericapsular osteotomy of the ilium for treatment of congenital subluxation and dislocation of the hip. *J Bone Joint Surg Am* 1965;47:65-86.

103. Chiari K: Medial displacement osteotomy of the pelvis. *Clin Orthop Relat Res* 1974;98:55-71.

104. Sutherland DH, Greenfield R: Double innominate osteotomy of the pelvis. *J Bone Joint Surg Am* 1977;59:1082-1091.

105. Steel HH: Triple osteotomy of the innominate bone. *J Bone Joint Surg Am* 1973;55:343-350.

106. Ganz R, Klaue K, Vinh TS, Mast JW: A new periacetabular osteotomy for the treatment of hip dysplasias: Technique and preliminary results. *Clin Orthop Relat Res* 1988;232:26.

107. Shands AR: The care and treatment of crippled children in the United States. *J Bone Joint Surg Am* 1953;35:237-244.

108. Koop SE: *We Hold This Treasure: The Story of Gillette Children's Hospital*. Afton, MN, Afton Historical Society Press, 1998.

109. Poland J: *Traumatic Separation of the Epiphyses*. London, England, Smith, Eller and Company, 1898.

110. Bergenfeldt E: Beitrage zur kennntuis de traumatschen epiphysenlösungen an dem langen rohrenlöchen der extremitäten. *Eine Kinish-Roentgenologishe Studie Acta Chir Scand* 1933;73(suppl 28):1.

111. Aitken AP: Fractures of the epiphyses. *Clin Orthop Relat Res* 1965;41:19-24.

112. Salter RB, Harris WR: Injuries involving the epiphyseal plate. *J Bone Joint Surg Am* 1963;45:587-622.

113. Shapiro F: Epiphyseal growth plate fracture separations: A pathophysiologic approach. *Orthopedics* 1982;5:720-736.

114. Ogden JA: Skeletal growth mechanism injury pattern. *J Pediatr Orthop* 1982;2:371-377.

115. Peterson HA: Physeal fractures: Part 3. Classification. *J Pediatr Orthop* 1994;14:439-448.

116. Peterson HA, Madhok R, Benson JT, et al: Physeal fractures: Part 1. Epidemiology in Olmsted County, Minnesota, 1979-1988. *J Pediatr Orthop* 1994;14:423-430.

117. Peterson HA: Physeal fractures: Part 2. Two previously unclassified types. *J Pediatr Orthop* 1994;14:431-438.

118. Langenskiöld A: The possibilities of eliminating premature partial closure of an epiphyseal plate caused by trauma or disease. *Acta Orthop Scand* 1967;38:267-279.

119. Blount WP: *Fractures in Children*. Huntington, NY, Robert E. Kreieger Publishing Company, 1977, pp 26-43.

120. Kregor PJ, Song KM, Routt ML, Sangeorzan BJ, Liddell RM, Hansen ST: Plate fixation of femoral shaft fractures in multiply injured children. *J Bone Joint Surg Am* 1993;75:1774-1780.

121. Timmerman LA, Rab GT: Intramedullary nailing of femoral shaft fractures in adolescents. *J Orthop Trauma* 1993;7:331-337.

122. Hensinger RN: Changing expectations. Editorial. *J Pediatr Orthop* 2002;22:1.

123. Dunlop J: Transcondylar fractures of the humerus in childhood. *J Bone Joint Surg Am* 1939;21:59.

124. Swenson AL: The treatment of supracondylar fractures of the humerus by Kirschner-wire transfixion. *J Bone Joint Surg Am* 1948;30:993-997.

125. Ralston EL: *Handbook of Fractures*. St. Louis, MO, CV Mosby Company, 1967.

126. Pollen AG: *Fractures and Dislocations in Children*. Baltimore, MD, Williams & Wilkins Company, 1973, p 23.

127. Gruber MA, Hudson OC: Supracondylar fractures of the humerus in childhood: End-result study of open reduction. *J Bone Joint Surg Am* 1964;46:1245-1252.

128. Flynn JC, Matthews JG, Benoit RI: Blind pinning of displaced supracondylar fractures of the humerus in children: Sixteen years' experience with long-term follow-up. *J Bone Joint Surg Am* 1974;56:263-272.

129. Ramsey RH, Griz J: Immediate open reduction and internal fixation of severely displaced supracondylar fractures of the humerus in children. *Clin Orthop Relat Res* 1973;90:131-132.

130. Rang M: *Children's Fractures*, ed 2. Philadelphia, PA, JB Lippincott Company, 1983, pp 154-169.

131. Green NE: Fractures and dislocations about the elbow, in Green NE, Swiontkowski MF (eds): *Skeletal Trauma in Children*, ed 3. Philadelphia, PA, WB Saunders, 2003, p 272.

CHAPTER 4

FRACTURES AND DISLOCATIONS

The Tipping Point

Prior to World War I, orthopaedics played a relatively minor role in American medicine. The few men (there were no women) who called themselves orthopaedists restricted themselves largely to providing bracing, prosthetic, and other rehabilitative services. Their surgical practices dealt mostly with limited procedures in the extremities. A few more daring, tough-minded individuals ventured into spine surgery, arthroplasties, and the treatment of difficult fractures, but the books and journals of the first 15 years of the 20th century described safer, less daring pursuits. The table of contents of the 1913 *American Journal of Orthopaedic Surgery*, volume 10 ("being at the same time volume 25 of the *Transactions of the American Orthopaedic Association*") contained 48 articles. Only five addressed surgical treatment of an orthopaedic disorder. German surgeons wrote two of the articles: K. Ludoff, on open reductions of neglected congenital hip dislocations, and Adolf Stoffel, on tenotomies in spastic contractures of the lower limbs. Americans wrote the remaining three articles: Arthur T. Legg of Boston reported on two patients with flat feet in whom he had transferred the tibialis anterior tendon from the first metatarsal to the scaphoid; James Watkins of San Francisco wrote about several cases of claw foot, in which he had performed tenodeses of the long toe extensor tendons to the metatarsal heads; and Leonard Ely of Denver published a very brief report on a patient with "Volkmann's paralysis" in whom he had proposed a percutaneous tenotomy of several fingers to correct the flexion contractures. Only one paper, by Bryson Patterson of Hallville, Ontario, concerned the treatment of fractures; he described a method of applying vigorous traction to correct the deformity of an impending malunion of a fractured femur. Thus, in this journal, the precursor to the *Journal of Bone and Joint Surgery* (*JBJS*), only three American orthopaedic surgeons managed to publish papers concerning surgical procedures—all very minor and essentially percutaneous operations.

Changes came for orthopaedics as an independent surgical discipline during the Great War of 1914–1918. America did not enter the conflict until 1917, when on April 6 of that year Congress passed a joint resolution formally declaring war on Germany.[1] By the end of the war in November 1918, almost 1 ½ million American men were under arms. These huge numbers posed terrible problems for physicians in general, especially when a mutant flu virus swept through crowded camps, killing thousands of soldiers and civilians. However, orthopaedic surgeons saw relatively little action, since the army had only a few months of independent service during the conflict. After the collapse of the czarist forces on the Eastern Front in late 1917, the Germans had hundreds of thousands of extra soldiers available for a major offensive against the British and French forces in the west. To support the Allies in resisting the German advance, the American High Command under General John J. Pershing dispersed newly arrived American units among Allied troops defending Paris against the last great German offensive. The Americans conducted independent operations with their own medical departments and services for only a few months after the offensive failed—from September 1918 until the armistice on November 11, 1918.

During the early months of America's involvement in World War I, the Surgeon General of the Army relegated only a minor role to orthopaedic surgery, defining the duties of orthopaedists as follows: "The derangements and disabilities of joints, including ankylosis; deformities and disabilities of the feet, such as hallux valgus, hallux rigidus, metatarsalgia, painful feet, flat or claw foot; fracture malunions or nonunions; injuries to the ligaments, muscles, and tendons; tendon transplantation, or other treatment for irreparable destruction of nerves, nerve injury complicated by fractures or stiffness of joints; and conditions requiring surgical appliances, including artificial limbs."[2] Even this limited role was challenged; when Major John Ridlon, an orthopaedic surgeon, began to treat malunions and nonunions, a general surgeon named Major Edward Martin objected. The Surgeon General himself had to intervene. He determined that "if a soldier was to have the best possible care, he must not be referred automatically to one group of surgeons or another, since the only reasonable basis of distribution is individual fitness, and this must be determined by local conditions . . . While a large number of orthopaedic surgeons possess the greatest skill in this difficult work, some did not. Similarly, while many general surgeons showed preeminent skill in fracture work, many who possessed the highest ability in certain lines of general surgery had neither interest nor skill in fractures."[3]

Despite these restrictions on their level of military practice during World War I, the culture of orthopaedics changed as a result of the war. This happened in part because of proactive efforts of the American Orthopaedic Association (AOA) in 1916. Realizing that America could enter the conflict at any time, the AOA at its annual meeting voted to appoint a preparedness committee to consider the needs of military hospitals from an orthopaedic standpoint. The AOA then voted to send their committee's report to the Surgeon General of the Army, who was impressed enough to act on it. After further consultation with members of the AOA, he created a division of orthopaedic surgery and directed it to "plan for the proper personnel, both in France and in the United States; to arrange for the necessary hospital equipment overseas . . . for the development of orthopaedic reconstruction in the United States, and for the work of orthopaedic surgery in the Army." To increase the number of doctors in the orthopaedic division, the army recruited general surgeons and "many young practitioners." They were trained in the necessary skills at hastily arranged courses at Harvard, New York University postgraduate medical school (Bellevue Hospital), the University of Pennsylvania, Oklahoma City Bone and Joint Hospital, and the army medical school in Washington. Later, the army added courses in orthopaedics in Chicago and Los Angeles, training nearly 700 physicians in the necessary methodologies of orthopaedics for the prevention and treatment of deformities, healing of nonunions, fitting of prostheses, and vocational rehabilitation.

The impetus for all of this, including the initiative of the AOA, probably came from Sir Robert Jones. In the middle of the war, before the United States entered the conflict, he found himself overwhelmed with casualties sent to him in England from emergency surgery at the front. No British orthopaedic surgeons could help him because the British army had ordered them all to France. Major General Jones thus found himself confronting "a ghastly array of derelicts" without the medical and surgical personnel to care for them. He requested help from the Americans, who sent a group of 20 young orthopaedic surgeons to the rescue. Jones described them as "keen, enthusiastic, and well trained."[2] The final report of the medical department after the war sounded more matter of fact than that, declaring that "these men were endeavoring to show that orthopaedic surgery had its contribution to make to acute general surgery; deformity, if it was to be prevented, must be recognized as a potential deformity in the early stages of wound healing. The contribution was not a conspicuous one, but nevertheless a real and considerable one."[2]

American orthopaedic surgeons came out of World War I with considerable experience in treating trauma-related deformities and disabilities. Robert Osgood described this new perception and reflected on the confidence and optimism of orthopaedists in an address he gave in 1919, published in the *Journal of Orthopaedic Surgery*. He noted:

> The war has suddenly brought into
> promise a young specialty. It is fair to say
> that many honest surgeons believe too
> great prominence. Will it remain a spe-
> cialty? Probably yes. We believe that the
> specialty has rendered a great service to
> the soldier and the nation by insisting that
> locomotive, wage-earning function, con-
> served and increased, is the chief end of
> life-saving surgery. It has maintained that
> a small group of surgeons were specially
> fitted to direct this conservative repair . . .
> it was not being done without them, and
> it is being done with them.[4]

In the same 1919 volume that carried Osgood's remarks, there are almost 400 articles or abstracts compared with the 48 papers published by the same journal in 1913; of these articles, 24 were fracture related. The experiences of World War I jolted the small community of orthopaedic surgeons in the United States, prompting them to change how they perceived themselves.

In the years between World War I and World War II, orthopaedic surgeons developed an even greater interest in the treatment of musculoskeletal trauma, whereas in the community of general surgeons, this interest diminished. It is difficult to measure such trends, but a comparative review of papers published in orthopaedic and surgical journals confirms this impression. From 1919 to 1938, papers related to extremity and spine fractures virtually disappeared from the *Annals of Surgery*, which was the official journal of the American College of Surgeons (ACS) and the American Surgical Association (ASA). In 1936, the *Annals* published one paper on a fracture-related subject; in 1937, it again published only one paper; and in 1938, it published three papers on fractures. The papers related to fractures in *JBJS*, the official journal of the American Academy of Orthopaedic Surgeons (AAOS) and the AOA, increased over that same 20-year period and averaged 31 papers a year in the late 1930s. The rising interest in fractures and the increasing sophistication and quality of the published articles began to draw patients and referring physicians to orthopaedic surgeons for treatment of musculoskeletal injuries.

The tipping point came with the appointment of Norman Kirk (Figure 18) to the position of Surgeon General of the Army in 1943.[5] Early in his administration he firmly decreed that orthopaedic surgeons would henceforth care for all fractures and dislocations. The historical record of orthopaedic surgery in World War II, compiled by Colonel Mather Cleveland, notes that General Kirk had based this decision on orthopaedic surgery's long-term involvement in treating fractures. The army asked William Darrach, Professor of Surgery at Columbia University, and Fremont Chandler of Ohio, a member of the American Board of Orthopaedic Surgery (ABOS), to evaluate the personnel available to provide orthopaedic care in the zone of the interior (the mainland United States). Darrach and Chandler used a four-level classification system for orthopaedic surgeons in service, with those in group A being the most qualified (professors or associate professors in medical schools) and those in group D the least qualified, having had 30 days of orthopaedics training in an army hospital. They found 907 men serving as orthopaedists in military hospitals in the continental United States in 1943. Only three of these were in group A and only 15 were in group B. Furthermore, at that time there were only 660 diplomates of the ABOS and only 110 members of the AOA.

Darrach emphatically questioned whether all extremity wounds should be assigned to orthopaedic sections. In his report he noted that, in light of his personal experience in World War I, "80 percent of all wounds would involve the arms and legs." He suggested that the 907 surgeons classified as orthopaedists (some of these with questionable credentials) would simply not be able to care for the exorbitant number of casualties. He strongly suggested that the Surgeon General go back to the World War I system of assigning all acute extremity injuries to general surgeons. Darrach reported, "This advice was not followed." Darrach was a general surgeon who at that time headed the Fracture Service at Columbia University.[5]

The army overcame this problem of voluminous patient load by compartmentalizing the levels of care for injured soldiers and assigning qualified orthopaedic surgeons primarily to the general hospitals, where they would do the most good. Once a man was wounded in combat, he would pass through a battalion aid station, followed by a collecting station, then a clearing station, and finally a field hospital. An extremity wound (even multiple extremity injuries) usually relegated the injured man to a secondary priority status because chest and abdominal wounds or an obstructed airway—given their life-threatening nature—required immediate treatment. Unless the extremity wound occurred in conjunction with a life-threatening condition (e.g., profuse bleeding, deep shock, or a serious abdominal or chest wound), soldiers with injuries limited to the extremities had to wait at the clearing station level until mortally wounded soldiers received lifesaving care. At the field-hospital level, the wounded soldier would receive only emergency splinting of fractures or dressings of extremity wounds, along with emergency débridement to control the bleeding. Definitive care did not begin until the injured soldier reached the station-hospital level or, more often, the general hospital level. There, "fractures were reduced" and other definitive care provided (Figures 19, 20, and 21).[6]

The Surgeon General and his consultant orthopaedic surgeons established a rigidly controlled treatment plan for specific injuries at each level; departure from the protocol could result in serious trouble for a physician who flouted it. For example, open fractures could never be closed primarily in the field hospitals; definitive reduction, closure, and fixation had to wait until an orthopaedist could provide treatment at the appropriate hospital level. The army therefore managed to stretch the supply of available orthopaedic surgeons and maximize their effectiveness. These policies also meant that trained orthopaedic surgeons were responsible for educating general practitioners, general surgeons, and partially trained orthopaedists in proper orthopaedic procedures. This aspect of an orthopaedist's life in the service, along with administrative duties imposed from above, made it difficult for some to sort out their priorities in wartime. The official histories of the medical department published after the war acknowledged this, but not sympathetically:

> If the chief of the orthopaedic service
> were to perform his duties competently,
> he had to exercise his supervisory and
> executive functions to the fullest extent.
> They were not so exercised when he dis-
> sipated his time and effort by assuming
> the duties of a ward officer on any special
> ward. It was essential, instead, that he
> keep his time free for ward rounds, super-

> vision of junior officers, emergency con-
> sultations, observation of seriously ill sol-
> diers, and operating room duties. At times
> he had to spend the entire day in the
> operating room. The best section chiefs
> were those who utilized their time in this
> fashion.[7]

The Surgeon General's office required much from its orthopaedic surgeons but apparently gave relatively little guidance on how to do all that was required. Nevertheless, this community of physicians—consisting of orthopaedic surgeons, general surgeons who were usually young and partially trained when assigned to fracture wards, junior ward officers who were generalists with little or no surgical training, and enlisted technicians—provided outstanding service. These physicians and their assistants, when they returned to civilian life after such incredible experience, decided on orthopaedic surgery as a lifetime career choice. The maturation of the discipline, in addition to the policies implemented by Norman Kirk as the newly appointed Surgeon General of the Army, took orthopaedics to a higher level of importance.

Dr. Norman Kirk

In the early months of 1943, General James C. Magee, a specialist in preventive medicine by training and Surgeon General of the Army, was struggling. The General Staff had reorganized the medical department, making it a responsibility of the Supply Division of the General Staff. This meant that General Magee no longer reported directly to the Chief of Staff (General George Marshall), and he had to go through a full extra layer of Army bureaucracy to enact orders transmitted to him from the Supply Division. Nor could he report directly to General Marshall on the many problems he had in trying to maintain the health of over 3 million soldiers and provide care for their wounds. The possibility of a 1918-like epidemic of influenza, typhus, malaria, or syphilis apparently worried him constantly; he may have complained that the high command should be more concerned about his problems. Furthermore, the medical arm of the Army Air Force began to operate independently, flouting his directives and regulations. He found himself unable to control the air force's constant encroachment on his budget, hospitals, and personnel. Nonetheless, Magee served honorably and when his 4-year term in office ended, he most likely considered himself a candidate for reappointment and evidently hoped to be selected by the president and approved by Congress to serve again. General Marshall, who was responsible for recommending and nominating the prospective Surgeon General to the president, however, chose someone else. In late February 1943, Marshall selected Brigadier General Albert W. Kenner, the theater surgeon in North Africa, whose record of service with General Patton had impressed him.

General Marshall passed General Kenner's name on to Secretary of War Henry L. Stimson for consideration by President Roosevelt. Stimson and Marshall praised Kenner to the president, describing his North African campaign service and his appointment to Brigadier General status by General Eisenhower. They both urged prompt action on President Roosevelt's part so that Kenner might quickly familiarize himself with the problems of his new post. Kenner, in fact, returned to Washington to do just that. The president demurred, complaining to General Marshall that no physician sits in on the meetings of the general's staff. Several days later, President Roosevelt wrote Secretary Stimson: "I want you to reconsider the tentative selection made two or three weeks ago for Surgeon General of the Army. My best advice is that he is a good doctor, but that he would not be regarded as an outstanding choice by the medical profession. As you know, I am in much closer touch with the medical profession and all its ramifications than most people are, and I believe that some other selection could be made which would do more credit to all of us." President Roosevelt strenuously objected to pressure placed on him by subordinates, urging him to appoint a particular candidate to a given office; the more the pressure, the "greater his determination not to yield, regardless of the merits of the candidate involved." He "liked to make up his own mind."[8] Secretary Stimson replied that Kenner was his first choice and that he had acquired unique experience in World War I and in the North African campaign in 1943. If, however, the president wanted another name, he would give him that of General Norman Kirk, who at the time was commanding officer of the Percy Jones General Hospital in Battle Creek, Michigan. Stimson noted that Kirk had a good reputation as an orthopaedic surgeon and as an energetic, aggressive administrator. General Marshall concurred, commenting on Kirk's "vigor, initiative, and aggressiveness, all the qualities which were at present most needed in the administration of the Surgeon General's office."[9]

Norman Kirk was an orthopaedic surgeon. President Roosevelt's polio had caused him to spend a good deal of time in Warm Springs, Georgia, under the care of another orthopaedic surgeon, Michael Hoke. A friendship developed between the two men; Roosevelt's recorded remarks, delivered at a Thanksgiving dinner at the Georgia Warm Springs Foundation, reflected the respect and affection he had for Hoke. Roosevelt said of Hoke: "He is a man dear to my heart . . . he is our friend and understands what he can do and what he can accomplish . . . and he is a very old friend whom we recognize as a great leader, not only of American medicine, but of American progress . . . social progress, and economic progress in every branch."[10]

The fact that Hoke and Kirk were colleagues in the specialty of orthopaedic surgery and members of the AOA, where they inevitably would have met and socialized, may have influenced the president. Roosevelt himself was a "cripple." By the time he had endured his acute polio, with postinfection depression and the final realization that his paralysis was permanent, he had gained an insight into the medical profession. His experience with Hoke made him believe that orthopaedists cared more about an individual's outcome than whether they merely lived or died. This quality of orthopaedics and the nature of the specialty made its practitioners at that time regard "crippled" persons in a different light. This gave people hope that they could bounce back from an illness or injury, earn a living, and live with self-respect. Roosevelt manifested that attitude with cheerful optimism and hope—qualities that resonated with people and contributed to his popularity. Roosevelt's appreciation for the work of orthopaedic surgeons may have influenced the president to appoint one of them to this high position.

Roosevelt's appointment of Norman Kirk as Surgeon General of the Army had immediate consequences for orthopaedic surgery. Despite the same frustrations and difficulties that had beset Magee, Norman Kirk had a successful tenure. On his watch, the army medical corps grew from 1,200 doctors to 47,000, plus 15,000 dentists and 500,000 other personnel who cared for more than 15 million patients. The death rate from disease dropped from 165 per 10,000 patients in World War I to 60 per 10,000 in World War II. President Harry Truman selected Kirk as his personal physician at the important Potsdam Conference in 1945. Kirk published many books and articles on orthopaedic subjects, including *Amputations*,[11] which went through several editions.

Norman Kirk was born in 1888 on a farm in Rising Sun, Maryland, going straight from high school to medical school at the University of Maryland. He served in the military from 1912 to 1947, when he retired from the army. Then he settled in the eastern tip of Long Island, New York (Montauk Point), and became the small town's family doctor. He actually had all of the qualities ascribed to him during the selection process for the post of Surgeon General of the Army, being brusque, assertive (if not aggressive), intimidating, energetic, feisty, and demanding. At the same time, he was also humorous and kindly when required by circumstances. He died of a ruptured abdominal aneurysm on August 6, 1960, after being operated on at the Walter Reed Hospital by Michael DeBakey.[12,13]

Post-WWII Growth in Orthopaedic Trauma Care

In 1956, 11 years after the war had ended—when Kirk was no longer Surgeon General and had retired from the army—Colonel Mather Cleveland completed a three-volume series of books on the practice of orthopaedic surgery in the Mediterranean Theater, European Theater, and the Theater of the Interior (the homeland of the United States). The books recount the role of orthopaedics in North Africa, Europe, and the homeland during the war. In the book about the European Theater, Charles Odom reviewed the casualties sustained by the Third Army over a six-month period in late 1944. He stated that Third Army hospitals treated 64,389 wounded men during that time. Of these, 43,348 (67.3 percent) had injuries of the extremities or buttocks. This high number—and the devastating character of the wounds themselves—presented many problems. The accompanying nerve lesions, vascular injuries, trunk injuries such as pneumothorax and lacerated viscus, and the high possibility of multiple extremity injuries in a single patient strained the capabilities of the medical department. Even so, for men with wounds of the extremities in Third Army hospitals, fewer than 1 percent died, compared to a mortality rate of nearly 3 percent of all admissions. Odom attributed this successful outcome to policies of the Surgeon General's office, which mandated that orthopaedic surgeons perform a radical débridement for all open fractures and not close any extremity wounds until the danger of infection had completely passed. The army by that time had established a policy that the wounded would receive "chemotherapy," consisting of sulphonamides early in the war and penicillin after it became available in sufficient amounts. The army had also established policies regarding fracture care after the acute treatment of the wound. A report prepared by Cleveland, finally published in 1956, detailed how physicians should apply traction, splints, or casts, and how to immobilize fractures or dislocations for patients being transferred from station hospitals to general hospitals.

Several kinds of orthopaedic problems deserve special mention. One relates to the "ideal plan of management" for "battle-incurred injuries of the hip joint." This list was prepared by Marshall Urist for *Orthopaedic Surgery in the European Theater*.[7]

1. Initial surgery should consist of débridement, arthrotomy, exploration of the joint, irrigation, and primary closure if loss of substance does not prevent it.

2. The approach is preferably the anterior iliofemoral, described by Smith-Petersen, or the posterior approach, described by Kocher.

3. The operation should be performed as soon as possible after wounded, but sepsis does not contraindicate its delayed performance.

4. Débridement should consist of complete excision of blood clots, devitalized muscle, adipose tissue, bone fragments, foreign bodies and other foreign material along the track of the wound . . . the surgeon must use his judgment in deciding how much chiseling, scraping, and curetting are necessary to secure clean bleeding bone surfaces . . . all tissues, including bone, which has no remaining circulation, must be excised to eliminate soil for infection.

5. The deeper parts should be closed over the joint, but the skin wound should be left open to be closed within 4 to 10 days by primary suture.

6. The extremity should be extended by skeletal traction for 8 to 12 weeks.

7. Arc of motion should be begun, in traction as early as possible.

8. When sepsis is established, if treatment as above fails, excision of the joint by Girdlestone's method or disarticulation should be done. Operation should not be unduly delayed if sepsis is severe, since the patient's condition deteriorates rapidly in these circumstances.

9. Whole blood and other supportive measures should be used when indicated.

10. Penicillin and sulfadiazine should be used parenterally—not locally. Both drugs are adjuncts to surgery, not a substitute for it.

11. In occasionally carefully selected cases, reconstructive procedures with internal fixation may be employed four to six weeks after successful delayed primary suture of the wound.

This description of an ideal management plan reveals the grave concern that experienced military orthopaedic surgeons had about infection complicating war wounds and the low priority they assigned to a perfect reduction held together with internal fixation devices.

Among other issues during Kirk's administration was the development of policies for treatment of internal derangements of the knee. The medical department report of orthopaedic surgeons in World War II goes into considerable detail on the initial overtreatment of medial meniscal injuries by newly inducted orthopaedic surgeons. The report states that civilian orthopaedists generally had good results with medial meniscectomy in young, healthy individuals who had meniscal injuries due to minimal trauma or relatively mild athletic injuries. The orthopaedic surgeons found it very difficult to understand why vigorous young men in a military setting who had the same injuries did so poorly after surgery. The report suggested that a return to the rigors of active military duty produced far greater stresses on a knee postoperatively and that long marches, heavy packs, violent exercise, and other forms of physical endeavor overwhelmed the structures in the knee. "The comparison of soldiers returned to combat with football players returned to the game were particularly unrealistic."[7]

The final army report after the war cited other factors contributing to the poor results of knee surgery. "The diagnoses were sometimes in error, and too often operations were performed indiscriminately by medical officers who, in some instances, were also knife-happy." The report also cited "secondary neurotic considerations" in keeping men from returning to duty after knee surgery, suggesting that some men exaggerated existing organic symptoms and others manifested a conversion hysteria, reporting knee symptoms in the absence of an organic lesion.[7]

As a result of the epidemic of bad results following meniscectomies in these patients, the Surgeon General mandated policy changes and limited surgery in soldiers with noncombat injuries.

A preoperative diagnosis of arthritis was a contraindication to surgery. The decision to perform a meniscectomy on an active-duty soldier usually required review by a superior medical officer. A patient who had a painful knee with a presumed meniscal injury before induction in the Army would not qualify for surgery unless he had special military value other than serving only in combat. Otherwise, the orthopaedist should declare that the patient was not physically fit for service. The Army reviewed several large series of these patients: Colonel R. Soto-Hall presented a review of 500 meniscal injuries from six hospitals and Major Vernon Luck presented an analysis of a series of 1,132 men with the same diagnoses. Colonel Mather Cleveland, who reviewed and reported on these series of patients with meniscal tears, manifested some skepticism in his report about indications for the surgery and possibly also regarding the surgical technique. He believed that the nearly 10 percent incidence of hypermobile meniscus without a meniscal tear actually meant that the operating surgeon had made a wrong diagnosis 10 percent of the time. He also noted the high prevalence of associated lesions, such as chondromalacia patellae, loose bodies, osteochondritis dissecans, and diffuse arthritis with tears of the cruciate and/or collateral ligaments, probably would have precluded surgery if identified properly beforehand. Colonel Cleveland's report devoted many pages to the history of symptoms, physical examinations, radiographic examinations, differential diagnosis, and indications for surgery in these patients, and he inveighed against performing such operations on active-duty Army personnel.

Surgeons during World War II did not do these procedures arthroscopically, of course. They had to make at least one and sometimes two skin incisions, each at least 2 inches long. They also had to make similar cuts through the capsule and synovium to enter the joint and locate the pathology. Colonel Cleveland gave due deference to differences of opinion regarding whether all or only part of the meniscus should be excised and did not offer an opinion of his own.

Alfred Shands, Jr., collaborated with Colonel Cleveland in writing the sections of the postwar report for the medical department on the subject of military shoes. Chief of Staff General George Marshall returned from a tour of American forces in North Africa early in 1943 expressing dissatisfaction with the footwear that soldiers wore in combat in the North African desert. The shoes had proved satisfactory for small-scale maneuvers of the early prewar training period but fell apart after only 2 or 3 weeks of actual combat maneuvers. Shortages in rubber and leather contributed to this poor level of quality. As a result of General Marshall's concerns, development of World War II army shoes became a high priority. The final model had flesh-side-out upper leather and arches higher than the previous model, with a cuff and buckle instead of laces. The sole consisted of thick synthetic rubber. The Army developed an elaborate foot-measuring and shoe-fitting platform for providing soldiers with adequate footwear, and theoretically, combat troops were to be given five pairs of shoes per year. Podiatrists (called "chiropodists" in the army reports) and cobblers were in high demand and were assigned to the Sanitary Corps to work with the orthopaedic division.

James Callaghan wrote the section on march fractures in the postwar medical department report. He described how these injuries occurred in the absence of actual combat violence, appearing as linear cracks in normal metatarsals after prolonged marching—almost always in unseasoned soldiers. He also noted that physicians saw these injuries infrequently in World War I because training was much less intense than in the World War II (6 to 8 weeks as opposed to 17 to 18 weeks). Furthermore, World War I training consisted mostly of marching in formation over soft, level ground. In World War II, march fractures incapacitated a lot of soldiers, and several orthopaedic surgeons studied large series of men with these kinds of injuries. Lieutenant Colonel Clarence Hullinger and Major William L. Tyler collected the names of 1,157 and 207 patients, respectively, with these injuries. The great majority of the fractures involved the metatarsals, but they did occur elsewhere—in the os calcis, proximal tibia, distal fibula, supracondylar portion of the femur, femoral neck, and inferior pubic ramus. After analyzing their earlier experience with march fractures, the army determined that plaster casts, rest, and crutches could not adequately serve either the patients or the army. The final report prepared by Callaghan did not indicate whether a directive came from the Surgeon General's office on the subject, but the orthopaedists treating patients with metatarsal fractures came to use a metal bar riveted to the outside of the sole of the shoe in the non–weight-bearing portions. Callaghan reviewed the results of the various forms of treatment of march fractures of the foot and found that this method provided the best results.

It is interesting to compare the World War I and World War II reports made by the army medical department with those made about subsequent conflicts. By 1944, there were standardized policies of thorough débridement of wounds. Antibiotics were widely used, particularly the newly discovered penicillin. There were official recommendations that surgeons use blood transfusions freely to restore blood volume after wounding. The military also implemented universal immunizations, especially for tetanus. As a result, many men lived who in other wars would have died from pyogenic infections, gas gangrene, lockjaw, irreversible shock, and other conditions. During the Korean War, the Army medical department could investigate other issues.[14] Papers published in 1954 had titles such as "Hepatic Function Following Wounding and Resuscitation with Plasma Expanders,"

"Muscle Metabolism and Catabolism and Endogenous Creatinine Clearance in Combat Casualties," and "A Study of Plasma and Erythrocyte Cholinesterase Activity in Combat Casualties," which illustrate the direction of this research activity. The Website of the army medical department in the first decade of the 21st century, during wars in Afghanistan and Iraq, describes telemedicine, neuroprosthetics, virtual reality, handheld computers, and robotics, among other issues.

The Evolution of Fracture Care After World War II

The Revolution in Imaging

Prior to December 28, 1895, the diagnosis of a fracture depended on a history and physical examination. The history usually, but not always, included the recounting of the injury; the physical examination generally included the observation of swelling, bruising, and deformity. Sometimes, in doubtful cases, the limb could be put through a range of motion to elicit crepitus as the fragments of bone rubbed against each other.

That all changed when William Conrad Roentgen (1835–1913) presented a paper on a "new kind of ray" at a meeting of the Sitzungberichter der Wurzburger Physic-Medic Gesellschaft. During his demonstration, he called the previously unknown ray an "x-ray" "for the sake of brevity." In December 1895, Roentgen performed an experiment in which he passed a high-voltage electrical charge through a vacuum tube covered with dark paper. Several other physicists had performed similar studies, but Roentgen's purpose was to observe the effect of any electromagnetic energy produced by the electrical discharge in the vacuum tube on a fluoroscopic material. He noted that paper coated with barium platinocyanide glowed under the influence of the rays produced by the electrical discharge. He further observed that dense materials such as metals or bone absorbed the rays so that the fluorescent material did not glow in the shadow of these substances. He tried the same experiment using photographic plates and actually created photographic images of coins and other metal objects as well as the bones in his wife's hand. In his presentation of these phenomena on January 23, 1896, he created a similar x-ray photograph of a hand of an audience member, Professor Albert Rudolph von Kölliker. Those in attendance realized that they were witnessing one of the most remarkable occurrences in the history of medicine, agreeing with von Kölliker's suggestion that the rays Roentgen had called x-rays should henceforth by called roentgen rays. Roentgen refused to seek any personal profit from this discovery, and he eschewed any patents or royalties. He did accept the Nobel Prize, which was the first ever presented, and he lived comfortably on his professor's salary until his retirement. Between the wars, the rampant inflation of the Weimar Republic destroyed the value of Roentgen's savings, and he died in poverty.

Roentgen's discovery enjoyed huge and immediate success. Every serious physician, quack, and businessman, including such American entrepreneurs as Thomas Edison, Walter Westinghouse, and George Eastman, got in on the action. In the United States, as in every country in Europe, roentgen rays became the rage. On February 3, 1896, less than 3 weeks after Roentgen gave his epochal demonstration, Professor Edwin Frost produced the first clinical roentgen plate in America in the physics laboratory at Dartmouth College. His brother, Dr. Gillman Dubois Frost, had a patient with a painful swollen wrist; Gillman asked Edwin to photograph the bones in the wrist to determine if there was indeed a fracture. The patient, Ed McCarthy, was a student at the college.

It did not take long for the hazards of working with x-rays to become apparent. Despite skin cancers and x-ray burns, however, the use of Roentgen's rays swept the world and became an indispensable modality in modern medicine.

The legal profession also quickly comprehended the usefulness of Roentgen's discovery. In December 1896, the case of James Smith versus W. W. Grant came before Judge Owen LeFevre in Denver, Colorado. Smith had accused Grant of malpractice because Grant had failed to diagnose Smith's femoral fracture. Smith had sought a second opinion from another Denver physician, Tennant. Tennant obtained an x-ray picture of Smith's leg, which confirmed that Smith had sustained a fracture. Judge LeFevre accepted the evidence of the x-ray picture and ruled for the plaintiff. A similar case in Nottingham, England, also had been decided on the basis of an x-ray picture of a fracture in a patient's foot. That case was decided in June 1896, only 2½ months after Roentgen announced the discovery. It took American lawyers only a few more months to bring Roentgen's rays into the courtroom.[15]

Although Roentgen's discovery revolutionized orthopaedic surgery, it had its limitations. Static images—frontal, lateral, and oblique views—clearly helped localize foreign bodies and define the nature of fractures and dislocations. But using the rays continuously in fluoroscopy proved too difficult and dangerous during surgery. It was necessary to place the patient between the operator and the vacuum tube, and the operator had to look directly at the x-ray beam, This led to dangerously high levels of exposure. This method of fluoroscopy also produced very faint images, necessitating prolonged dark adaptation of the eye, with the wearing of red glasses between procedures. In the 1950s, the development of image intensification overcame these problems and led to a dramatic change in the way fracture surgeons treated musculoskeletal injuries. In past years, the surgeons performing operations had to rely either on the limited capabilities of fluoroscopic guidance or obtain multiple x-ray pictures during the procedure. Each individual photograph required repositioning of the x-ray tube and careful placement of a photographic plate against the patient. This was followed by development of the plate, usually at a place distant from the operating room, and redraping, when the x-ray technician finally produced a suitable picture. Relatively straightforward procedures could take many hours under these circumstances. In the late 1970s, however, development of modern image intensification eliminated these deficiencies and led to a renaissance in fluoroscopy. With an image intensifier, the x-ray beam passing through the patient was focused on to a small radiosensitive plate, producing the image. A television camera viewed the image and transferred it to a remote monitor or screen. With the vacuum unit on a rotating C-arm and draped into the surgical field, a fracture surgeon could quickly, easily, and safely perform procedures almost unthinkable without this technology. These devices have transformed modern fracture care.[16]

Fixation Technology

Examinations of skeletons recovered from archeological excavations of ancient gravesites reveal that human beings have suffered fractures and dislocations since the species Homo sapiens first appeared on Earth. Furthermore, books and atlases relating to medical history carry numerous pages of illustrations that depict how the practitioners of a given time or era corrected the deformities caused by such injuries. In addition, numerous texts have described how the deformities can be kept stable until enough healing has occurred to prevent recurrence of the original malalignment. These descriptions frequently mention the materials used to create devices that will stabilize a broken limb. Practitioners have used such obvious devices as flat boards and metal splints secured with linen bandages to support a broken extremity. To avoid the problems associated with rigid non-conforming devices, techniques were developed for stiffening wrappings with materials such as honey, egg yolk, wax, moss, pitch, glue mixed with flour, or lead acetate. Plaster of Paris, so-called because of the large gypsum deposits beneath the city of Paris, has a remarkably long history of use in this application. Physicians in the 10th century discovered that by heating gypsum, they could produce a substance able to rehydrate with the addition of water. The powdered material resulting from the original heating would set into a hard homogeneous material that could conveniently reinforce bandages. This knowledge was lost until the early 19th century when Dutch, German, and Russian physicians rediscovered it in 1814, 1816, and 1831, respectively.[17] Initially, the fractured limb was placed in a box and liquid plaster that had yet to harden was poured in. Applying grease to the skin before using the plaster prevented it from sticking to the skin, but removing these casts must have been incredibly difficult.

Antonius Mathijsen,[18] a Dutch surgeon, wrote the first paper describing the use of plaster of Paris incorporated into strips of gauze in 1832. Used in this way, plaster of Paris was easy to apply, quickly hardened while the deformed limb was held in the corrected alignment, and the surgeon could easily mold it to conform to the contours of the limb. It also had the advantages of easy storage. It was lightweight, strong enough to prevent breakage under most circumstances, and inexpensive. If the cast was properly applied with sufficient padding over bony prominences, it could be worn comfortably for a long time or at least as long as was necessary. Initially, removal of these casts proved difficult, requiring the use of heavy, long-handled shears. The fracture surgeon had to labor long and hard to force the shears to bite through the heavy plaster, advancing the jaws of the device a little at a time. The invention of the lightweight oscillating saw by an orthopaedic surgeon named Homer Stryker changed that; with its advent, fracture surgeons could now remove casts and change them with relative ease.

In the mid-1970s, manufacturers began to produce and supply casting material reinforced with fiberglass instead of plaster of Paris.[19] This material, which has had a remarkably successful run, consists of a monomer that can be catalyzed by water. The fiberglass material hardens quickly and has many of the qualities of plaster of Paris. It is lightweight, easy to use, and comfortable, but it costs more. Surgeons also have at least some difficulty in molding it as well as they can mold plaster of Paris to the contours of the limb. It is stronger than plaster of Paris, however, and perhaps most important, it does not crumble or fall apart when it gets wet.

Splints and casts are methods of purely external fixation. They encase a limb as rigidly as possible but provide no real fixation of the fracture fragments themselves. They often need changing as swelling subsides, or as dressings or sutures beneath them need to be removed or changed. The immobilization they produce is relatively incomplete, and stiffness and muscle atrophy often develop, which might require years of rehabilitation. These occur because the patient cannot move the limb when a cast or rigid dressing immobilizes joints above and below the fracture site.

Treating fractures with casts or splints, or with prolonged traction and bed rest, is based on the theory that a little deformity may not interfere with function or cause pain—at least in the short term. Initially, this treatment strategy assumes that if a nonunion or unacceptable deformity does result, surgical intervention with bone grafting and internal fixation can salvage the unsatisfactory outcome. Some surgeons have argued that more strict criteria regarding assessment of outcomes would persuade orthopaedic surgeons to use open surgical reduction and internal fixation more often. One of the first to embrace this viewpoint was William Arbuthnot Lane of Guy's Hospital in London.[20] Lane began the practice of open surgical reduction and fixation of fractures in the early 1890s. First, however, he had to ensure himself, his patients, and his superiors at the hospital that postoperative sepsis would not automatically follow in the most cases. To that end, he assiduously improved and refined Lister's antiseptic technique, turning antisepsis into asepsis. In his words:

> In aseptic surgery, the great object . . . is
> that everything that comes into contact
> with the wound shall be absolutely free
> from germs which are pathogenic to Man
> or which are putrefactive. In antiseptic
> surgery, the wound was kept in an anti-
> septic state by irrigation or spray, so the
> germs getting in the wound might be
> killed. [20]

Lane used towels and drapes sterilized with dry methods rather than soaking them in carbolic acid, and he sterilized his instruments with the same methods. He also used a no-touch technique in which only sterilized instruments actually came in contact with the patient's tissues. In addition, Lane had consummate skill and could perform surgery quickly and atraumatically. At first, in 1892, he began using a wire suture, a method he referred to as an internal splint. By 1893, he had switched to wires and screws, and by 1902, he had devised the Lane plate.

In 1909, Lane visited America as a guest of the ASA. Their annual meeting that year convened at the Bellevue Stratford Hotel in Philadelphia. Minutes of that meeting published in the *Annals of Surgery* describe "a paper of the controversial W. Arbuthnot Lane of Guy's Hospital, London." In the paper, Lane described the pathology of the "allusory condition" of chronic intestinal stasis, how he had performed surgery for release of adhesions (which he called "Lane's bands"), and how in some cases he had performed partial bowel resection. The secretary of the meeting noted acidly that at the end of his paper Lane gave no further statistics and no further details. The reviewers of Lane's paper found it unacceptable and made several unkind remarks about it.

Later that same evening, John B. Walker, a surgeon at the Bellevue Hospital and Hospital for the Ruptured and Crippled in New York, presented a paper stating that 75 percent of damage suits against physicians were against surgeons—65 percent of them being fracture cases. He noted that the public "fortified by x-ray pictures holds strong views on the subject of fractures." He went on to suggest that too much of surgeons' attention had been devoted to the relatively new subject of abdominal surgery and that patients with fractures therefore had been neglected. Walker then proceeded to exhibit the radiographs of eight fractures that he had opened and fixed with wire sutures. These had all healed in good alignment.

Lane then rose to claim that he had never seen a case in which he could not achieve perfect alignment of the fragments and that he had advocated this kind of treatment for nearly 15 years. He had, however, abandoned wire sutures for fixation and had moved on to the use of "very strong plates with small screws which would stand the strain of 448 pounds, and the method will hold anything." Several other members, including Charles H. Mayo, also rose to comment on Lane's remarks. All spoke favorably about Lane's skill and his results in caring for patients with fractures. Those in attendance held Lane in high regard as a fracture surgeon, but less so as an abdominal surgeon.

William Arbuthnot Lane and Sir Robert Jones both influenced American orthopaedics, but in very different ways. Jones was essentially a reconstructionist regarding musculoskeletal injury and deformity. Neither of his books published after World War I addressed acute fractures and dislocations. Jones spent most of his time during World War I treating wounded soldiers sent from France to England, where he worked to prevent deformities and rehabilitate the wounded. He supervised the fitting of tens of thousands of prostheses and arranged for splinting of paralyzed limbs, grafting of nonunions, and retraining of wounded men in "curative workshops." He hoped after the war to keep the orthopaedic hospitals open to civilians for the same purpose. For a time, he considered calling them "special surgery hospitals," but eventually decided to keep the term "orthopaedic." His kindness and affable personality made him a favorite among American orthopaedists, and he came to America often.

Lane, on the other hand, projected an entirely different persona. He was sarcastic, a master of the putdown, but he was a brilliant surgical technician given to virtuoso performances in the operating room. He also had an extensive network of influential friends whom he exploited whenever the need arose. During World War I, he came out of retirement to perform plastic surgery on men with facial deformities resulting from their wounds. He entertained a steady stream of American visitors at his hospital during that time, but he apparently had little to do with fracture surgery and the use of his Lane plate during and after the war.

Although Lane popularized open reduction and internal fixation with plates, cables, and screws in the United States and Great Britain, several European surgeons had already performed this kind of surgery. In their 1947 book on the internal fixation of fractures, Charles S. Venable and Walter G. Stuck credited a German surgeon named Hauffman with the "original idea for bone plates and screws."[21] Alvin Lambotte, a Belgian, also began experimenting with these techniques in the first decade of the 20th century, about the same time as Lane. Lambotte tried several kinds of metal, such as aluminum, silver, and brass, but finally settled on soft steel, plated with gold or nickel, 1- to 1.5- mm thick, wider in the middle than at the ends, curved to the shape of the bone, and pierced with screw holes every 5 mm.[22] Lambotte had the same obsessive concern about asepsis as Lane, reporting very few infections using these devices. Robert Danis, also a Belgian, modified plate fixation to include the possibility of applying compression to the fracture to increase the likelihood of bone union. This gave rise to the concepts promulgated by the AO group.[23] D. L. Griffiths, who reviewed Danis' book *Théorie et Pratique de l'Ostéosynthèse* for the British volume of *JBJS* in 1951, presciently stated: "This is an important book."[24]

Lane himself used high-carbon steel in his plating system, a material that metallurgists now regard as too brittle for this application. Furthermore, the design of Lane's plate predisposed it to break easily. It was widened at the site of the screw holes and tended to fail there. His greatest contribution was probably his emphasis on aseptic technique, which made this type of surgery possible.

Venable and Stuck[21] devoted two chapters of their 1947 book, *The Internal Fixation of Fractures*, to stainless steel and cobalt-chromium, alloys that are still widely used. They described the gradual evolution of stainless steel and discussed the effects of varying amounts of chromium, carbon, vanadium, nickel, molybdenum, and other elements on the physical properties of objects manufactured from these alloys. In their early application, devices made of stainless steel then available failed frequently due to multiple causes that were poorly understood. Poor technique and postoperative infection, electrolysis, breakage, and loosening made many orthopaedists reluctant to use these methods. During the early years following World War I, surgeons instead tried such materials as ivory plates, beef bone xenografts, and plates made of horn. It was a general rule that any kind of internal fixation should be allowed to remain in place only as long as necessary for the bone to heal. After that, the surgeon was obligated to remove it. When Venable and Stuck published their text, orthopaedists and metallurgists still had not overcome the problems inherent in placing stainless steel in the body and leaving it there indefinitely.

By the late 1940s, Vitallium came into use in orthopaedic surgery. Metallurgists at the Austenal Laboratories in New York had developed it for use in dentistry in 1929, but Venable and Stuck did not begin to use it in fracture surgery until 1936, when they secured an ivory plate to a patient's femur with Vitallium screws. The fracture healed and the screws did not appear to cause any reaction, a finding that was consistent with their experiments in rabbits. They persuaded Willis Campbell of Memphis, Frank Dickson of Kansas City, and Melvin Henderson of Rochester to join in further clinical investigations. The war intervened, but Venable and Stuck were about to report large series of fracture cases fixed internally with Vitallium plates and screws in the 1940s. The results were quite good, and Vitallium did not appear to cause any harmful tissue reactions.

Vitallium is an alloy of 65 percent cobalt, 30 percent chromium, and 5 percent molybdenum. It is extremely resistant to corrosion, very hard, and not particularly malleable. Since its introduction, it has had multiple applications in orthopaedics. However, as metallurgical improvements have been made, stainless steel has regained some favor for use in fracture fixation over the harder, more rigid Vitallium. Biocompatibility, electrochemical reactions in metal, and consequent bone destruction are issues that continue to concern metallurgists and orthopaedists.

With the passing of time, orthopaedic surgeons have found that certain fractures almost always require open reduction and plate fixation, and that treating them otherwise exposes patients to the likelihood of deformity, pain, and prolonged disability. Both-bone fractures of the forearm, especially in its midportion, fall into this category. It is interesting to trace the history of the management of these injuries over the past century. Older textbooks document the problem of treating this injury, but only with closed techniques. Philip D. Wilson of Harvard Medical School and William Cochran of the University of Edinburgh published a text on fractures in 1928.[25] In the section on forearm fractures, they noted that the reduction needed to be as accurate as possible to avoid loss of pronation and supination with "resulting diminution of the usefulness of the hand." The fact that the surgeon had to reduce "not two but four fragments" made reduction difficult, but closed treatment always should be attempted before open reduction because "all too frequently open surgery is likely sooner or later to result in disaster." They also described how reduction maneuvers require that the surgeon take into account the effect of the attached muscles on the position of the fragments and how the distal fragments should always be manipulated into alignment with those more proximal. If the reduction is

adequate, the patient should be placed in a long arm cast for a minimum of
ten weeks; if the initial reduction is not acceptable, or if it is lost during that
ten-week period, the forearm should be put in traction. The patient would
be required to remain supine in bed while traction kept a pull on the forearm through adhesive tape strips on the patient's skin and a glove glued to
the hand. The physician had to apply countertraction to the upper arm to
keep the extremity from being pulled up off the bed. Even with this treatment, angulation can persist, and with traction, the patient risks circulatory
interference and a possible Volkmann's contracture.

By 1955, ten years after the end of World War II, the perception of the
best treatments of this injury had not changed. In his popular book on the
treatment of fractures, Sir Reginald Watson-Jones[26] once again carefully
and at length described manipulation under anesthesia, "the tricks for
closed reduction and the need for prolonged immobilisation in a long-
armed cast." He did devote two paragraphs to the open method but claimed
that open surgery resulted in nonunions in 10 percent of patients. He wrote:
"If I was one of the 10 percent of patients who developed a nonunion of the
fracture, requiring even yet another operation and a complicated bone grafting procedure, I would have no interest in the other 90 percent. I would be
indignant to pay such a penalty for their small prize." Ten years later, in
1966, Edward L. Compere, Sam Banks, and Clinton Compere, all of
Northwestern University in Chicago, published their *Pictorial Book of
Fracture Treatment*.[27] Their illustrations of the reduction techniques for
radial and ulnar shaft fractures included traction with countertraction, angulation "in the direction of the displacement of the lower fragment until the
ends lock," followed by straightening the forearm and placing it in a long
arm cast. If these reduction techniques failed, open surgery with fixation
secured by plates and screws or Rush pins or other intramedullary rods
(Figure 22) could be considered. The authors warned that "open reduction
is a difficult task, hence should be attempted only by the experienced surgeon . . . occasionally it may be preferable for the inexperienced surgeon to
use metal pin fixation above and below the fracture site." The surgeon could
then incorporate the pins into the cast. Closed techniques, however, too
often resulted in delayed or nonunions and late deformity, due to angulation
of the fractures.

Twenty-five years later, L. D. Anderson and Frederick Meyer of the
University of Alabama wrote in Rockwood and Green's *Fractures in Adults*
that even with a successful closed reduction, patients required frequent cast
changes, prolonged immobilization, very careful continued assessment of
position with radiographs because of the slow healing of the fracture, and
watchful assessment of the circulatory status of the arm.[28]

Anderson and Meyer's primary indication for open treatment was "all
displaced unstable fractures of the radius and ulna in adults." In describing
methods of internal fixation for these fractures, they discussed
intramedullary rods and plates and screws. Several innovative orthopaedic
surgeons had attempted to fix these fractures with intramedullary devices,
but early results generally did not justify the continuation of this practice.

100

Reports of large series of patients treated with these devices revealed intra-operative technical problems, as well as high rates of malunions and nonunions. F. P. Sage[29] had devised an intramedullary rod for fixation of various fractures. The rod was triangular, semiflexible, and prebent to accommodate the double bowing structure of that bone. His technique required an open reduction of the fracture and retrograde insertion of the rod from the radial styloid just above the wrist. The surgeon had to guide the rod carefully through the fracture site into the upper fragment, with gentle taps on the rod from below. Technical difficulties arose, such as selecting a rod that was too long, too short, or too thick. This could result in the radius exploding and having the rod stick in the shaft, resisting all attempts to remove it or change its position. In addition, rods could not be used in several kinds of fracture patterns, thus limiting their utility. Orthopaedic surgeons have largely abandoned intramedullary devices for forearm fractures, and have accepted plating technology as the better method to treat these injuries.

Fracture surgeons observed the technical difficulties of intramedullary fixation just when dramatic improvements of plate technology were occurring. The Eggers slotted plate, larger and stronger than its predecessors, theoretically permitted the plate to slide on the bone, so that the fracture fragments could come together in impaction, decreasing the chance of delayed union or nonunion.

The current, strongly supported opinion regarding fractures of the forearm is that they are best treated surgically, and "this has been most predictably accomplished with plate fixation." The revolutionary concepts of William Arbuthnot Lane, Alvin Lambotte, and Robert Danis have triumphed.

Although plating methods of the shoulder, forearm, elbow, and wrist can prevent pain and deformity, fracture fixation with plates and screws for treatment of fractures between the trochanters of the femur can extend a patient's life. These injuries occur in elderly people who tolerate fractures with great difficulty. Elderly individuals also frequently have life-threatening comorbidities that hip fractures impact adversely, changing stabilized illnesses (such as diabetes mellitus, mild congestive heart failure, arteriosclerotic heart disease, and early dementia) into a catastrophic cascade of multiple system failures. The well-documented experiences of orthopaedic surgeons over the past 50 years have shown that the elderly have the best chance of survival with prompt surgical reduction and stabilization of the fracture. The well-reduced and stabilized hip fracture eliminates the pain caused by the uncontrolled motion of the fragments in the patient's upper thigh, allowing mobility instead of virtual recumbency for six or eight weeks, during which time the fracture consolidates. Without internal fixation, the fractures often heal in a deformed alignment, leaving the patient with short and badly rotated limbs; the prolonged inactivity exposes the patient to the risks of decubitus ulcers, thrombophlebitis, and pulmonary emboli.

Fracture surgeons recognized the need to improve the treatment of hip fractures more than 100 years ago. Roland Bissell published a paper in the

Philadelphia Journal of Medicine in 1903 on his review of 450 elderly patients with hip fractures in New York hospitals.[30] He observed all the above problems in these patients, leading to death associated with multiple comorbidities. He recommended that surgeons consider treating these injuries more aggressively, even "cutting down" on them to achieve reduction and stabilization.

During the first half of the 20th century, orthopaedic surgeons did not consistently apply the evolving principles of plate technology to intertrochanteric hip fractures. One of the most popular orthopaedic fracture texts in 1946, *Fractures and Joint Injuries* by Sir Reginald Watson-Jones, devoted little more than a page to the subject of intertrochanteric hip fractures. He acknowledged "the dangers and inconveniences" associated with "three or four months' immobilisation in plaster" required for treatment of these injuries and wrote that "whenever possible the fracture should be nailed." If, however, comminution made the fracture unsuitable for nailing, if nailing had failed, or if the patient was "too old for treatment in plaster, or in a frame" he recommended that well-leg traction be used instead. This method required a long leg cast on the noninjured side, with an outrigger attached to the sole of the foot. From the outrigger attached to the sole of the leg cast on the normal side, traction was applied to a pin in the distal tibia on the fractured side. A short leg cast would hold the pin in place. The normal limb, encased in the long leg cast, then provided the support for the traction on the injured side. Watson-Jones recommended this kind of treatment for up to six months in slow-healing fractures.

In his next edition, published nine years later in 1955, Watson-Jones still strongly recommended nonsurgical treatment of intertrochanteric hip fractures in the elderly.[26] He acknowledged that "many think that despite the proved success of conservative treatment when skilled nursing is available, it is better to perform internal fixation of the fracture . . . there must be a plate with four screws into the femoral shaft." He illustrated this point by showing a radiograph of a healing intertrochanteric fracture secured with a McLaughlin nail and side plate. Watson-Jones objected to the surgery because of the operation's effect on the elderly patient.

Few, if any, orthopaedic surgeons now regard nonsurgical treatment as the preferred method in managing intertrochanteric fractures, even in the elderly. The device Watson-Jones used in his illustrations, that is, a plate to which a triflange nail is rigidly attached, had certain disadvantages. It prevented impaction of the fragments so that if impaction did occur, the nail would cut through the femoral head and damage the socket. If the nail succeeded in preventing impaction, it would prevent contact within the major fragments and delay or prevent healing. Several models of these devices, featuring the fixed-angled rigid nail-plate junction, were introduced from the 1950s through the 1970s. Several surgeons reported on their various attempts to overcome these basic problems. However, a fixed-length nail attached to a side plate, secured to the lateral cortex of the proximal femur, had a basic design flaw. No matter how the fracture was reconfigured with osteotomies and various displacements of the fragments, bone absorption and at least some collapse and impaction almost always occurred.

A reasonable solution to these problems came with the development of the sliding compression screw and side plate. This required the heavy reinforcement of the upper end of the side plate and its modification to include the creation of a large screw hole in the reinforced upper end. Modification also included the extension of the plate up into the femoral neck. The extension of the plate up into the hollow femoral neck had a barrel or tubular configuration so that a surgeon could pass a heavy threaded screw through it into the femoral head. By tightening a lag screw, the surgeon could impact the fracture fragments during the operation because the large threaded screw could slide in the barrel of the modified plate.

Improved preoperative preparation and anesthesia, the widespread use of antibiotics and transfusion, and pinpoint-accurate surgery made possible by image intensification have helped the plates originally conceived by Lane, Lambotte, and Danis become essential to modern fracture surgery in ways not previously imagined.

Intramedullary Fixation

In 1945, orthopaedic surgeons on active duty in the U.S. Army inherited a large number of patients from their German counterparts. Some were American prisoners of war who had sustained wounds, including fractures of the femur, before capture. When the American physicians reviewed their new patients' histories and radiographs, they expressed concern that German surgeons had treated many femur fractures in American prisoners by inserting steel rods into the medullary canals to achieve fixation. American orthopaedists, accustomed to reduction with prolonged skeletal traction followed by mobilization in a walking spica cast, regarded the German preference for intramedullary fixation as experimental, verging on a war crime. They soon realized, however, that the femur fractures treated with rods healed more quickly and with fewer complications. Far from being experimental, intramedullary fixation in femur fractures in 1945 logically followed earlier attempts to stabilize these injuries with an implant inside the bone as opposed to a plate on the outside. In fact, Leslie Rush of Meridian, Mississippi, began using Rush semiflexible stainless steel rods in 1936 to secure fixation of long bones.[31] From 1937 to 1968, he used Rush rods in the treatment of 211 consecutive cases of femoral shaft and condylar fractures. Rush rods, however, eventually wound up outside the mainstream of intramedullary fixation techniques as better and more stable devices supplanted them. Gerhard Küntscher, who supervised the treatment of Allied prisoners' femur fractures, also began work on intramedullary fixation in the late 1930s. German investigators attempted intramedullary fixation with ivory pegs or rods of bone, but infection, breakage, and fracture nonunion plagued these efforts. Küntscher was determined to devise a better method. His technique and the concerns he addressed in 1940 set the stage for future improvements in fracture care with intramedullary rods. Küntscher's method has survived essentially intact for over 65 years. He established the principles for intramedullary fixation of blind nailing with radiographic guidance without direct exposure of the fracture, and the use of strong, semiflexible nails large enough to fill the canal of the bone to control alignment, rotation, and translation.[32]

These principles, simple enough at the outset, required ingenuity and considerable time to put into practice. The blind nailing with radiographic guidance in the 1940s posed too many difficulties for most orthopaedists, and when Küntscher nails first came to the United States in the postwar years, almost all of the surgeons who used them employed open techniques in which an incision was made over the fracture, the nail driven out through the greater trochanter, and then retrograded back down into the distal fragment. Küntscher did not have the advantage of using modern image intensification, instead relying on multiple intraoperative radiographs or the use of fluoroscopy during surgery. A surgeon could step out of the operating room during the exposure of an x-ray plate, but fluoroscopy in that era required wearing a fluoroscopy headpiece or using a hand fluoroscope. Surgeons had to stand directly in front of the x-ray beam, suffering radiation burns or worse as a result. The images lacked clarity, and obtaining multiple images took a great deal of time. Most surgeons thus preferred to accept the risks of open reduction and the possibility of a higher infection rate, more blood loss, and slower fracture healing. Küntscher and his rods gained a wide following in the 1960s and 1970s because they produced such good results, but the open surgery carried serious risks.

Küntscher's other principles regarding the size, shape, and physical properties of the nail also led to widespread experimentation by orthopaedic surgeons eager to devise a better and more marketable device. Küntscher maintained that the nail should fill the canal of the femur; this requirement mandated that the surgeon ream the canal to make it possible to insert the largest diameter nail possible. His experiments showed that the damage to endosteal circulation caused by reaming did not slow fracture healing because of the transience of the effect. Several American models involved soft broaching, with less satisfactory canal filling and stability. In addition, Küntscher's original open cloverleaf design was modified considerably. Other orthopaedists attempted to use solid rods, diamond-shaped rods, and other devices of varying configurations. An enormous improvement on Küntscher's original design, however, came about with the development of interlocking screws in the 1980s.[33-36] The insertion of these devices, made possible only through the development of excellent image-intensification fluoroscopy, allowed the expansion of Küntscher's techniques and their indications well beyond his original intentions. Before development of the interlocking screws, Küntscher rods had their best chance of success only in stabilizing femoral shaft fractures at the isthmus (or the narrowest part) of the femur. Below the isthmus, the femur flares out into a trumpet-like configuration; even with reaming, the rod cannot fill the hollow bone. In the upper part of the femur, the wide femoral canal diameter similarly makes stability difficult to achieve without supplementing the rod with transverse screws, plates and screws, or cerclage wires.

Lorenz Böhler, who published several fracture texts before and after Küntscher, described the use of Küntscher's concepts in the treatment of bones other than the femur. Interestingly, intramedullary fixation of the humerus, radius, ulna, and even the clavicle was attempted and mostly failed to withstand the scrutiny of modern evidence-based medicine. Küntscher rods, as well as their successors, have survived in the treatment of the femur and the tibia, however. They have found wide application in treating fractures of these bones. The most recent articles and texts carefully describe reaming and interlocking techniques for these injuries. The advent of closed intramedullary rodding of femur fractures supplemented by interlocking screws led to a revolution in the care of these injuries.

J. O. Lottes, an American, reported excellent results in the treatment of tibial fractures with a bent, slightly flexible, triangular intramedullary nail he developed in the early 1950s.[37-39] He used a blind technique, but without image intensification. He inserted his rod into the upper end of the tibia through a small incision on the medial side of the knee at the level of the tibia tubercle. The slight flexibility of the nail made it possible for him to guide it across the fracture line into the distal fragment. The Lottes nail achieved a good deal of popularity during those years.

Other orthopaedic surgeons have modified Küntscher's nail to extend its indications and improve its results. Robert Zickel[41] of New York began work on a "combined intramedullary rod and a triflanged nail" in the mid-1950s, 20 years after Küntscher's first reports on his development of a workable intramedullary nail. Zickel's discussion of his own device alluded to the failures of nail-plate combinations in treating fractures of the femur in a subtrochanteric location. The mechanical stresses in that part of the femur often overwhelm the screws in the plate used for fixation, causing the plate to break or pull away from the outer cortex. Alternatively, the junction of the nail and the plate often snapped, causing the fracture to become displaced again. The morbidity associated with these events in elderly patients with chronic illness had the potential for resulting in the patient's death. Zickel devised a nail bent into two planes to accommodate entry through the normal configuration of the upper femur. He made the upper portion of the rod quite large (17 mm in diameter), big enough to fill the upper end of the femur and contain a tunnel through which a triflange nail could be passed into the femoral neck and up into the femoral head. A set-screw inserted in the nail from the upper end of the rod secured the fixation. Ten years after his preliminary report, Zickel presented his experience with "this appliance" in the treatment of 84 patients with nonpathologic fractures in the subtrochanteric region of the femur. His ingenious application of intramedullary nail technology proved successful; the fractures in the 75 patients united uneventfully. He did, however, describe sobering intraoperative technical problems, including comminution of the greater trochanter and difficulty in passing the guidewire into the femoral head and neck for insertion of the triflange nail. Despite these difficulties, Zickel's basic design has gained in popularity, although modified extensively by those who have adopted it. The Gamma nail, Russell-Taylor nail, Alta intramedullary nail, and the Trofix nail, for example, have all expanded Küntscher's original concepts. These changes made possible fixation of high femoral fractures, which previously were very difficult to secure effectively. Küntscher's semirigid intramedullary rod was also modified by J. Ender, an Austrian, in the mid-1970s.[35] Ender devised nails that were thin and quite flexible. His technique required the introduction of multiple rods (three to five) into the femoral canal from below, that is, at the level of the femoral condyles. Many North American orthopaedic surgeons used Ender's nails after he first reported on his success with them, particularly in the treatment of hip fractures. The method achieved relatively poor fixation, however, and was tedious to perform. As a result, it has largely fallen out of favor in the United States.

External Fixation

American orthopaedic surgeons had little experience or interest in external fixation techniques before World War II. Jean François Malgaigne, Alvin Lambotte, Raoul Hoffman, and Henri Judet in Europe, as well as Roger Anderson and Otto Stader in America, published papers on their inventions, which at the time seemed too far out of the mainstream for general use.[42-44] Roger Anderson's devices required the use of heavy smooth pins that could be inserted at divergent angles to maximize stability and prevent them from backing out of the bone.[42] Stader pins had thin threaded tips for insertions through one cortex of the bone and into the cortex of the opposite side.[44] Neither of these constructs stood up well in actual use. Anderson's heavy smooth pins too frequently loosened and became infected. Stader, a veterinarian, had devised a system for use in animals, mostly dogs, and it did not adapt well to use in human patients.[45]

External fixation methods performed so poorly that the Surgeon General of the army prohibited their use during World War II. The report of the medical department of the U.S. Army concerning orthopaedic surgery in the Mediterranean Theater of Operations states, "Almost as soon as the method began to be used, it became evident that its indiscriminate use in military surgery was attended with pitfalls and hazards and that it must be rigidly restricted . . . drainage from the sites of the pins was fairly frequent. In the great majority of cases, combat-incurred fractures were much better managed by other methods and there was little or no need for apparatus for this method in the theater of operations."[6] As a result, American orthopaedic surgeons essentially abandoned external fixation for nearly 20 years.

In the mid-1970s, during the early development of trauma center hospitals, trauma surgeons at the University of Maryland resurrected the concept of external fixation for use in civilian trauma at that institution. Early results supported enthusiasm for the method, and through multiple presentations, publications, and courses, the concept of external fixation regained respectability. Surgeons selected the Hoffman apparatus for the procedure. This system, because of the size of the pins and their strategically spaced and tapped threads and rigid stainless steel metallurgy, worked well in civilian use. Exhaustive analyses of the mechanics of these systems have been published, and the Hoffman apparatus ranks high in these studies.[46] The

Hoffman apparatus subsequently has been widely used for the treatment of extremity and pelvic fractures in the United States.

In the late 1970s and early 1980s, American orthopaedic surgeons became aware of the work of Gavriil Ilizarov. Ilizarov had radically altered the concept of external fixation by switching from heavy 5-mm pins to thin 1.5-mm wires. Instead of spearing the fragments of bone with heavy pins and attaching the pins to thick rods, Ilizarov's method supported the bones from a circular or half-circle frame the way the thin wire spokes of a bicycle wheel support the bicycle and rider from the wheel rim. The method used by Ilizarov, fine transosseous wires attached to a circular frame, probably originated in the late 19th century. Nathan Parkhill devised a wire circular frame apparatus for the treatment of fractures in 1898.[47]

Ilizarov lived and worked in Kurgan, more than 1,000 miles east of Moscow in Siberia. Americans had limited access to his work during the more restrictive days of the Cold War, a fact that possibly explains the short shrift initially given him by American orthopaedic surgeons. In his 1983 text, Dana Mears noted, "In the USSR, surgeons lack the ability of a wide variety of sophisticated devices . . . Russian medical engineering has lagged substantially behind its Western counterpart . . . and while the Ilizarov design provides an academic curiosity for potential innovators, it would not appear to be of interest for Western surgeons."[48] Two other texts on external fixation published in 1982 and 1983 (at the same time Mears released his *External Skeletal Fixation*) did not mention Ilizarov.[47-49]

Ilizarov, however, achieved extraordinary success not only in treating routine fractures but also in treating complex malunions, nonunions, and bone infections. He also devised ways to lengthen bones. The Wagner apparatus (a derivative of the Hoffman system) had also achieved success in limb-lengthening procedures, but the Ilizarov methodology appeared to shorten the process and reportedly was more predictable. As a result of this achievement, Ilizarov became widely known in communist countries, and orthopaedic surgeons who worked behind the Iron Curtain began to use his transosseous fixation methods. News of the successes began to leak out. In northern Italy, Spinelli and Monticelli, who had seen the results of using the Ilizarov technique on injured Italian tourists returning from Yugoslavia, employed the technique and soon received international recognition as experts in treating problem fractures. Fidel Castro sent 30,000 Cuban soldiers to Angola in the attempted communist takeover of that country during the 1970s and early 1980s; the wounded Cubans who had been treated with Ilizarov's methods appeared to do so well that Latin American orthopaedists also became interested in the technique. American orthopaedic surgeons who knew about the potential of transosseous wire fixation methods actually wanted to visit Ilizarov in Kurgan, but Soviet bureaucracy and the closed nature of Soviet society precluded this. Stuart Green of the Rancho Los Amigos National Rehabilitation Center in Downey, California, finally made contact with Ilizarov, who wrote back that he "had no objection" to a visit from Green. Finally, after prolonged wrangling with Soviet immigration officials, Green secured the necessary visas and became the first U.S. citizen to visit Ilizarov in the spring of 1987. He had learned to speak Russian especially for the trip and stayed there for several weeks. Victor Frankel of New York and several others soon followed.

American orthopaedists were intensely interested in having Ilizarov lecture and demonstrate his methods at their institutions. The Soviet authorities, however, initially denied his requests to leave the Soviet Union. Eventually, however, a Soviet cultural delegation, including Ilizarov, received orders to fly to New Orleans to demonstrate Soviet goodwill in scientific, medical, and cultural exchanges. Ilizarov lectured at medical schools in New Orleans, Tulane University, and Louisiana State University.

In December 1988, Ilizarov lectured at an international conference hosted by Victor Frankel and Dror Paley at the Hospital for Joint Diseases in New York. As a Canadian citizen, Paley had been able to visit Kurgan and Ilizarov before the Americans. Stuart Green also provided "editorial assistance" to Ilizarov in the publication of an 800-page text, *Transosseous Osteosynthesis: Theoretical and Clinical Aspects of the Regeneration and Growth of Tissue.* Gavriil Ilizarov, professor and director of the Kurgan All-Union Center for Restorative Traumatology and Orthopaedics, died in 2005.[50-52]

The Trauma Societies

Orthopaedic Trauma Association

As must happen often with the foundation of a professional society, the Orthopaedic Trauma Association (OTA) began as a friendly conversation over lunch.[53] Edwin Bovill and Michael Chapman had hosted Ramon Gustilo of the Hennepin County Hospital in Minneapolis on the occasion of Gustilo's visit to the San Francisco General Hospital in late January 1977. The three men discussed the problems they encountered as orthopaedic traumatologists working in large, underfunded public hospitals while trying to meet their responsibilities related to teaching, administration, and research. They decided to meet again and invite other orthopaedists who they knew were in the same situation. They called their nascent organization the Orthopaedic Trauma Center Study Group (OTCSG).

They held their first formal meeting at the Los Angeles County Hospital in 1978, with J. Paul Harvey as host. They devised no organizational structure and consequently had no bylaws or officers. They merely met at an agreed location for two days, sharing papers and case presentations. In addition to Gustilo, Bovill, Chapman, and Harvey, early members included Sigvard (Ted) Hansen of the Harborview Medical Center in Seattle, Renner Johnston of Denver General Hospital, Arsen Pankovitch of Cook County Hospital in Chicago, David Segal of Boston City Hospital, Edward Habermann and Michael Distefano of Montefiore Hospital in New York, Bruce Browner and Andrew Burgess from Maryland Shock Trauma Center in Baltimore and several members from the Parkland Hospital in Dallas.

The society held annual meetings thereafter, changing its name in 1979 to the Orthopaedic Trauma Hospital Association (OTHA). In 1985, when the AAOS developed the Council of Musculoskeletal Specialty Societies (COMSS), the OTHA developed bylaws, officers, statements of mission and goals, and in 1983 changed its name to the Orthopaedic Trauma Association. The focus changed from institutional members to individuals. Gustilo served as the first president of the OTA, followed by Chapman, who completed incorporation in 1985. By this time, the OTA had money in the treasury, a valuable set of minutes and transactions, industry support, a trauma registry and fracture classification. The first educational meeting was held in 1987 in Baltimore under the leadership of Charles Edwards and Alan Levine.

The OTA began publishing a specialty journal devoted to orthopaedic traumatology, the *Journal of Orthopaedic Trauma* (*JOT*), in 1987. Phillip G. Spiegel of the University of South Florida College of Medicine in Tampa served as the editor-in-chief, with Michael Chapman and Christopher Colton of Nottingham in the United Kingdom serving as deputy editors. The list of editorial board members numbered 23 from the United States and 15 from other countries.

Today, *JOT* also serves as the official journal of the International Society for Fracture Repair, the Belgian Orthopaedic Trauma Association, the Japanese Society for Fracture Repair, the Canadian Orthopaedic Trauma Society, and the Argentine Association of Orthopaedic Trauma. *JOT* also publishes in association with the Deutsche Gesellschaft für Unfallchirurgie and the Association for the Rational Treatment of Fractures.

In 1991, under the leadership of the seventh president, Richard F. Kyle, the OTA established a Research and Education Fund to collect contributions from members and corporate partners and fund research into orthopaedic trauma. The fund has grown through the years and now awards over $500,000 in research grants annually. Several multicenter prospective clinical studies, as well as many basic science projects which subsequently received NIH grants, had their start as OTA-funded projects.

As part of its goal to become the primary source of orthopaedic trauma education, the OTA began in 1992 to offer trauma update courses for the practicing orthopaedic surgeons of the United States and Canada. The first such course was initiated by Richard F. Kyle, and was offered in Vail, Colorado. The OTA continues to sponsor surgeon education courses each year in partnership with the AAOS, and to offer additional education at the Annual Meeting and during Specialty day. At the OTA annual meeting in Tampa, Florida, in 1995, the society began to offer a course for orthopaedic residents in basic fracture care. The course was directed by Robert A. Winquist, the eighth OTA President.

Resident education has become a high priority for the OTA, and two resident courses are currently offered each year. A complete resident curriculum of lectures on trauma and fracture care has been produced by OTA with Paul Tornetta, III, the twenty-first OTA President, as developer and editor of the original lecture series and is available to download from the Website.

The OTA today is seen as the premier source of commercial-free, trauma-related orthopaedic education, and a leader among specialty societies in its educational offerings.

In addition to promotion of research in trauma and fostering education, the OTA is involved in a wider variety of advocacy and leadership activities. The Fellowship and Career Choices Committee provides career mentoring for residents, educational symposia, and a coordinated platform for applying to and interviewing for fellowships. There are currently 46 North American orthopaedic trauma fellowship programs with spots for 77 orthopaedic trauma fellows. The Practice Management Committee is involved in the process of reviewing relative values and promoting new CPT codes, a process that was begun in collaboration with AAOS by M. Bradford Henley, the sixteenth president of OTA. The Health Policy Committee is actively involved in a variety of advocacy activities and interfaces with a variety of organizations to influence health policy issues.

American College of Surgeons Committee on Trauma (ACSCOT)

The ACSCOT is the primary body within the ACS which deals with trauma. Their activities include verification of trauma centers in the United States, running the Advanced Trauma Life Support (ATLS) course, producing a variety of trauma related publications, promoting trauma research, helping states to develop trauma systems, and advocacy. The ACSCOT is composed of a large number of general surgeons with special expertise in trauma, as well as surgical specialists—orthopaedic surgeons, neurosurgeons, and pediatric surgeons.

The ATLS course was first offered by the ACS in 1980. The course was developed in response to a tragedy involving an orthopaedic surgeon who was involved in a private plane crash in rural Nebraska. His wife was killed, and he and his children sustained serious injuries. He recognized that the trauma care which his family received during the first few critical hours was inadequate primarily due to lack of training for the providers. This recognition led to the development of a course involving lectures and skills training for trauma care under the auspices of the Committee on Trauma of the Nebraska chapter of the ACS. From that beginning, the ATLS course has grown to approximately 1,100 courses each year, training about 20,000 doctors in lifesaving trauma skills. The approach to the injured patient that is taught in ATLS involving the ABCs of trauma care has saved the lives of countless patients.

In 1976, the ACSCOT, in order to improve trauma care in the United States, devised criteria for a classification of hospitals that provide trauma care into levels from 1 to 4. A level I trauma center is the highest designation, and denotes a center with specialized capabilities and personnel. A level I trauma center "provides comprehensive trauma care, serves as a regional resource, and provides leadership in education, research, and system planning." A level I designation requires that the hospital have trauma surgeons immediately available along with anesthesiologists, subspecialists, nurses, and resuscitation equipment. In addition, level I trauma hospitals must treat "1,200 admissions a year or 240 major trauma patients per year."[54] Levels II, III, IV, and V trauma hospitals have different requirements. A level II hospital, for example, must meet level I all standards except for the volume quota and participation in education and research. Since 1976, 35 states have adopted these standards, and the physicians and surgeons working in hospitals with levels I and II category designations have achieved an 8 percent decrease in deaths from motor vehicle accidents and up to a 50 percent decrease in deaths caused by trauma overall. Hospitals are designated with regard to trauma center level by their appropriate state, and the ACS provides verification services to those hospitals who wish to have that service.

The provision of appropriate care to injured patients is an ongoing challenge in the United States. Because the burden of trauma falls disproportionately upon the young and poor, and because trauma care is very expensive, recent years have seen many trauma centers closing due to financial pressures. In addition, the lack of surgeons and surgical specialists to take calls at trauma centers coupled with increasing demands for care through hospital emergency departments has created unique challenges to the ongoing provision of care. Only through cooperation and commitment of surgeons, hospitals, and government can these problems be solved.[55-56]

AO Foundation and AO North America

The AO Foundation was formed in Switzerland in December 1958.[57] Four surgeons, Maurice Müller, Robert Schneider, Hans Willenegger, and Martin Allgöwer had established social and professional ties as a result of their service in the Swiss army. Müller, Schneider, Willenegger, and Allgöwer came from different cities in Switzerland, but all had matured professionally in the tradition of Lambotte, Küntscher, Böhler, and Robert Danis, the master surgeons of the previous generation who strived to perfect the art and science of the care of the injured. Müller and his associates initially proposed founding a school for teaching surgical technique in the tradition of European fracture treatment. They organized themselves into a group which they called "Arbeitsgemeinschaft für Osteosynthesefragen" (AO), ("Association for the Study of Internal Fixation.") The group quickly expanded and began to hold meetings on improving their practices. In February 1958, the group met at the Canton Hospital in Chur, Switzerland. The members of the group presented their ongoing work in a two-day session, critically evaluating their methods and techniques. They reviewed the materials and instruments that were currently available for internal fixation and realized the were inadequate. They selected Maurice Müller to be in charge of developing new instrumentation, which they would later evaluate for approval or rejection. Müller, realized that they would need the expertise of engineers and metallugists and obtained the consultation of a manufacturer, Robert Mathys, who had founded a company that specialized in manufacturing stainless steel products.

The AO group, also established the Laboratory for Experimental Surgery in Davos, Switzerland. Allgöwer negotiated the acquisition of the building, at that time owned by the Swiss Research Institute for High Mountain Medicine and occupied by the Institute of Pathological Anatomy. He obtained funding from the AO group, staffing and equipping the building after modifying it to suit the group's needs. By the end of 1959, the group had established bylaws and officers, developed and approved numerous implants and devices, and collected data on nearly 1,000 cases treated with them. The AO had organized this information meticulously, an effort that required analysis, documentation, and storage of almost 10,000 radiographic images.

AO improved the quality of instruments and implants available for the treatment of fractures. Leaders in documentation and record keeping, one of the earliest principles of the group was that the implants would not be provided to other surgeons or centers without training in how to use them. In accordance with this principle, AO began presenting courses in Davos in the 1960s. The large attendance there suggested the need for additional courses in other countries. The first AO course in the United States was in Columbus, Ohio, in 1973. Synthes began the independent distribution of AO-approved fracture equipment and orthopaedic implants shortly thereafter. The AO Group's research, clinical documentation, and educational imperatives, coupled with the precision of the products has made AO a major force in orthopaedic surgery worldwide. (P. Rothenberg, personal communication, 2005). As AO teaching became a worldwide process, the need to decentralize became evident, and AO North America was formed in 1992 to focus on education and research on the North American Continent.

In the early years of AO, the close collaboration of surgeons, engineers, and manufacturers allowed rapid advances in materials and techniques. The profitability of the implant business provided large amounts of money for teaching and research. As the business of surgery became more sophisticated and market driven, however, the continued tight linkage between the AO and the manufacturers (including Synthes) became a problem. To maintain credibility as teachers and researchers, the AO (particularly in North America) realized it must separate itself from the commercial aspect of the business. This process, which has begun, will no doubt take some time, as all involved try to preserve the best aspects of this fruitful collaboration. In the meantime, AO courses for surgeons and operating room personnel set the standard for hands-on technical instruction in fracture surgery.

References

1. Morison SE, Commager HS, Leuchtenburg WE: *A Concise History of the American Republic.* New York, NY, Oxford University Press, 1977, p 556.

2. Weed FW, McAfee L: *The Medical Department of the United States Army in the World War.* Prepared under the direction of Maj Gen M. W. Ireland. Washington, DC, Government Printing Office, 1927, section II: Orthopedic Surgery, 1927, pp 429, 549-748.

3.   Request for information in cases of fracture, 15 August 1918. Letter to the Commandant, Camp Greenleaf, Fort Oglethorpe, GA (through Division of General Surgery and Brig Gen T. C. Lyster) Surgeon General's Office. In the Medical Department of the United States Army in the World War. Washington: Government Printing Office, 1233, vol. 1, 1927, pp 1135-1136.

4.   Osgood R: The orthopedic outlook. *J Orthop Surg* 1919;1:1-6.

5.   Cleveland M, Shands AR, McFetridge EM: *Surgery in World War II: Orthopaedic Surgery in the Zone of the Interior*. Washington, DC, Medical Department: United States Army, Office of the Surgeon General, Department of the Army, 1970, p 7.

6.   Coates JB, Cleveland M, McFetridge EM (eds): *Surgery in World War II: Orthopedic Surgery in the Mediterranean Theatre of Operations*. Washington, DC, Medical Department: United States Army, Office of the Surgeon General, Department of the Army, 1957, p 14.

7.   Coates JB, Cleveland M, McFetridge EM (eds): *Surgery in World War II: Orthopedic surgery in the European Theater of Operations*. Washington, DC, Medical Department: United States Army, Office of the Surgeon General, Department of the Army, 1956.

8.   Documents collected by Dr. Zachery Freidenberg, including letters signed by Secretary of War Stimson, extracts from Stimson's diaries, biography of General Kirk, memoranda from FDR; provided by K. Moody. The FDR Library currently holds the originals.

9.   Parrish T: Roosevelt and Marshall: *Partners in Politics and War*. New York, NY, William Morrow and Company, Inc, 1989, p 96.

10. Address of President Roosevelt: Thanksgiving Dinner, November 30, 1933, Warm Springs, Georgia. Available at http://www.cviog.uga.edu/Projects/gainfo/ FDRspeeches/FDRspeech33-6.htm. (Accessed March 16, 2007)

11. Kirk NT: *Amputations, Operative Techniques*. Washington, DC, Medical Interpreter, 1924. Republished as monograph by WF Prior Co, Hagerstown, MD, 1942.

12. Norman Thomas Kirk: Available at http://history.amedd.army.mil/tsgs/kirk.htm. (Accessed March 16, 2007)

13. Duryea EA: General's Journey—Norman T. Kirk. Available at http://history.amedd.army.mil/tsgs/Kirkstory/Kirkstory.html. (Accessed March 16, 2007)

14. Howard JM, Hughes CW (eds): *Battle Casualties in Korea: Studies of the Surgical Research Team*. Washington DC, Army Medical Service Graduate School, Walter Reed Medical Center, 1954.

15. Grigg ERN: The *Trail of Invisible Light from X-strahlen to Radio(bio)logy*. Springfield, IL, Charles C. Thomas, 1965, p 25.

16. Wolbarst AB: *Physics of Radiology*. Norwalk, CT, Appleton & Lange, 1993, p 5.

17. Bick EM: *Source Book of Orthopaedics*. New York, NY, Hafner Publishing Company, 1968, pp 279-329.

18. Mathijsen A: *Du Bondage Plâtre et de son Application Dans le Traitement des Fractures*. Liege, Belgium, Grandmont-Donders, 1854.

19. Kowalski KL, Pitcher JJ, Bickley B: Evaluation of fiberglass versus plaster of Paris for immobilization of fractures of the arm and leg. *Mil Med* 2002;167:657-661.

20. Layton TB: *Sir William Arbuthnot Lane: An Enquiry into the Mind and Influence of a Surgeon*. Edinburgh, Scotland, ES Livingston Ltd, 1956.

21. Venable CS, Stuck WG: *The Internal Fixation of Fractures*. Springfield, IL, Charles C. Thomas, 1947.

22. Lambotte A: *L'Intervention Opératoire dans les Fractures Récentes et Anciennes*. Paris, France, Moloine, 1907.

23. Danis R: *Théorie et Pratique de l'Ostéosynthèse*. Paris, France, Masson et Cie, 1949.

24. Griffiths DL: Book review of Théorie et Pratique de l'Ostéosynthèse, by Robert Davis. *J Bone Joint Surg Br* 1951;33:144.

25. Wilson PD, Cochrane WA (eds): *Fractures and Dislocations: Immediate Management, Aftercare, and Convalescent Treatment With Special Reference to the Conservation and Restoration of Function*. Philadelphia, PA, Lippincott, 1925, pp 215-249.

26. Watson-Jones R: *Fractures and Joint Injuries*, ed 4, vol II. Baltimore, MD, Williams & Wilkins, 1955, pp 560-587.

27. Compere EL, Banks SW, Compere CL (eds): *Pictoral Book of Fracture Treatment*. Chicago, IL, Year Book Medical Publishers, 1966, pp 120-221.

28. Anderson LD, Meyer FN: Fractures of the shafts of the radius and ulna, in Rockwood CA, Green DP, Bucholz RW (eds): *Fractures in Adults*, ed 3, vol I, 1991, pp 679-738.

29. Sage FP: Medullary fixation of fractures of the forearm: A study of the medullary canal of the radius and a report of fifty fractures of the radius treated with a prebent triangular nail. *J Bone Joint Surg Br* 1959;41:1489.

30. Bissell JH: The treatment of fracture of the neck of the femur at Bellevue, St. Vincent's, and New York Hospitals. *Philadelphia Medical Journal* 1903;11:900-903.

31. Rush LV, Rush HL: Evolution of medullary fixation of fractures. *Am J Surg* 1949;78:324.

32. Bick EM: The intramedullary nailing of fractures by G. Kuntscher: Translation of *Arch Klin Surg* 200:443, 1940. *Clin Orthop Relat Res* 1968;60:5-12.

33. Brumback RJ, Uwagie-Ero S, Lakatos RP, Poka A, Bathon GH, Burgess AR: Intramedullary nailing of femoral shaft fractures: Part II. Fracture-healing with static interlocking fixation. *J Bone Joint Surg Am* 1988;70:1453-1462.

34. Kempf I, Grosse A, Beck G: Closed locked intramedullary nailing: Its application to comminuted fractures of the femur. *J Bone Joint Surg Am* 1985;67:709-720.

35. Ekeland A, Thoresen BO, Alho A, Stromsoe K, Folleras G, Haukebo A: Interlocking intramedullary nailing in the treatment of tibial fractures: A report of 45 cases. *Clin Orthop Relat Res* 1988;231:205-215.

36. Bone LB, Johnson KD, Weigelt J, Scheinberg R: Early versus delayed stabilization of femoral fractures: A prospective randomized study. *J Bone Joint Surg Am* 1989;71:336-340.

37. Lottes JO, Hill LJ, Kay JA: Closed reduction plate fixation and medullary nailing of fractures of both bones of the leg: A comparative end-result study. *J Bone Joint Surg Am* 1952;34:861-877.

38. Lottes JO: Medullary nailing of the tibia with the triflange nail. *Clin Orthop Relat Res* 1974;105:53-66.

39.   Sedlin ED, Zitner DT: The Lottes nail in the closed treatment of tibia fractures. *Clin Orthop Relat Res* 1985;192:185-192.

40.   Zickel RE: A new fixation device for subtrochanteric fractures of the femur: A preliminary report. *Clin Orthop Relat Res* 1967;54:115-123.

41.   Ender J, Schneider H: Subtrochantere brüche des oberschenkels: Behandlung mit federnägeln. *Actuelle Chir* 1974;9:359.

42.   Anderson R: Castless ambulatory method of treating fractures. *J Int Coll Surg* 1942;5:458.

43.   Vidal J: External fixation: Yesterday, today and tomorrow. *Clin Orthop Relat Res* 1983;180:7-14.

44.   Lewis KM, Briedenbach L, Stader O: The Stader reduction splint for treating fractures of the shafts of long bones. *Ann Surg* 1942;116:623.

45.   Shaar CM, Kreung FP, Jones DT: End results of treatment of fresh fractures by the use of the Stader apparatus. *J Bone Joint Surg* 1944;26:471.

46.   Coppola AJ, Anzel SH: Use of the Hoffman external fixator in the treatment of femoral fractures. *Clin Orthop Relat Res* 1983;180:78-82.

47.   Brooker AF, Cooney WP, Chao EY: *Principles of External Fixation.* Baltimore, MD, Williams & Wilkins, 1983.

48.   Mears DC: *External Skeletal Fixation.* Baltimore, MD, Williams & Wilkins, 1983, pp 1-41.

49.   Uhthoff HK: *Current Concepts of External Fixation of Fractures.* New York, NY, Springer-Verlag, 1982.

50.   Ilizarov GA: The tension-stress effect on the genesis and growth of tissues: Part II. The influence of the rate and frequency of distraction. *Clin Orthop Relat Res.* 1989;239:263-285.

51.   Ilizarov GA: The tension-stress effect on the genesis and growth of tissues: Part I. The influence of stability of fixation and soft tissue preservation. *Clin Orthop Relat Res* 1989;238:249-281.

52.   Ilizarov GA: Nonunions with bone defects, in Coomly R, Green S, Sarmiento A (eds): *External Fixation and Functional Bracing.* London, England, Arthrotext, 1989, p 189.

53.   The Orthopaedic Trauma Association: Available at http://www.ota.org/about/history.html. (Accessed March 16, 2007)

54.   MacKenzie EJ, Hoyt DB, Sacra JC, et al: National inventory of hospital trauma centers. *JAMA* 2003;289:1515-1522.

55.   Rodriguez JL, Christmas AB, Franklin GA, Miller FB, Richardson JD: Trauma/critical care surgeon: A specialist gasping for air. *J Trauma* 2005;59:1-7.

56.   Rogers FB, Osler T, Hrashford SR, Healey MA, Wells SK: Charges and reimbursement at a rural level I trauma center: A disparity between effort and reward among professionals. *J Trauma* 2003;54:9-15.

57.   Matter P: History of the AO and its global effect on operative fracture treatment. *Clin Orthop Relat Res* 1998;347:11-18.

CHAPTER 5

THE TOTAL JOINT REVOLUTION AND THE NEW SCIENCE OF BIOMATERIALS

The Beginnings of Joint Surgery

Débridement

Anesthesia and antiseptic surgery permitted the evolution of operations on joints during the late 1800s and early 1900s. Tuberculosis of the musculoskeletal system provided surgeons with considerable experience in performing procedures such as resections, débridements, fusions, and osteotomies. By the mid-20th century, orthopaedic surgeons began applying these methods to the treatment of musculoskeletal pain caused by the various forms of noninfectious arthritis. Paul Magnuson of Northwestern University,[1] for example, described joint débridements in patients with osteoarthritis. His papers, published in the 1940s, included lengthy descriptions of preoperative selection, surgical technique, and postoperative care. The operation itself consisted of removing whatever looked abnormal from a hip or knee—menisci, osteophytes, loose bodies, thickened synovium, sometimes all or part of the patella, or any hyaline cartilage that appeared fibrillated or worn. The patients had to remain recumbent for a few days, but Magnuson warned them before the operation that he would require them to move the knee almost immediately postoperatively. He reported that he would not perform an operation on a patient who appeared to lack the strength of character and stoicism to endure early active and passive motion the day after surgery. Magnuson had great confidence in his outcomes, stating, "The results for traumatic and hypertrophic arthritis of the knee or hip are among the most satisfactory of any form of joint surgery." He accompanied his description of the operation with several photographs confirming the patients' quite severe osteoarthritic changes in their knees. By the late 20th century, these individuals would have undergone total joint arthroplasties, but Magnuson took his surgical procedure only up to the point at which present-day surgeons would have cut the femur and tibia for implantation of a knee prosthesis. In the hip joint, he merely excised osteophytes and loose bodies without replacing the femoral head and resurfacing the acetabulum.

Synovectomy of joints with rheumatoid arthritis and débridement of osteoarthritic joints have fallen out of favor among orthopaedists and rheumatologists. Thirty-five years ago, orthopaedic surgeons performed both operations in large numbers and reported on them in their papers and presentations. In 1971, for example, Chitranjan Ranawat and his colleagues at the Hospital for Special Surgery in New York critically evaluated 12 of their synovectomy patients by performing synovial biopsies six months to six years after the original procedure.[2] They reported synovial tissue regenerated in all of their patients, with microscopic evidence of inflammatory changes that "were quantitatively less severe than those observed in the original specimens." Ranawat followed this limited endorsement of synovectomy in rheumatoid arthritis with a much stronger affirmation two years later. In 1975, he reported on 32 knees in 26 patients followed for three years; a total of 69 percent experienced pain relief and controlled inflammation, and the operation preserved the articular cartilage in 71 percent of patients.[3] Ranawat tempered his enthusiasm for the "cleanout" of rheumatoid knees, noting that "by longer followup, the disease, with loss of articular cartilage, will recur in a large number of cases." He emphasized that he had performed the operation on patients with chronic synovitis but no deformity, normal motion, no instability, and no loss of articular cartilage.

In 1973, Jay Graham and R. G. Checketts[4] also reported somewhat disappointing outcomes over time, even after limiting open synovectomy to patients with early rheumatoid arthritis. Nine years after the operations, 55 percent of their 107 patients reported continued pain relief, but this relief occurred in only those patients whose rheumatoid arthritis had improved overall with medical treatment. Graham and Checketts reviewed the literature and referenced 15 papers on open synovectomies for rheumatoid arthritic knees up to that time. The orthopaedic surgery community has gradually moved away from this operation, especially as medical treatment has improved. With the advent of arthroscopy, accounts of open synovectomy for the treatment of rheumatoid arthritis of the knee have all but disappeared from the medical and orthopaedic journals.

Osteotomy

The standard textbooks of the first half of the 20th century did not discuss realignment. Arthur Steindler, Paul Colonna, and Willis Campbell (whose first edition of *Campbell's Operative Orthopaedics* was published in 1939) did not even reference tibial osteotomy for the treatment of painful osteoarthritis of the knee. In 1961, J. P. Jackson and W. Waugh of Mansfield, England, published one of the first papers on this subject.[5] They referenced previous literature on the potential benefit of osteotomies about the hip for osteoarthritis, but they alluded to no previous papers on realignment of the knee. They reported that the operation had been performed in Liverpool and other centers, but they were not aware of published results relating to its use in the treatment of the osteoarthritic knee joint. Jackson and Waugh did the procedure by creating a ball-and-socket convex cut through the tibia at the level of the tibial tubercle, manipulating the leg into varus or valgus alignment to correct for either type of deformity. They also found that in performing the osteotomy at that level, they had to cut through the fibula to manipulate the tibia into the corrected position. They used no internal fixation, instead employing a long leg cast for 8 to 10 weeks, permitting weight-bearing in the cast at about three weeks after surgery. At follow-up 31 months later, all ten of their patients told them that they were "considerably, if not completely, relieved." Jackson and Waugh learned from this series of patients that correction of bowleg deformities with tibial osteotomy had better outcomes than correction of knock-knee (valgus) deformities. They postulated that in case of valgus deformity, the angulation occurs at the lower end of the femur and that "osteotomy through the femur may seem the correct procedure." In any event, "the aim was to make the leg look straight."

American orthopaedic surgeons quickly adopted the idea of realigning the knee with an osteotomy of the tibia or femur for the treatment of painful osteoarthritis. Bauer and his colleagues at the Hospital for Special Surgery presented their paper on the subject in the *Journal of Bone and Joint Surgery* (*JBJS*) in 1969.[6] Mark Coventry of the Mayo Clinic published his article in *JBJS* in 1973,[7] followed by Kettelcamp and associates[8] in 1976. Papers on the subject of osteotomy about the knee for the treatment of painful osteoarthritis continue to appear in the literature. The combined experience of these individuals has helped to establish the best indications for the operation. Together they have shown that patients with unicompartmental arthritis do best with realignment procedures.

Whether closing wedge, opening wedge, internal fixation, or external fixation is used, the basic requirement of unloading the prematurely deteriorating compartment remains unchanged. Osteotomy about the knee came into the group consciousness of orthopaedic surgeons fairly recently, shortly before the sudden appearance of the dramatic and successful joint arthroplasty procedures. Unfortunate timing may have prevented the useful, conservative approach of osteotomy from receiving the recognition and use that it deserved.

Widespread use of femoral osteotomies specifically for the treatment of painful arthritis of the hip did not occur until the 1930s. Orthopaedic surgeons had previously become familiar with the techniques of upper femoral, acetabular, and pelvic osteotomies in the treatment of nonunions of femoral neck fractures and untreated or failed treatment of congenital hip dislocations. Realignment for osteoarthritis, however, began rather recently. In 1935, T. P. McMurray of Liverpool published an article in the *British Journal of Surgery* on osteoarthritis of the hip joint.[9] He had treated 89 patients with this condition over a period of 15 years. He reported that in early mild cases, manipulation and exercise produced pain relief for varying periods of time, but when the osteoarthritis was more advanced, he employed rest and immobilization techniques with braces or casts. The long-standing conflict between motion and exercise versus rest and immobilization persisted well into the 20th century.

When either or both of these methods failed, McMurray felt compelled to offer another kind of operation to his patients. He attempted an operation he called an arthroplasty that, according to his description of the technique, was a reshaping of the femoral head with removal of bone spurs and loose bodies. He also mentioned the possibility of interposition of some tissue such as fascia or fat, but found that regardless of the technique, arthroplasty yielded results that were "decidedly poor."

McMurray also performed a resection arthroplasty in four of these patients with removal of the femoral head. He found that these operations "invariably give motion, but there is an inevitable diminution of the voluntary power of the limb." Furthermore, the improved motion occurs "at the expense of a certain amount of stability." McMurray performed hip fusions on 17 patients in the series, all of which proved successful and reliable in achieving pain relief with stability. He acknowledged the disadvantage of transferring the stresses of body motion to the lumbosacral spine, which caused low back pain. He also noted that hip fusion takes longer and carries more surgical risk than the other procedures. He determined that the fusion operation, which required 40 minutes for him to complete, exposed patients to "shock," noting that "the question of shock must be very seriously considered." To avoid this problem, he hit upon the idea of a subtrochanteric osteotomy with medial displacement of the distal fragment so that the lower fragment lies about half an inch below the level of the head of the femur, just below the edge of the acetabulum. McMurray claimed that he could perform this operation "in a few minutes." His postoperative care consisted of immobilization of the hip in a cast for 4 to 5 months. By the time the osteotomy healed, the patient could have "complete freedom." McMurray performed this operation on 15 patients and reported excellent results in 12 patients. He found that the patients had no pain, with good but not full motion. He said, "In my opinion, the operation holds a very important place in the treatment of osteoarthritis of the hip joint." He referred to it as a "Lorenz bifurcation osteotomy." The McMurray osteotomy aimed to shift the line of weight bearing medially, transferring as much weight bearing as possible onto the medially displaced distal fragment.

Friedrich Pauwels[10] devised alternatives to the McMurray-Lorenz osteotomy: realignment procedures of the upper femur based on the biomechanical analysis of the forces transferred across the hip joint. He published a series of papers in the 1930s that defined the hip as a single-plane lever system. According to this analysis, joint reaction forces in the hip depend on moments of force developed by body weight, counterbalanced by forces generated by the abductor muscles. Since then, other orthopaedists have refined Pauwels' perceptions of femoral realignment procedures, placing more emphasis on realigning the femur to place remaining healthy articular cartilage of the femoral head in a position to bear the loading and compressive forces of weight bearing. These operations require internal fixation to maintain alignment while the osteotomy heals. European orthopaedic surgeons, such as Maurice Müller and his AO Group of Switzerland and Renato Bombelli of Italy, have taken the development of instrumentation for this operation to a very high level.[11,12]

Interposition Arthroplasty and Surface Replacements

Interposition arthroplasty of the hip, the so-called cup arthroplasty (Figure 23) had a 30-year run as the premier operation for most painful hip conditions. Marius Smith-Petersen created the concept in the late 1920s and published his first series in 1939.[13] Smith-Petersen died in 1953. Nine years later, his associate at the Massachusetts General Hospital, Otto Aufranc, published *Constructive Surgery of the Hip*,[14] in which he reported that he, Smith-Petersen, and others at Massachusetts General Hospital had performed more than 3,000 of these operations.

Smith-Petersen, one of the icons of American orthopaedics, merits special mention. His obituary, published in *JBJS* in 1953, states that he was Norwegian, born in Grimstad in 1886. He immigrated to this country in 1903 at 17 years of age and settled with his family in Milwaukee. He graduated from the University of Wisconsin but spent the rest of his life in Boston at Harvard and Massachusetts General Hospital. During World War I, he served with Harvey Cushing. He went to France in 1915 (along with Dr. Philip Wilson), returning to Boston after the war. By 1929, he had been appointed chief of the orthopaedic service at Massachusetts General Hospital.

Smith-Petersen conceived several procedures and innovative devices in orthopaedics that bear his name. One was the extended iliofemoral anterior exposure of the hip, which he allegedly developed because of "the frequent shock which followed hip surgery due to exsanguination" (as stated in his obituary). An efficiently executed Smith-Petersen anterior approach results in little blood loss because it takes the surgeon between muscles and neurovascular structures, not through them. He also developed the Smith-Petersen nail for the internal fixation of femoral neck fractures. The nail has a triflange configuration so that when driven through the lateral cortex of the upper femur, it will pass up through the neck and lodge solidly in the femoral head. Although Smith-Petersen put his heart and soul into developing the cup arthroplasty, it was a failure. Although 30 percent to 60 percent of patients reported pain relief initially after the early rehabilitation period, 70 percent had moderate to severe pain at ten years. Furthermore, the belief that the femoral head beneath the cup and the surface of the acetabulum developed hyaline cartilage was wrong. Fibrocartilage (or more often, no cartilage at all) appeared on these surfaces, which was discovered by orthopaedic surgeons only upon frequent revisions of the operation. Total joint arthroplasty proved to be the better idea, and today cup arthroplasty has a limited role, if any, in modern orthopaedics.

Smith-Petersen may have realized this. His memorialist describes Smith-Petersen's last clinic before the Robert Jones Club the April before he died as a "stirring demonstration . . . of a large group of patients upon whose hips he had performed . . . his Vitallium-mold arthroplasty. Throughout morning and afternoon he presented patient after patient whose gratitude . . . knew no bounds. More brilliant results have yet to be shown." One wonders why Smith-Petersen would have pressed so hard to prove his point. Perhaps he realized presciently that, within a decade, British, European, and even a few Americans would eclipse his operation with the new technology of total hip arthroplasty.

Smith-Petersen and Aufranc devised a set of special instruments to prepare the joint for the interposed Vitallium cup.[15] These consisted of ice cream scoop–shaped reamers, ranging from very small to very large. A spherically shaped socket was created with the male reamers, and a spherical head sized to fit into the socket was made with the female reamers. The surgeon had to choose a cup sized to fit loosely on the femoral head and loosely in the acetabulum to permit motion between the head and cup and the cup and socket. Surgeons found that these requirements often made for imperfect positioning of the cup, which would move unexpectedly into less than perfect alignment. Technical difficulties, uncertain outcomes, and a desire to make the operation the definitive procedure for painful osteoarthritis led Smith-Petersen to continually modify the technique. He began working on cup arthroplasties in the early 1920s, when he implanted a molded Pyrex cup into a series of patients with hip arthritis. Upon removing a piece of glass from a patient's back shortly after World War I, he observed that a fibrous envelope had developed around the glass foreign body. The patient had elaborated clear serous fluid about the foreign body, along with an envelope of fibrous tissue; it looked like the inside of a joint cavity. Observing this, Smith-Petersen thought that glass might serve as interposition material in joint reconstructions. Unfortunately, all the glass molds broke inside the patients. In his book on the subject published in 1962, Aufranc did not elaborate on these issues except to say, "The mold went through several stages of evolution, both in the shape and in the materials used. Vitallium became the final choice through a trial-and-error process."[14]

Smith-Petersen experimented with other materials before finally deciding on Vitallium.[16] Having settled the materials issue, he devised cups of various shapes and configurations. For a time, he inserted cups with an outwardly flared rim. Later he used hemispherical cups, and then nearly spherical cups. The inside cup configuration and edge of the cup (sharp, beveled, or squared off) all came under consideration. One cannot really conclude that all the concentrated effort and years of work that went into cup arthroplasty came to naught. American orthopaedic surgeons developed profound interest in hip arthroplasty, and Smith-Petersen's experimentation with cup arthroplasty set the stage for the total joint revolution.

Interposition arthroplasty of the hip has a long history. French and German surgeons experimented with the procedure in the 19th and early 20th centuries using skin, fascia lata, fat, wood, gold foil, and chromacized submucosa of pig bladder. From 1923 until the early 1970s, Boston surgeons made interposition with Vitallium the accepted method. Coincident with the development of Sir John Charnley's total hip arthroplasty, several surgeons continued work on interposition and resurfacing technology even when the majority embraced Charnley's techniques. Harlan Amstutz, for example, developed the THARIES (total hip acetabular replacement) technique combining elements of resurfacing with replacement.[17] This approach consisted of rounding off the femoral head with cylindrical reamers and chamfering the resultant cylindrical bone to permit application of a fitted cap cemented to the bony peg. A thin cup of high-density polyethylene on the acetabular side of the joint, also cemented with methylmethacrylate, completed the construct. The reports of early good results of the THARIES technique generated considerable enthusiasm, but these outcomes deteriorated markedly with time due to loosening and breakage of the components, osteonecrosis of what was left of the femoral head, and femoral neck fractures. Amstutz essentially abandoned the procedure. Numerous other surgeons worked on this problem, all more or less achieving the same unsatisfactory results. There is, however, a resurgence of interest in resurfacing in the hip. The key difference between the original THARIES hip technique and what is now proposed is the use of a thin metal acetabulum rather than one of thick polyethylene. The articulation is metal on metal to minimize the generation of wear particles in the joint, and the metal's thinness allows for minimal resection of bone from both the acetabulum and the femoral head.

Orthopaedists' interest in interposition arthroplasty did not end with the hip, of course. Throughout the mid-20th century, joint surgeons also attempted to place various tissues and materials between the tibia and femur as well as between the patella and femur to improve the results of débridement and synovectomy of the knee. Willis Campbell expounded on the subject at the prestigious Sir Robert Jones Lecture delivered at the Hospital for Joint Diseases in New York in 1930. Campbell described a group of his patients who underwent the operation and compared them with another group in whom "spontaneous arthroplasty" occurred. The surgical arthroplasties consisted mostly of débridements of severely arthritic knees, with interposition of fascia lata between the eroding joint surfaces. The "spontaneous arthroplasties" occurred in patients whose arthritic ankylosed joints improved spontaneously "through functional adaptation," that is, aggressive joint motion by the patient. Campbell biopsied all these joints, reporting that grossly and histologically they all looked about the same. All had dense fibrocartilaginous tissue on the bone ends and a fibrous tissue membrane lining the joint cavity. The joint also contained what looked like normal joint fluid. Campbell remarked that pseudarthrosis of long bone fractures had the same appearance.

In 1940, Campbell published a paper entitled "Interposition of Vitallium Plates in Arthroplasties of the Knee" in the *American Journal of Surgery*,[18] mentioning fascial interposition as "one of several important steps in the operative technique." He also alluded to previous failures of interposition arthroplasty in the knee using gold or silver foil, which he asserted led to their abandonment 50 years ago. He then cited Smith-Petersen's success with the new alloy Vitallium developed by the Austenal Corporation and used by Venable and Stuck. Campbell adapted it to the knee by developing a Vitallium plate that extended from the anterior surface of the distal femur, curving around the condyles of the femur posteriorly. Two flanges hooked into the back of the femoral condyles, and an anterior Vitallium screw secured the upper part of the plate to the distal shaft of the femur. Campbell reported that the patients did not achieve the range of motion he had hoped for. He noted further that fascial arthroplasty yielded such good outcomes that he was not ready to discard it for the Vitallium interposition.

Other orthopaedic surgeons also experimented with cellophane and nylon membranous materials for interposition in knee arthroplasty. Using nylon as an interposition material, John G. Kuhns,[19] at the Robert B. Brigham Hospital in Boston, found that 58 of the 70 knees he operated on had "good results" and 12 had "unsatisfactory results." Kuhns' operation consisted of a thorough joint débridement as described by Magnuson, followed by wrapping the entire distal end of the femur with a thick nylon membrane. He secured the membrane in position by stapling it with thin stainless steel staples.

Duncan McKeever[20] of Houston, Texas, used a cellophane membrane instead of nylon, but he did not cover the entire distal femur with it. His goal was simply to prevent arthrofibrosis from occurring after a joint débridement, in which case the quadriceps tendon and the rest of the extensor mechanism would scar down on the front of the distal femur. This had happened to several of his patients after he had performed synovectomies and débridements of their knees.

In 1956, Joseph Brown, W. H. McGaw, and Darrell Shaw of St. Luke's Hospital in Cleveland presented a paper at the American Academy of Orthopaedic Surgeons Annual Meeting entitled "Use of Cutis as an Interposing Membrane in Arthroplasty of the Knee." In their introduction, they remarked on "the fantastic foreign bodies" being used for interposition arthroplasty (Vitallium, rubber, nylon, cellophane, and chromacized pig bladder). They believed that an autogenous substance used as an interposing membrane would better serve the patient, citing prior use of this technique dating back to 1913. The technique of Brown and his associates consisted of harvesting a large full-thickness skin graft, splitting it so that the epidermis could be sutured down over the skin defect as a partial-thickness graft. The dermis and subcutaneous fat that remained served as interpositional material. They covered the anterior surface of the distal femur and the weight bearing surface of the femoral condyles with it, folding the remainder to cover the weight bearing surface of the tibia. The radiographs of the four patients undergoing this operation showed that this type of surgery was ineffective.

In the heyday of cup arthroplasty for hip arthritis, Smith-Petersen and his associates determined to extend the principles of that interposition technique to the knee. William Jones documented Smith-Petersen's experience with this technique in a 1969 *Clinical Orthopaedics and Related Research* commemorative issue.[21] Jones reported that Smith-Petersen had devised a "flat, cup-like mold" made of Vitallium, with fins that extended up into the intercondylar notch of the femur and down into the area between the medial and lateral tibial articulating surfaces. He hoped that this device would serve as a "free-moving mold." The operation did not work; it took almost 3 hours, and the patient lost a lot of blood. The knee remained stiff and painful. Smith-Petersen performed the first two of these operations in 1942 and delayed doing another for 8 years. The first mold covered only the area of the distal femur that would have borne weight when the knee was fully extended. The second mold nearly covered the distal femur, from the trochlear groove to the upper part of the posterior femoral condyles. It had no fins to stabilize it; Smith-Petersen intended it to move relatively freely in the knee joint. When the mold failed in practice, Smith-Petersen and his associate (Jones) mounted a 4 1/2-inch Smith-Petersen nail on it to provide at least some intramedullary fixation. Smith-Petersen, Jones, Aufranc, Morton Smith-Petersen (Smith-Petersen's son), and others participated in modifying the "MGH [Massachusetts General Hospital] femoral condylar mold" arthroplasty, using such improvements as a longer, stronger intramedullary stem, valgus alignment of the mold relative to the stem to provide for the normal mechanical axis of weight bearing, and modifications in the contours of the medial and lateral sides of the mold. In his paper describing the development of the MGH mold, however, Jones noted that in actual clinical use, "the results were far from good." Other orthopaedic surgeons in different parts of the country also pursued the goal of a functional femoral mold. Austin Moore and Emmet Lunceford in Georgia devised a femoral condylar mold fixed to the distal femur with "multiple small stems," and Dana Street of Memphis tried an "acrylic replacement prosthesis." In 1974, five years after William Jones had described the MGH efforts to devise a workable femoral condylar mold, David Murray and Salvatore Barranco[22] described their experience using this kind of interpositional device in 59 patients. They used a long U-shaped incision and reflected the tibial tubercle to gain access to the knee. They reshaped the femoral condyles to accept the Vitallium mold. Murray and Barranco did rather well in their application of the MGH femoral condylar mold to knee arthritis. They had 51 good-to-excellent results in their 59 patients and suggested that the operation might have some utility even in the age of total knee arthroplasty. They concluded, however, that "the indications for hemiarthroplasty in any joint have been gradually reduced to the vanishing point."

While interposition arthroplasty with femoral condylar molds went through its painful evolutionary stages, other orthopaedic surgeons attempted interpositions elsewhere in the knee. Duncan McKeever, one of the most innovative of these surgeons, invented patellar and tibial plateau resurfacing devices.[23] McKeever's tibial plateau operation entailed cleaning out and débridement of the arthritic knee and placement of a concave vitallium implant fitted as accurately as possible into a defect chiseled into the joint surface. Two vitallium fins protruded from the flat underside of the implant to provide stability and prevent undue rocking or rotation of the device in the cancellous bone of the upper tibia.[24] Theoretically, the femoral condyle would conform to the concavity of the tibial prosthesis throughout the arc of knee motion. McKeever's patellar prosthesis consisted of a V-shaped Vitallium cap which covered an arthritic patella. A transverse screw locked the device onto the patella. MacIntosh's tibial plateau prosthesis[25] had a roughened underside instead of fins for fixation of the tibial plateau prosthesis. MacIntosh's prosthesis required the surgeon to create a space in the articulating surface of the tibia for implantation of the device. Both the McKeever and MacIntosh tibial plateau resurfacing operations demanded exacting technique to prevent the devices from dislodging. Furthermore, significant angular deformity of the knee, stiffness, laxity of the collateral ligaments, muscle weakness, prior sepsis, subchondral cysts, and "poor patient motivation" all specifically contraindicated these operations. As expected, tibial plateau prostheses yielded fair results: 47 percent to 68 percent satisfactory in the various authors' series in patients with rheumatoid arthritis and 80 percent to 89 percent satisfactory in patients with osteoarthritis.[24,25]

More recently, there has been renewed interest in patellofemoral arthroplasty, as practiced by McKeever and others. Some patients with anterior knee pain have degenerative arthritic changes limited to the patellofemoral joint with no significant changes in the articulations between the femoral condyles and the tibial plateaus. When both the patellar and trochlear sides of the patellofemoral articulation are involved, resurfacing of both surfaces might offer significant relief.

Patellofemoral arthroplasty has an almost 30-year history. In 1979, Martin Blazina, who practiced in Los Angeles, and his associates reported the results of patellofemoral replacements in 85 patients.[26] Their procedure consisted of resurfacing the trochlear groove with a Vitallium plate on the femoral side. A high-density polyethylene button resurfaced the patella.

In the last decade, several surgeons revisited the subject and are now reporting on procedures of this type done in hundreds of patients. The patellofemoral devices in use now all have very similar appearances. Although large forces act on these implants, loosening and breakage occur infrequently and the results appear to justify the procedure in the short term. Alan Merchant of Stanford and Wayne Leadbetter of Rockville, Maryland, served as guest editors for a 2005 symposium on the subject published in *Clinical Orthopaedics and Related Research*. Despite the vast number of papers, books, and presentations related to total knee arthroplasty, a relatively small number of orthopaedic surgeons seem to have created a niche for a procedure that until recently was thought to be only of historical significance.

Hemiarthroplasty of the Hip

Fusions, débridements, synovectomies, osteotomies, resurfacings, and interposition arthroplasties had limitations that led to the development of hemiarthroplasty, the removal and replacement of the ball of the ball-and-socket joint with a prosthesis. Jean and Robert Judet,[27] Parisian orthopaedists, invented one of the first of these devices (Figure 24). In 1945, the Judets used femoral heads sculpted out of a block of acrylic, polished to a high finish. They mounted the acrylic heads onto a short stem that they impacted into the femoral neck from above after removal of the femoral head. The Judet prosthesis looked somewhat like a lightbulb with its round head and short stem. The acrylic femoral heads initially yielded excellent results, but they quickly broke or loosened and had to be removed. The Judets switched to Vitallium, hoping for better outcomes, but the concept of the short stem in the femoral neck was flawed and had to be abandoned. Charles O. Townley[28] devised a femoral head replacement that extended the Judet stem for a short distance down the medullary canal of the femur, but again, despite early success, this device proved inferior to later models. Harold Bohlman and Austin Moore[29] of Johns Hopkins University School of Medicine in Baltimore, Maryland, devised the technique for femoral head replacement that has survived the test of time (Figure 25). Their device consisted of a femoral head mounted on a long intramedullary stem. They inserted it into the femoral neck, but the shape of the stem made it possible for them to anchor it well down the femoral canal. Their design incorporated the feature of stem fenestration so that bone could grow into the prosthesis, fixing it even more solidly into the femoral canal. The device, which came to be known as the Austin Moore prosthesis, has since been extensively modified by numerous inventive orthopaedic surgeons, but the basic design has remained intact.

Moore and Bohlman published their first paper on hemiarthroplasty in the *JBJS* in 1943,[29] presenting a patient with a pathologic fracture through a giant cell tumor of the proximal femur. They fabricated a prosthesis with the intention of replacing the entire upper femur upon resection. "Calculations were made from roentgenograms of the bone, wax models were fashioned, and from these a mold was made, and a Vitallium mold of the upper end of the femur was finally produced." They made the distal part of the prosthesis hollow and in the shape of a pipe; this enabled them to slip it over the distal femur and engage it solidly enough to permit early weight bearing. Unfortunately, they underestimated the diameter of the bone, and the prosthesis would not fit. The bone then had to be reduced in size, and the outer cortex was "chiseled away." They found that "this was a serious mistake." However, despite an infection of the wound and an extrusion of a sequestrum, the surgical site finally healed and a heavy involucrum formed over the prosthesis. This rendered the limb stable, and the patient could walk bearing full weight and virtually no pain 2½ years later. At that time, the patient had an acute fatal myocardial infarction. Moore and Bohlman removed the prosthesis at autopsy. They found that the Vitallium was "unaffected by its period of service in the body. It was just as bright and shiny as the day it was inserted, and at no point was there any evidence of corrosion."

The editors of *JBJS* included an interesting footnote at the bottom of the first page of the Moore-Bohlman article. They wrote: "This case was presented to the Columbia Medical Society of Richland County, South Carolina, December 14, 1942, and has been reported in *The Recorder* of the Columbia Medical Society, VI, 12, December 1942. It is contrary to the policy of *The Journal* to reprint material, but, since this publication is not available to many readers of *The Journal*, an exception has been made in this case."

Harold Bohlman's interest in Vitallium femoral prostheses predated his collaboration with Austin Moore. He made femoral head replacements out of Vitallium and buried them in his garden along with prostheses fabricated out of other materials and metals. Bohlman found that even after prolonged periods, the Vitallium had not corroded, so he used these devices clinically with considerable success. Despite the technical difficulties noted in his paper written with Austin Moore, he proved the utility of a new kind of artificial hip implant and essentially created the concept of the hemiarthroplasty. It caught on quickly, and other orthopaedic surgeons began to use it in large numbers.

Austin Moore, Bohlman's partner in performing the first reported upper femoral prosthesis operation, developed his own modifications of technique and design. Because he found that the anterior Smith-Petersen approach to the hip had proved difficult, he developed a modification of the Gibson[30] posterior approach to facilitate the insertion of the Austin Moore prosthesis. Gibson had described a long posterior incision, which included removing the attachments of the gluteal tendons to the greater trochanter. It provided more exposure than necessary, however, and left the patient with weak abductors, even if the surgeon repaired them properly. Moore's surgical approach, which he termed "the southern exposure," came into the hip joint much lower than Gibson's incision and left the abductor muscles intact. It also was shorter and involved much less dissection and tissue injury. Moore's first prosthesis had a slightly curved, solid stem that fit down the canal of the femoral shaft. With time, he increased the curve of the stem and fenestrated it for a bone ingrowth for better fixation. Moore also devised techniques for reaming and broaching the upper femur that still serve as the basis for methods now in wide use. In 1957, he published a definitive paper on his developments and use of the Austin Moore prosthesis. He employed it mostly for patients with acute fractures of the femoral neck but also used it in the treatment of more than 30 patients with osteonecrosis or arthritis. The usual set of complications accompanied this series of 159 operations, such as acute infections, but only two dislocations of the prosthesis occurred postoperatively. Moore also noted that in a few patients, the prosthesis loosened after a few years or settled within the femoral shaft.

American orthopaedic surgeons became intensely interested in femoral head replacement using Moore's prosthesis and others designed along the same lines. Frederick R. Thompson,[31] for example, created a femoral head prosthesis with a somewhat longer neck and a solid curved stem, which also came into wide use at about the same time. The topic became so important that the American Academy of Orthopaedic Surgeons (AAOS) organized a Committee on Scientific Investigation[32] to study preferred prostheses and methods. In the summer of 1952, the committee sent a questionnaire to all AAOS members, asking, "Are you now using femoral head prostheses? Yes or No? If so, what kind?" (Choices included Judet, Eicher, Moore, Thompson, Naden-Rieth, Collison, Judet acrylic, Judet stainless steel, and other types, totaling 37 [Figure 26].) The questionnaire also asked what members thought about indications, surgical approach, contraindications, and complications. It did not ask for results, stating: "We feel it is far too early to ask for results."

The committee concluded in part that (1) too many prostheses were being used, (2) the trend was toward abandonment of the Judet prosthesis made of acrylic, and (3) there was increased use of intramedullary types.

They also noted that the Gibson approach was the most popular, and that complications were in excess of what was acceptable.

In discussing the issue of complications, the committee stated: "The complications listed in this preliminary survey have been appalling and if a procedure cannot be done with fewer complications . . . something is wrong."

The report went on to recommend that the survey "should be correlated with the Committee on Instruments and Gadgets," noting that AAOS members probably had first seen these prostheses in the "gadget exhibit" at the Annual Meeting. Finally, the Committee on Scientific Investigation concluded: "The promiscuous use of this device should be curtailed, and we should discipline the manufacturers and salesmen until better evaluation has been made." Because that was difficult to do, members agreed—off the record—that orthopaedic surgeons should discipline themselves.

Two years later, AAOS revisited the matter. Serving as members of the Committee for the Study of Femoral Head Replacement Prostheses were Claude Lambert, Chairman, Lee Ramsey Straub, and Donald King.[33] Lambert and King had served on the Committee for Scientific Investigation two years earlier. Lambert, Straub, and King disclosed that despite the caveats of the 1952 investigation, the membership had implanted 8,354 femoral head prostheses since then. Per the 1952 report, the entire academy membership had up to that time performed only about 6,000 of these procedures. Clearly, then, femoral head replacement with a prosthesis had become a very profitable and successful operation. Numerous orthopaedic inventors and innovators modified the earlier designs, but the membership indicated that it used the Austin Moore or Frederick Thompson models more than any other.

Several members of the Academy rose in dissent at the meeting during which the committee presented its findings. Carl Badgley of Ann Arbor, Michigan, objected strenuously to replacing the femoral head with a metal ball, stating: "Metal replacement introduces a new, and to me, a frightening period of experimental surgery. One must call it a 'mechanistic period,' certainly it is not biological." He much preferred a cup arthroplasty for osteoarthritis because the cup served as "an intervening material . . . molding the joint surfaces so as to adapt them to the transmission of stresses."

Philip D. Wilson of New York also voiced objections to femoral head replacement in principle. He said: "It involves a new and as yet unproved principle—that of substituting the metallic or plastic counterpart for a portion of the skeleton and fixing it in place." Nevertheless, Wilson could report on 150 patients who had been given femoral head prostheses at his hospital over the previous four years. A third of these had done very poorly because they had received acrylic Judet femoral heads with very short stems. Thereafter, the Hospital for Special Surgery used mostly Vitallium prostheses with short-stem fixation. Mark Coventry of the Mayo Clinic reported that at his institution the staff had abandoned the Judet prosthesis made of either acrylic or Vitallium. The surgeons there adopted instead "the intramedullary type developed by A. T. Moore," which has "proved a valuable adjunct to restoration of hip function."

Within ten years of this meeting, the use of Austin Moore and Frederick Thompson prostheses had become routine among American orthopaedic surgeons. They had identified the best indications, surgical approaches for varying hip abnormalities, rehabilitation protocols, surgical tricks, how to avoid complications, and what to do for complications. This set the stage for the total joint revolution.

Total Hip Arthroplasty

Total hip arthroplasty (THA) is one of the major achievements of modern orthopaedic surgery. Thousands of patients with osteoarthritis who would have had disabling hip pain without effective treatment can now expect excellent prolonged relief because of this operation.

In past years, many patients with hip pain had rheumatoid arthritis, but the medical treatment of this disease has improved greatly and fewer patients with rheumatoid arthritis now have hip pain severe enough to require replacement surgery. Rheumatologists have developed therapeutic interventions with drugs such as methotrexate, gold salts, imuran, cytoxin, cyclosporin, plaquenil, penicillamine, and sulfasalazine, which can modify rheumatoid arthritis effectively. These so-called disease-modifying antirheumatic drugs (DMARDs) in conjunction with nonsteroidal anti-inflammatory drugs (NSAIDs), and even the judicious limited use of steroids, have decreased the numbers of patients needing hip replacements for rheumatoid arthritis.

Osteonecrosis of the femoral head resulting from alcoholism, steroid use, sickle cell disease, fractures, or other diseases or injuries can cause death of bone tissue within the femoral head and collapse of the ball of the ball-and-socket joint in numerous patients. Surgical treatment of osteonecrosis with drilling and decompression of the femoral head or with free vascularized fibular grafting has the potential for revascularization of the head, thus preventing its collapse. Many patients, however, present with an advanced stage of femoral head deformity, making a good outcome from this type of surgery unlikely. These individuals and those whose drilling or grafting have failed usually require hip replacement.

The simplicity of the human ball-and-socket joint belies the difficulty of replacing it. The surgeons who devised the first successful total hip implants in the 1960s and early 1970s had to confront three major issues. First, they had to develop a basic design for the THA implant. Second, they had to replicate as nearly as possible the weight-bearing surfaces in a way that would result in minimal friction and wear. Third, they had to solve the problem of loosening.

The experiences of orthopaedists with hemiarthroplasties during the 1950s and 1960s established the fact that a femoral head prosthesis works best with a long stem inserted well down the medullary canal of the femur. The Moore and Thompson prostheses proved more stable and successful than the Judet prosthesis and its variants in which the lightbulb-shaped femoral head sits precariously on the femoral neck, secured only by a short stem inserted into the femoral neck. These were easy to insert, but the devices broke or loosened and failed too often for surgeons to continue their use. Intramedullary fixation required broaching and reaming, more blood loss, more time under anesthesia, and more loss of bone stock, but the stable surgical construct produced superior outcomes.

The first THA was probably done by Themistocles Gluck (1853–1942)[34] in the late 1800s. He used an ivory ball-and-socket prosthesis fixed with nickel-plated screws and secured in some cases with a mixture of plaster of Paris, powdered pumice, and resin. His results were poor, forcing him to give up. Philip Wiles,[35] a renowned British orthopaedist, devised a femoral head prosthesis consisting of a stainless steel ball mounted on a short stem that traversed the entire length of the femoral neck. The stem was anchored in the lateral cortex of the upper femur and had to be long enough to pass through the cortex into a lateral plate, which Wiles bolted to the femoral shaft. Wiles intended that the stem of the prosthesis could slide in the plate, if or when the femoral neck resorbed. He inserted eight of these into patients who also received a prosthetic acetabulum made from stainless steel, but he had poor outcomes. "The results could be regarded as tolerably satisfactory in 2 patients only." He abandoned the procedure.

The shape of the native acetabulum accommodates the nearly spherical femoral head well. It would appear that the creation of a design to replace it would be easy. Indeed, all of the early acetabular prostheses had a cup-shaped socket, which could be made to fit over the femoral head, but securing the artificial socket into the real one led to a variety of configurations. Peter Ring,[36] for example, invented a stainless steel cup with a long, heavy threaded bolt mounted on the apex of the cup. Its proper insertion into the iliac portion of the hemipelvis required extensive dissection inside as well as outside the pelvis to ensure correct alignment. Other designs featured barbed spikes for pelvic fixation or short pins to prevent rotation; others featured metal flanges designed to engage acetabular bone in the depths of the socket.

Several surgeons looked for ways to anchor prostheses or other implants into bone using glue, adhesive, or cement. Edward Haboush of the Hospital for Joint Diseases in New York first used methylmethacrylate for this purpose; he described his results in a lengthy paper published in 1953.[37] Haboush devised a true total hip with a femoral head replacement and a prosthetic acetabular cup. He experimented with several designs and settled on a proximal femoral replacement that consisted of a Vitallium head on a narrow curved stem passing down the medullary canal of the femur. He secured the stem in the femoral canal with polymethylmethacrylate, which he mixed and prepared on the operating table. He reported that "the liquid monomer is sterilized under vacuum by passing through a sterile Burkfeld filter. The powdered polymer is sterilized by fractional sterilization." He pushed the methacrylate down the canal just before the insertion of the prosthesis and allowed it to set, holding the prosthesis in proper alignment while the cement hardened. Haboush designed a femoral head replacement that differed markedly from the Judet or Thompson/Moore replacements. He recontoured the femoral head and neck into the shape of a truncated cone on which he mounted a femoral head, the inside of which was shaped to fit closely over the reshaped femoral head and neck. He also extended a Vitallium "cloak" down from the rim of the prosthetic head. This encased the femoral neck as far distally as the intertrochanteric line. Haboush's femoral head prosthesis looked like a helmet and cuirass portion of a medieval suit of armor. Haboush also cemented a thin acetabular Vitallium shell into the socket as part of his operation. In the conclusion of his paper, he wrote: "The use of fast-setting dental acrylate, relatively non-toxic, is introduced in this paper. This may open a new avenue in definitive orthopaedic surgery."

Haboush performed this operation on four patients. He emphasized that the facing surfaces of the femoral and acetabular components should conform to the same level of precision used in the manufacture of ball bearings and that the surgeon should use methylmethacrylate to rigidly fix the components onto the osseous portions of the hip joint. Despite his scientific approach to replacing painful hips, he had questionable results—one dislocation, one patient with acetabular erosion and an early protrusio, and one patient with profound intraoperative bleeding and shock. Only one patient had an uncomplicated and successful recovery from surgery. Haboush appears to have been the first orthopaedist to report on the use of methylmethacrylate in the fixation of the components of the total hip prosthesis and one of the first to consider the physics of wear, lubrication, and motion. The design flaws of Haboush's prosthesis precluded wide use of his devices, and other orthopaedic surgeons had to come forward with better ideas and better outcomes. Chief among these was Sir John Charnley (Figure 27), who considered the issue of THA during the 1950s and 1960s at the Wrightington Hospital in Wigan, near Manchester, England.

In the mid-1950s, Charnley experimented with Haboush's design. He described how he reshaped the upper femur to make it look like a spigot and how he capped this with a cup-shaped device designed to fix snugly on the spigot, which was all that remained of the femoral neck. He reported that this design failed because it removed the blood supply to the femoral head and upper neck and resulted in osteonecrosis and fracture. Charnley published a paper in the British volume of *JBJS* in 1960,[38] reiterating what Haboush discovered, namely that methylmethacrylate cement can anchor a femoral head prosthesis solidly onto the upper femur. Charnley made reference to "amine-cured ethoxyline resin as reported by Bloch (1958)." Bloch suggested that the resin adhered directly to bone and that bone would grow into it with the passing of time. Charnley noted, however, that methylmethacrylate cement functioned only as a "grouting agent," which would function as part of a prosthesis to extend the contact of the prosthesis into the interstices of cancellous bone throughout the entire upper part of the femur. Charnley stated that the physical properties of the cement did not really matter and that "the strength of the material is not the most important feature." As a grouting agent, all it needed to do was resist compression; Charnley suggested that plaster of Paris would have done as well. In his 1960 *JBJS* article, Charnley reported that he used this method of fixation in 29 patients successfully, "and the general quality of the results appear superior to that in cases in which the plastic anchorage had not been used."

G. K. McKee and J. Watson-Farrar[39] of Norwich, England reported on their experience with cement fixation in 1966. They devised a Vitallium acetabular prosthesis with a straightforward dome-like configuration. They studded the outer surfaces of the cup with small metal projections. McKee and Watson-Farrar implanted this device into an acetabulum that they reamed to conform to the cup size required by the patient's anatomy, then cemented in a Thompson femoral head prosthesis that fit the cup precisely.

Thus, by the mid-1960s, British orthopaedists hit upon the basic design of a successful total hip implant. The designs differed in several important ways, but they were the same in relying on an intramedullary femoral component solidly anchored in the femoral shaft and a well-aligned acetabular component rigidly contained and cemented within the socket. The differences between the two designs, however, are important and of considerable interest with regard to the third important consideration in THA, mainly the weight-bearing surface (Figure 28).

McKee and Watson-Farrar's design consisted of a large femoral head that articulated with an acetabular component of essentially the same size, machined to fit perfectly. Both the ball and the socket were made of Vitallium. McKee and Watson-Farrar stated that the metal-on-metal design using hard, highly polished and perfectly matching components would not wear out over a patient's lifetime and that wear particles would not cause trouble. They also noted that the large diameter of the femoral head would provide a much larger surface for weight bearing, a design element that would lessen wear even more. The large head also would make the hip more stable.

Charnley had a different approach. After he abandoned the spigot-trunion configuration and adopted cemented fixation and the basic intramedullary femoral component, he worked toward developing a new kind of prosthetic acetabulum. Charnley's early efforts centered around the fabrication of a prosthesis made of polytetrafluorethylene, also known as Teflon. This material appealed to him because it had a very smooth, slippery surface that would provide good boundary lubrication between the metal of the femoral head and the Teflon of the socket. He began to use Teflon acetabular prostheses in 1958 with (in his words) "spectacular early results." Teflon had poor resistance to wear, however, and led to "disastrous complications." McKee and Watson-Farrar[40] also used the word "disastrous" to describe poor results with Teflon, adding a remark about how Teflon wear particles could "wreck a good hip." They used Charnley's experience as justification for their support of a metal-on-metal surgical construct. Charnley, however, sought to understand why Teflon failed so quickly (two or three years after implantation). He found that the large wear particles of Teflon (up to 300 um in size) led to the development of large granulomatous masses. He thus needed to find material that would wear more slowly and generate much smaller wear particles. By 1962, Charnley decided on ultra-high molecular weight polyethylene (UHMWPE) as the best alternative to Teflon. During this time of experimentation, he developed to a high level the science of tribology as applied to hip prostheses. Tribology, the science of the mechanisms of friction, lubrication, and wear of interacting surfaces in relative motion, led him to perform multiple experiments analyzing hip joint motion, as reported in his 1979 book on low-friction arthroplasty.[41] He also noted in his 1961 paper in *Lancet* that up to that time, only he and E. S. Jones—nearly 30 years previously—had concerned themselves with the coefficient of friction in normal animal joints and how joint surfaces are lubricated. He described how arthroplasties such as the Smith-Petersen cup, Judet acrylic femoral head, and the various American Vitallium models often squeak during motion, and offered theories to explain this phenomenon. Basically, he thought that the resistance that developed between the surfaces moving against each other grew so great that the surfaces seized together to produce the audible squeaking sound. He found that metal on Teflon had a coefficient of friction that came close to that of normal cartilage, and he decided that the boundary lubrication mechanism also operated when these two materials moved on each other as in a normal joint. The synovial fluid does not act as a lubricant but is "rather a product of the activity of joints." When Teflon failed so badly and Charnley moved on to UHMWPE for replacing the acetabular side of the joint, he found that the coefficient of friction between UHMWPE and metal rose fivefold. He expressed concern that this would lead to excessive wear, but he believed that his concept of a low-friction arthroplasty obviated those worries.

By the time Charnley completed this work, he had enlisted the support of the Manchester Regional Hospital Board in the development of laboratories and a research workshop where "a fitter and turner" made the implants. He also established productive working relationships with the Manchester University Department of Engineering, and with the support of the Regional Hospital Board he established the Center for the Surgery of the Hip Joint at Wrightington Hospital in Wigan, England. His application of engineering principles and materials research resulted in good surgical outcomes in those early years. Patients came to him for evaluation and treatment of their painful hip joints in increasing numbers. To minimize risk of surgical infections, he devised filtration systems to ensure clean air in operating rooms and developed "body exhaust" techniques in which surgeons wore impervious gowns with a headpiece that covered the entire head and neck. Clean room air and body exhaust systems greatly reduced, and often eliminated, the amount of bacteria that could colonize the incisions used for the prosthesis implantation. This lowered the chances of infection postoperatively to 0.05 percent or less. Charnley also devised rigidly standardized techniques for performing the surgery and controlling all stages of surgical care. In his 1979 book,[41] he discussed intraoperative antibiotics, control of postoperative thromboembolic phenomena, and the postoperative rehabilitation methods that he employed.

By the late 1960s, Charnley was performing a tremendous number of hip replacements under these improved conditions.[42] Orthopaedic surgeons from around the world flocked to the Wrightington Hospital in the small town of Wigan to observe his techniques. In 1968, Frank Stinchfield, then chairman of the Department of Orthopaedic Surgery at Columbia University in New York, visited Charnley. Stinchfield was enormously impressed. Shortly after he returned home, he gathered a small group of hip surgeons, suggesting they convene an organization to be called The Hip Society.[43] Stinchfield's infectious enthusiasm and the intense interest of these American leaders in orthopaedic surgery (along with public interest in Charnley's achievements) swept the rest of their surgical colleagues into the total hip revolution. Many American orthopaedic surgeons visited Charnley, and those who did before 1970 came back to perform cemented hip replacements on large numbers of eager patients. In 1971, however, the FDA determined that it had not certified methylmethacrylate as a safe material for use in the human body. It further determined that those orthopaedic surgeons who used it before 1970 could continue to do so, but all others would have to wait until its safety had been investigated more thoroughly. It took the FDA 3 years to decide that polymethylmethacrylate (PMMA) was indeed safe and that all orthopaedic surgeons could use it legally in hip implantations. Those who visited Wigan before 1970 and started using PMMA before that year often developed very large joint arthroplasty practices, at the expense of those who had delayed doing so.

John Charnley was a pivotal figure in modern orthopaedics. He had what appeared to be limitless energy and determination. He generated a steady flow of new ideas and devised a way to pursue them. Charnley was born in Bury, England, in 1911 and was educated at Manchester University. After his army service in the Middle East in World War II, he returned to Manchester, where with the help and guidance of his mentor, Sir Harry Platt, he embarked on his remarkable career. Commander of the British Empire, Knight Bachelor, Fellow of the Royal Society, and winner of the Lister Medal, Sir John Charnley died in 1982.[44]

Charnley's career peaked in the mid-1970s, and he dominated the way orthopaedic surgeons thought about hip replacement surgery in those days. With the passing of time, several issues arose that somewhat dampened the enthusiasm for his methods. For example, polyethylene wear, osteolysis, and loosening became increasingly evident in patients treated with cemented metal-on-polyethylene components. In addition, patients who had had dramatic relief from hip pain either suddenly or gradually experienced a recurrence that sometimes brought worse discomfort. American surgeons who performed large numbers of Charnley or Charnley-Müller (a close copy) total hip replacements found themselves increasingly involved with equally large numbers of difficult revision operations with potentially uncertain and unpredictable outcomes. As a result, surgeons searched for new ways to anchor implants into bone, beginning with the implantation of total hip components with weight bearing surfaces that differed from Charnley's. The acetabular cup, for example, now has a new structure consisting of metal backing of the polyethylene weight bearing surface, and Charnley's original all-polyethylene cup has largely disappeared, at least in the United States. Materials experts have proposed new kinds of polyethylene such as highly cross-linked or carbon-fiber reinforced. The latter, however, demonstrated excessive wear and has been abandoned.[45] Surgeons also have tried a bewildering array of prosthesis shapes and configurations. The surfaces of the components matter more now. Surgeons and manufacturers have developed roughened surfaces into which bone grows, depending on the pore size of the surface. Prosthetic surfaces might have a wire mesh, plasma-sprayed, or sintered coating. Scores of orthopaedists have presented thousands of papers at meetings large and small, and the major journals and, minor journals have included hundreds (if not thousands) of papers on modifications of the original design.

The Hip Society

The education of American orthopaedic surgeons in the new science of THA evolved rapidly after Stinchfield returned from his 1968 meeting with John Charnley. The Hip Society, a small group with restricted membership founded in 1968, convenes two meetings a year—one closed, and one open meeting on Specialty Day at the AAOS Annual Meeting. The AAOS also devotes a significant time at its Annual Meeting to subjects related to THA. In 1985, David Hungerford of Johns Hopkins, started a new journal called the the *Journal of Arthoplasty*. Lawrence Dorr of the University of California at Irvine, Jorge Galante of Rush University in Chicago, Dennis Lennox of Johns Hopkins, Chitranjan Ranawat of Cornell, and Richard Scott of Harvard were the members of Hungerford's original editorial advisory board. In the mid-1990s, Hungerford relinquished his position as editor-in-chief at the journal, to be replaced by Richard Rothman. In 1995, the *Journal of Arthroplasty* became the official journal of the American Association of Hip and Knee Surgeons (AAHKS). AAHKS[46] was founded in 1991 by members of The Hip Society and The Knee Society. The intention was to create a large organization that would serve the research and educational needs of numerous orthopaedists in a way that the other small and rather exclusive societies could not.

The Hip Society has published papers presented at its meetings annually in a special issue of *Clinical Orthopaedics and Related Research*. The multiple organizations and journals interested in total joint arthroplasty have led to a virtual avalanche of information, and hip surgeons have explored almost every conceivable aspect of it. In a "specialty update" published in *JBJS* in 2005, Michael Huo and Nathan Bilbert observed that between April 2004 and April 2005, THA was the subject of 55 articles in *JBJS* (American volume), 140 in the *Journal of Arthroplasty*, and 68 in *Clinical Orthopaedics and Related Research*. These 263 peer-reviewed articles represent thousands of hours invested by several hundred authors and reviewers.[47-52]

Revision THA has developed into a modern orthopaedic specialty. Most of these operations are necessary because of osteolysis related to dissemination of polyethylene wear particles throughout the hip joint or possibly to mechanical causes related to the interfacial environment.

Total hip arthroplasty is rapidly evolving; one wonders where Sir John Charnley's operation has taken orthopaedic surgery. Quantifying the results of this surgery has proved to be difficult but necessary.[53-56] "Walks with perfect freedom" and "excellent outcome," terms used in the past, are unacceptable today. Orthopaedic surgeons have had to devise hip scoring systems to give numeric credibility to the results of their efforts.

Total Knee Arthroplasty

Until the 1960s, patients with osteoarthritic or rheumatoid arthritis of the knee who could not achieve sufficient pain relief with medical treatment had four options. If pain and deformity were severe enough, they could undergo knee fusion. Otherwise, they could select a surgical cleaning out (débridement) of the knee or, if the arthritis was limited to only one compartment, an osteotomy to realign the joint. More recently, they could select an interposition or resurfacing procedure in which metal, plastic, or biologic implants are placed between the joint surfaces.

The surgeons who performed these operations claimed some success. Fusions gave good pain relief and stability but at the cost of severe functional impairment. Realignment with an osteotomy had limited application and could be used only if the arthritis was limited to one compartment. Furthermore, the beneficial effect usually lasted for only a few years. Débridement and synovectomies had poor results overall; many surgeons avoided them because of the likelihood that symptoms would recur after the operation. The same held true for interposition procedures, including the MGH condylar mold (Figure 29) and the various designs of patellar prostheses and tibial plateau prostheses.

In the 1950s and 1960s, orthopaedic surgeons in Europe and the United States explored more aggressive approaches to surgery for the arthritic knee, using prostheses to replace the joint. The early models were fixed hinges. Majnoni d'Intignano, for example, devised a hinge made of acrylic in the late 1940s and reported on it in 1950.[57] The device failed, and he used it only once. Börje Walldius[58,59] of the Karolinska Institute expressed hope in 1953 that he could build on the record of the Judet acrylic hip prosthesis (more than 300 done at the Karolinska Institute with good results at that time) and make an acrylic hinge joint for the knee. His prosthesis had a "femoral part and tibial part joined together by a stainless steel transverse axle." He tested this device through repetitions equivalent to walking continuously for 273 miles bearing almost 200 pounds of weight. He used it on eight patients between 1951 and 1953. All had been "total invalids" preoperatively, who had "everything to gain and little to lose by operation."

Walldius described spectacular results using this acrylic, completely constrained hinge joint, having followed one patient for 18 months and the others for less than a year. He expressed optimism about the operation, but asked, "How will the joint look after five to ten years?"

A British orthopaedic surgeon, L. G. B. Shiers,[60] developed a similar device in the early 1950s, reporting in 1954 on how it worked in four patients. His stainless steel prosthesis had a fixed hinge that connected the femoral and tibial components. Each of these components connected to a stem that extended up into the femoral canal on the femoral side and distally down into the tibia on the tibial side. After describing his prosthesis and the excellent outcomes in three patients, he concluded that he could not "draw definite conclusions from less than, say, 50 cases followed up for at least two years."

W. Russell MacAusland[61] of Boston developed a similar device in 1956, implanting it bilaterally in one patient. His implant was made of Vitallium and, like the others, consisted of a femoral rod and tibial rod, each mounted on a hinge mechanism that articulated at the level of the knee joint.

Despite all of the time and effort orthopaedic surgeons put into designing fixed-hinge knee arthroplasties, almost all these devices failed and have disappeared from the marketplace. The knee does not function like a rigid fixed hinge. The completely constrained devices (Walldius, Shiers, MacAusland, Young,[62] Witvoet,[63] and others) require removal of menisci, cruciate ligaments, and possibly the collateral ligaments, concentrating all of the stresses of knee motion and weight bearing on the axle and bolt of the device. It is no small wonder that these break, and that the femoral and tibial stems whipsaw in their respective bony canals, causing loosening, bone loss, fracture, and infection.

When the fixed hinges failed so dramatically, several orthopaedists attempted to use devices they hoped would compensate for the complexity of knee motion but at the same time provide the stability of a fixed hinge. In 1973, Larry Matthews, David Sonstegard, and Herbert Kaufer[64] of the University of Michigan devised the so-called spherocentric knee with these concepts in mind (Figure 30). The device consisted of the tibial component, with a flat tray resting on the tibial plateau and a stem going down into the tibial medullary canal for fixation. The tibial tray had two slots for the insertion of polyethylene tracks. The striking feature of the tibial component was the metal peg coming up from the posterior half of the tray. Matthews and his associates mounted a metal ball on the peg. The metal ball fit up into the inside of the femoral component and presumably provided for rotation between the femur and tibia, as well as for flexion and extension in the sagittal plane, with slight rocking in the coronal plane. The bearing surfaces consisted of Vitallium on polyethylene; methylmethacrylate was used to secure fixation of the implants into the bones. The spherocentric unit was large and bulky, necessitating the removal of large amounts of bone. This ultimately doomed it to fail in the orthopaedic marketplace.

Frank H. Gunston designed the first nonhinged prosthesis in 1968 (Figure 31). Gunston developed the device at the Wrightington Hospital in close association with John Charnley. Charnley, however, did not have his name on the Gunston prosthesis, preferring to give all the credit to his more junior associate. Gunston's device consisted of Vitallium or stainless steel runners inserted into the femoral condyles and polyethylene tracks cemented into the tibial plateaus. Gunston's prosthesis preserved the cruciate ligaments and required resection of very little bone. It had several disadvantages, however. Most surgeons found it technically difficult to use. It came with a complex set of jigs and alignment guides, but even with these it was very hard to align the tracks and runners exactly right. In addition, the bearing surfaces were quite small, and the polyethylene tracks tended to sink into the soft bone of the tibial plateaus. In 1973, Gunston reported the results obtained in 43 patients over two to five years.[65] He found that 38 polycentric arthroplasties were considered satisfactory. Also in 1973, Richard Bryan and associates[66] at the Mayo Clinic described their experience with a much larger number of patients (450). They emphasized the technical difficulty of the operation and said that they had seen early loosening, fracture, and dislocation postoperatively in their patients. They suggested that the polycentric total knee implant had many contraindications.

As the hinges and the polycentric knee and its derivatives began to fail in rather large numbers, orthopaedic surgeons struck off in new directions of prosthetic design (Figure 32). An earlier variant was the "geometric" TKA,[67] which entered the market in the early 1970s and had a run of around ten years. A team designed it (Mark Coventry of the Mayo Clinic, Jackson Upshaw of Corpus Christi, Lee Riley of Johns Hopkins, Gerald Finerman of UCLA, and Roderick Turner of Harvard Medical School), producing a design that was somewhat like the polycentric device, although more constrained. The tracks and runners were much wider on the tibia and femur, respectively, and each half of the respective components was connected with a crosspiece. Thus, instead of four units there were only two, one for the femoral runners and one for the tibial tracks. The operation, as described by Coventry,[68] consisted of complete débridement of the joint and insertion of the components adjusting for a knock-knee or bowleg deformity (valgus-varus) by removing bone to correct the malalignment. The components were then secured in position with methylmethacrylate. The components covered only the weight bearing part of the femur in full extension and did not address any potential patellofemoral arthritis. Loosening, early wear, and other complications plagued the geometric total knee and similar prostheses such as the Duocondylar (Chitranjan Ranawat and John Shine)[69] and the design by Theodore Waugh and associates[70] of the University of California at Irvine. Nevertheless, several of these devices were commercial successes for several years.

Michael Freeman began using his prosthesis in 1971. It consisted of a metal U-shaped femoral component that was higher in the back than in front and spanned the intercondylar notch of the femur, thus sacrificing the cruciate ligaments. The polyethylene tibial component covered the entire surface of the tibial side of the knee. It had a slight elevation front to back to conform to the shape of the femoral component, but otherwise the relationship between the components was unconstrained. The Freeman-Swanson prosthesis[71] (Swanson was an engineer who assisted in the design) was the essential breakthrough for later, increasingly successful modifications.

In 1976, John Insall, Chitranjan Ranawat, Norman Scott, and Peter Walker[72] of the Hospital for Special Surgery in New York described the total condylar knee replacement prosthesis, which was the next step in the evolution of TKA. The prosthesis lengthened the anterior surface of the Vitallium component to cover the entire joint surface. Insall and his associates also used a dome-shaped polyethylene button on the articular surface of the patella, and the all-plastic tibial component had a short peg that impacted into the proximal tibia to provide stability in that part of the total knee component. All the components were cemented with PMMA. The group also devised jigs and alignment guides for making precise cuts into the femoral and tibial surfaces.

Some patients with implants made according to the early total condylar prosthetic designs had difficulty walking up stairs, and many felt unstable while participating in activities that required deep flexion. Insall and his colleagues reported that instability in flexion resulted from removal of too much of the proximal tibia, but they had to acknowledge that gauging the flexion space correctly at the time of surgery was difficult. Furthermore, if the patient had had prior surgery, an excessive amount of tibia might already have been removed. Thus, when the tibia was brought into a 90° relationship with the femur, it might be loose and unstable even when a thicker tibial prosthesis had been implanted. To address this issue of posterior instability, Insall and Burstein devised a posterior stabilized condylar prosthesis in 1978. The modification replaces the posterior cruciate ligament with a "central polyethylene spine on the tibial component and a transverse cam on the femoral component." The polyethylene tibial spine thus projects into the femoral component with the prosthetic medial and lateral femoral condyles on each side. When the knee is extended, the tibial spine is located just in front of the transverse bar between the prosthetic femoral condyles. When the knee flexes, however, the transverse cam pushes the tibial spine forward so that the contact point between the femur and tibia moves posteriorly during full flexion. This facilitates femoral rollback. This combination of circumstances also lengthens the moment arm developed by the patellar tendon during extension; therefore, the patient generates somewhat less force in the quadriceps muscle to walk up stairs or rise from a chair.[73]

By the time surgeons at the Hospital for Special Surgery began to report large numbers of patients using the Insall-Burstein prosthesis, they had also developed their knee rating scale. In evaluating and comparing results of total condylar prostheses with posterior stabilized prostheses, they found that 76 percent of patients in the latter group had normal function postoperatively compared with 22 percent of those who had total condylar prostheses. These good results encouraged many other orthopaedic surgeons to perform knee arthroplasty using posterior stabilized prostheses. Other clinical rating systems have been devised subsequently.[74-77]

Modifications of the basic design continued with the addition of metal backing to the tibial component in the early 1980s. Frederick Ewald of Boston and his associates[78] reported on this modification in 1984. They found both clinically and with bench testing that "a metal-backed tibial component might transmit force more favorably to the underlying methylmethacrylate and bone." More discussion of the metal-backed tibial component was included in an overall evaluation of the "kinematic total knee" replacement, which differed from the Insall-Burstein knee in that the kinematic device retained the posterior cruciate ligament. Metal backing of the tibial component, in which the plastic polyethylene rests on a rigid metal tray, has been adopted almost universally and is now a feature of most total knee prostheses. This is similar, of course, to the development of metal backing for the acetabular components in THA. The metal backing contains and supports the soft plastic, facilitating more even distribution of weight-bearing forces to the underlying bone. As a result, the metal-backed plastic components tend to loosen more slowly and less often; thus, patients with these implants tend to have better outcomes. The issue of preservation of the posterior cruciate ligament is a less settled matter. Debate continues over cruciate ligament preservation versus the use of a posterior stabilized prosthesis.[79]

In the 1990s, innovators and high-volume surgeons established TKA as a reliable and effective operation that could reverse the crippling effects of advanced osteoarthritis and rheumatoid arthritis of the knee for up to 20 years. They defined the best basic design, and the number of orthopaedists interested in knee arthroplasty began to grow. Many of these innovators published several papers describing important but less elemental issues related to prosthetic design. Topics included such concerns as TKA after high tibial osteotomy, venous thrombosis after TKA, what combination of antibiotic prophylaxis to use, wear patterns, autologous blood transfusions, postoperative pain control, the best anesthesia, challenges associated with very elderly patients, what to do about fractured or unstable patellae, and TKA in obese patients. Tackling these issues improved methodologies and patient care but largely did not affect the way the prostheses were actually designed.

Cementless TKA was discussed during the early 1980s, but porous ingrowth of bone into knee prostheses did not occur as reliably as in total hip prostheses. Most surgeons still used PMMA to secure fixation of the implant into bone. The cement versus cementless issue remains somewhat controversial, however.[80,81]

Frederick Beuchel of New Jersey resurrected the design issue with the development of a prosthesis that had mobile bearings. Beuchel's concept considered the effect of the medial and lateral semilunar cartilages on knee flexion. These semicircular fibrocartilaginous structures, wedge-shaped in cross section, are normally interposed between the rounded femoral condyles and the flatter tibial articulating surface. They move freely during

knee motion, the lateral more than the medial. None of Beuchel's predecessors' designs considered the role of the menisci.[82]

Beuchel and his associate, M. J. Pappas, first published their experience
with the "New Jersey knee" in 1986 in a relatively obscure journal, The
Archives of Orthopaedic Trauma Surgery. The New Jersey knee challenged
the rationale and accepted wisdom of the fixed-bearing designs such as the
Install-Burstein, the kinematic, the Whiteside Ortholoc, Miller-Gallante,
and others. As it turned out, with the Beuchel knee there were reports of dislocations of the mobile bearings and mechanism failures. One of the most
recent papers on the subject published in *JBJS* reported that midterm results
of the Insall-Burstein 2 total knee and the New Jersey knee did not differ.[83]

The clinical success of total knee prostheses led to similar concepts such
as replacing just one side of the knee joint. In reports from 20 years ago,
unicompartmental total knee prostheses did not fare as well as the total
condylar knees then available. Premature loosening, breakage, and recurrent
knee pain occurred in series by Insall and Aglietti,[84] Laskin,[85] and Mallory
and Damfi.[86] These authors found sobering deterioration of initially good
outcomes in their patients with unicompartmental prostheses. Since then,
surgeons have refined the indications for unicompartmental TKA and
tweaked the designs of the prosthesis sufficiently to justify this kind of
surgery in the opinions of many orthopaedists.

Another issue of concern is revision of worn out or failed arthroplasties.
The survivability of a TKA largely depends on the alignment that was
achieved at the time the prosthesis was implanted. Lawrence Dorr of
Downey, California, edited a *Techniques in Orthopaedics: Revision of Total
Hip and Knee* in 1984, only nine years after Gunston's original report. The
authors of the chapters on knee revisions in Dorr's book all had participat-
ed actively in the development of total knee technology only a few years
earlier. Three years later, in 1987, Norman Scott (at that time chief of the
Joint Implant Service at Lenox Hill Hospital in New York) edited *Total
Knee Arthroplasty*.

The Knee Society

Orthopaedic surgeons involved heavily, if not exclusively, in TKA naturally
had a desire to discuss concerns about this surgery with their peers. Many
who participated in the evolution of the various designs, methods and techniques of knee replacement therefore decided to form The Knee Society.[87]
This limited-membership organization, whose annual meeting is open only to
members, announces on its Web site that it proposes "to advance the knowledge of the knee joint in health and disease, to create an optimum environment to enhance education, research and treatment of arthritis of the knee
joint, . . . [and] to promote and maintain professional standards to provide the
best care . . ." The society achieves its goal of education and dissemination of
information by publishing the papers presented at its closed annual meeting
in a special issue of *Clinical Orthopaedics and Related Research*. The Knee

Society also participates in Specialty Day at the Annual Meeting of the AAOS.

American Shoulder and Elbow Surgeons

Surgeons have the propensity for forming organizations, study groups, and small societies to meet with people who share an intense interest in their specialty. The Hip Society, The Knee Society, and AAHKS all serve as examples of this phenomenon. It is thus no surprise then that upper extremity orthopaedists established the American Shoulder and Elbow Surgeons (ASES) group,[88] which held its inaugural meeting in 1982. Carter Rowe (Harvard) and Charles Neer (Columbia-Presbyterian Hospital in New York) represented the senior orthopaedic surgeons. The ASES holds a closed annual meeting and participates, like most other orthopaedic subspecialty societies, in the AAOS Specialty Day. The ASES also serves as a clearinghouse for fellowships for training beyond the 4-year orthopaedic residency. In 1991, the ASES began publication of he *Journal of Shoulder and Elbow Surgery*. The creation of ASES, fellowships for specialized training, and a journal have led to increasing subspecialization in this area.

Total Shoulder Arthroplasty

Charles Neer of Columbia University College of Physicians and Surgeons and the New York Orthopaedic Hospital at Columbia-Presbyterian Medical Center devised an implant for humeral head articular surface replacement in 1953. It had an intramedullary stem much like an Austin Moore or Thompson femoral head prosthesis, with an attached rounded humeral head component. Neer originally recommended its use for humeral head fractures but soon expanded its indications for rheumatoid and osteoarthritic shoulders. By the mid-1970s, about 20 years after Neer's shoulder arthroplasty prosthesis appeared, he and other shoulder surgeons devised ways to replace the glenoid with polyethylene as well. The indications for shoulder arthroplasty have grown beyond osteoarthritis and rheumatoid arthritis to include rotator cuff tear arthroplasty, old sepsis, prior fusions, osteonecrosis, and previous trauma.

The glenoid, or socket, has a shallow saucer-like configuration, which causes problems in resurfacing or replacing that side of the shoulder joint. Unlike the hip joint, in which the surgeon can easily implant the cup into a deep socket, a shoulder surgeon must devise a way to attach the socket to a small, nearly flat surface with very little solid bone available for anchoring. This problem has led to some very imaginative designs, including reversing the natural ball-and-socket mechanism of the shoulder, thus attaching a socket to the upper humerus and a ball to the glenoid. Total shoulder arthroplasty has become a very specialized area of orthopaedics; relatively few articles on the subject appear in the general orthopaedic literature. Furthermore, those papers that are published often sound a cautionary note. For example, in 1995, *JBJS* published only two papers on the subject. One of these emphasized the importance of selecting appropriately sized humeral heads but stated further: "Our results . . . point to the variables of shoulder arthroplasty that the shoulder surgeon must master."[89] The other article addressed complications of fractures of the humerus both intraoperatively and postoperatively.[90] In 1996, *JBJS* again published only two articles related to shoulder arthroplasty compared with numerous articles on hip and knee replacements. One of the shoulder arthroplasty articles by Michael Wirth and Charles Rockwood[91] had the intimidating title, "Complications of Total Shoulder Replacement Arthroplasty." Presented as a Current Concepts Review, the 13-page article featured disturbing radiographs showing shoulder prostheses that had dislocated, disengaged, or otherwise failed catastrophically.

The technology of shoulder arthroplasty has not reached the point at which non-shoulder specialists should feel secure in doing this operation. Most shoulder surgeons who have experience in total joint arthroplasty report good to excellent results in many patients. However, serious complications, a surprising number of failures, practical difficulties, and unresolved issues regarding component structure and design have dampened enthusiasm for many nonspecialists. Shoulder replacement surgery has not reached the level of THA or TKA in terms of volume, outcomes, and acceptance by many orthopaedists.

Total Elbow Arthroplasty
Only a small number of patients have the kinds of arthritic diseases that justify total elbow arthroplasty. Consequently, these devices have less of a track record than total hip, knee, and even shoulder components. Currently, the most commonly used device for elbow replacement is the Coonrad-Morrey total elbow. Elbow arthroplasty surgery went through the same developmental phases as the other joints, and it is of interest that the elbow is one of the few joints in which interposition arthroplasty actually worked. Surgical débridement of rheumatoid elbow joint with synovectomy and excision of damaged joint surfaces give some patients both pain relief and functional mobility. Surgeons have experimented with various materials and tissues for interposition just as in hip and knee interposition arthroplasty, using, for example, skin, fascia lata, plastic membranes, and pig bladder. The cutis interposition elbow arthroplasty has the best record and probably the least morbidity, according to the literature.[92]

In the late 1970s, R. W. Coonrad of Duke University in Durham, North Carolina, described a total elbow prosthesis that featured a loosely constrained hinge connecting cemented intramedullary extensions into the humerus proximally and the ulna distally. The metal cross-bar axis of the hinge articulated loosely with a polyethylene cylinder. Despite the cement fixation, the humeral component tended to rotate. Bernard Morrey of the Mayo Clinic modified Coonrad's design by adding a flange to the anterior aspect of the humeral component.[93] The idea was that the intramedullary stem and the anterior flange would grip the anterior cortex of the distal humerus to neutralize rotational forces. The looseness and slight toggling of the Coonrad-Morrey prosthesis tend to negate the problems encountered with fixed hinges.

Experience with fixed hinges in the knee joint showed that the moments of force operating across the joint are so great that they can prematurely overcome the bond between the implant and the bone. The looseness of the elbow hinge has extended the period of useful function for the implants.[94]

Elbow replacement with a device such as the Coonrad-Morrey prosthesis has the potential for the same kinds of complications seen in hips, knees, and shoulders. Polyethylene wear, osteolysis, and loosening almost inevitably occur over time. In addition, the associated bone atrophy seen in conjunction with osteolysis so weakens the humerus or ulna that periprosthetic fractures often develop in these patients. These fractures can produce daunting degrees of comminution, which make for a difficult reconstruction, requiring extensive bone grafting and the use of custom-made devices. Nevertheless, elbow surgeons can now offer relief to patients with persistent pain and restore function in the joint. The design of the implant has improved gradually over years of trial and error and will continue to improve with further experience. Gill and Morrey[93] reported in 1998 that in a series of 69 patients with rheumatoid arthritis of the elbow, they had achieved a 92.4 percent ten-year survival of the prosthesis with 86 percent good-to-excellent results. Modern orthopaedic technology has progressed to the point at which a reasonably skilled implant surgeon could probably receive similar results.

Total Ankle Arthroplasty

Dr. Saint Elmo Newton invented one of the first total ankle prostheses in the United States in the early 1970s.[95] His design consisted of a high-density polyethylene tibial component, 1 cm thick, with a slightly concave surface for articulation with the convex talar component. The talar component, made of Vitallium, rested on the surface of the talar dome. The talar component also had a small peg for better fixation in the body of the talus, and both the tibial and talar components required cemented fixation.

The Newton prosthesis, the Oregon prosthesis, and others with similar designs developed the usual problems associated with metal on polyethylene— mainly wear, osteolysis, loosening, and failure. Other issues arose that were unique to the ankle. One of these was the relatively high rate of skin necrosis and infection after surgery.

The failure of these prosthetic designs and the difficulties inherent in improving on them have prompted highly negative assessments of ankle arthroplasty. In fact, the AAOS Instructional Course Lectures and texts such as *Campbell's Operative Orthopaedics* and the *Oxford Textbook of Orthopaedics and Trauma* advise against them.[96-98] In a recent edition of *Campbell's Operative Orthopaedics*, the authors of the chapter on ankle replacements stated: "At this time we do not think that the published short-term results of total ankle arthroplasty justify the widespread application for ankle arthritis outside of investigational centers."[97]

Most of the total ankle designs are hampered by the fact that ankle fusion offers a satisfactory alternative for most patients. Furthermore, in the past several decades, surgeons have simplified ankle fusions by using arthroscopic techniques and employing internal fixation with screws when possible to avoid cumbersome external fixators.

However, ankle fusion has several adverse consequences. Almost inevitably, patients must transfer the stress of motion onto the midtarsal joints, which eventually also deteriorate. In rheumatoids, arthritic involvement of the forefoot can make toeing off painful or impossible. Often, many patients with ankle fusions have difficulty walking on uneven surfaces, or even up stairs.

Accordingly, it is not surprising that orthopaedic surgeons continue to work toward the development of a stable, long-lasting total ankle. A 2004 symposium on the subject published in *Clinical Orthopaedics and Related Research* contained 20 papers on total ankle arthroplasty. The numerous authors discussed cementless fixation, mobile bearings, metal-backed tibial components, ceramic prostheses, wear patterns, and numerous design modifications and changes. Despite proscriptions, ankle arthroplasty may well find a niche in orthopaedics in coming years.

References

1.   Magnuson PB: Technique of debridement of the knee joint for arthritis. *Surg Clin North Am* 1946;26:249.

2.   Ranawat CS, Straub LB, Freyberg R, Granda JL, Rivelis M: A study of regenerated synovium after synovectomy of the knee in rheumatoid arthritis. *Arthritis Rheum* 1971;14:117-125.

3.   Ranawat CS, Desai K: Role of early synovectomy of the knee joint in rheumatoid arthritis. *Arthritis Rheum* 1975;18:117-121.

4.   Graham J, Checketts RG: Synovectomy of the knee joint in rheumatoid arthritis: A long-term follow-up. *J Bone Joint Surg Br* 1973;55:786-795.

5.   Jackson JP, Waugh W: Tibial osteotomy for osteoarthritis of the knee. *J Bone Joint Surg Br* 1961;43:746-751.

6.   Bauer GCH, Insall J, Koshino T: Tibial osteotomy in gonarthrosis (osteoarthritis of the knee). *J Bone Joint Surg Am* 1969;51:1545-1563.

7.   Coventry MB: Osteotomy of the knee for genenerative and rheumatoid arthritis. *J Bone Joint Surg Am* 1973;55:23-48.

8.   Kettelkamp DB, Wenger DR, Chao EY, Thompson C: Results of proximal tibial osteotomy: the effects of tibiofemoral angle, stance-phase flexion-extension, and medial-plateau force. *J Bone Joint Surg Am* 1976;58:952-960.

9.   McMurray TP: Osteoarthritis of the hip joint. *Br J Surg* 1935;22:916.

10. Pauwels F: *Atlas zur Biomechanik der gesunden und kranken Hufte. Prinzipien, Technik, und Resultate einer kausalen Therapie.* Berlin, Germany, Springer-Verlag, 1973.

11. Müller ME, Allgower M, Salineider R, Willenegger H: *Manual of Internal Fixation. Techniques Recommended by the AO Group*, ed 2. Berlin, Germany, Springer-Verlag, 1979.

12. Bombelli R, Santore RF, Poss R: Mechanics of the normal and osteoarthritic hip: A new perspective. *Clin Orthop Relat Res* 1984;182:69-78.

13. Smith-Petersen MN: Arthroplasty of the hip. *J Bone Joint Surg* 1939;21:269-288.

14. Aufranc O: *Constructive Surgery of the Hip*. St Louis, MO, CV Mosby, 1962.

15. Smith-Petersen MN: Evolution of mould arthroplasty of the hip joint. *J Bone Joint Surg Br* 1948;30:59.

16. Smith-Petersen MN: Lessons learned from fourteen years' experience with mould arthroplasty of the hip joint. *J Bone Joint Surg Br* 1952;34:714.

17. Amstutz HC: The THARIES hip resurfacing technique. *Orthop Clin North Am* 1982;13:813-832.

18. Campbell WC: Interposition of Vitallium plates in arthroplasties of the knee: Preliminary report. *Am J Surg* 1940;47:639.

19. Kuhns JG: Nylon membrane arthroplasty of the knee in chronic arthritis. *J Bone Joint Surg Am* 1964;46:448-449.

20. McKeever DC: The use of cellophane as an interposition membrane in synovectomy. *J Bone Joint Surg Am* 1943;25:576-580.

21. Jones WN: Mold arthroplasty of the knee joint. *Clin Orthop Relat Res* 1969;66:82-89.

22. Murray DG, Barranco S: Femoral condylar hemiarthroplasty of the knee: Review and follow-up study. *Clin Orthop Relat Res* 1974;101:68-73.

23. McKeever DC: Patellar prosthesis. *J Bone Joint Surg Am* 1955;37:1074-1084.

24. McKeever DC: Tibial plateau prosthesis. *Clin Orthop Relat Res* 1960;18:86.

25. MacIntosh DL, Hunter GA: The use of the hemiarthroplasty prosthesis for advanced osteoarthritis and rheumatoid arthritis of the knee. *J Bone Joint Surg Br* 1972;54:244-255.

26. Blazina ME, Fox JM, Del Pizzo W, Broukhim B, Ivey FM: Patellofemoral replacement. *Clin Orthop Relat Res* 1979;144:98-102.

27. Judet J, Judet R: The use of an artificial femoral head for arthroplasty of the hip joint. *J Bone Joint Surg Br* 1950;32:166-173.

28. Townley CO: Hemi and total articular replacement arthroplasty of the hip with the fixed femoral cup. *Orthop Clin North Am* 1982;13:869-894.

29. Moore AT, Bohlman HR: Metal hip joint: A case report. *J Bone Joint Surg Am* 1943;25:688-692.

30. Gibson A: Posterior exposure of the hip joint. *J Bone Joint Surg Br* 1950;32:183-186.

31. Thompson FR: Two and a half years' experience with a Vitallium intramedullary hip prosthesis. *J Bone Joint Surg Am* 1954;36:489-502.

32. Fahey JJ, King DE, Lipscomb P, Slocum DB, Lambert CN: Preliminary survey on femoral head prostheses by the Committee on Scientific Investigation of the AAOS. *J Bone Joint Surg Am* 1953;35:489-494.

33. Straub LR, King DE, Lambert CN: Symposium on femoral-head prostheses: Based on the report of the Committee for the Study of Femoral Head Prostheses as printed in the October (1954) issue of the Bulletin. *J Bone Joint Surg Am* 1956;38:407-420.

34. Gluck T: Referat uber die durch das moderne chirurgrohe Experiment genonnenen positiveen resultate, betreffend die nact und den Ersatz von Defecten höherer Gewebe Langeenberbs. *Arch Klin Chir* 1874;16:340-490.

35. Wiles P: The surgery of the osteo-arthritic hip. *Br J Surg* 1957;45:488.

36. Ring PA: Complete replacement arthroplasty of the hip by the Ring prosthesis. *J Bone Joint Surg Br* 1968;50:720-731.

37. Haboush EJ: A new operation for arthroplasty of the hip based on biomechanics, photoelasticity, fast-setting dental acrylic and other considerations. *Bull Hosp Joint Dis* 1953;14:242-277.

38. Charnley J: Anchorage of the femoral head prosthesis to the shaft of the femur. *J Bone Joint Surg Br* 1960;42:28-30.

39. McKee GK, Watson-Farrar J: Replacement of arthritic hips by the McKee-Farrar prosthesis. *J Bone Joint Surg Br* 1966;48:245-259.

40. Charnley J: Letter to Editor: Tissue reactions to polytetrafluorethylene. *Lancet* 1963.

41. Charnley J: *Low Friction Arthroplasty of the Hip.* New York, NY, Springer-Verlag, 1979.

42. Charnley J: Total hip replacement by low-friction arthroplasty. *Clin Orthop Relat Res* 1970;72:7-21.

43. The Hip Society: Available at http://www.hipsoc.org. (Accessed March 20, 2007)

44. John Charnley: In Memoriam. *J Bone Joint Surg Br* 1983;65:84.

45. Bartel DL, Bicknell VL, Wright TM: The effect of conformity, thickness, and material on stresses in ultra-high molecular weight components for total joint replacement. *J Bone Joint Surg Am* 1986;68:1041-1051.

46. American Association of Hip and Knee Surgeons: Available at http://www.aahks.org. (Accessed March 20, 2007)

47. Boutin P, Christel P, Dorlot JM, et al: Use of dense alumina-alumina ceramic articulation in total hip replacement. *J Biomed Mater Res* 1988;22:1203-1232.

48. Mahoney OM, Dimon JH: Unsatisfactory results with a ceramic total hip prosthesis. *J Bone Joint Surg Am* 1990;72:663-671.

49. Mittelmeier H, Heisel J: Sixteen-years' experience with ceramic hip prostheses. *Clin Orthop Relat Res* 1992;282:64-72.

50. Walter A: On the material and the tribology of alumina-alumina couplings for hip joint prostheses. *Clin Orthop Relat Res* 1992;282:31-46.

51. Park YS, Hwang SK, Choy WS, Kim YS, Moon YW, Lim SJ: Ceramic failure after total hip arthroplasty with an alumina-on-alumina bearing. *J Bone Joint Surg Am* 2006;88:780-787.

52. Davies AP, Willert HG, Campbell PA, Learmonth ID, Case CP: An unusual lymphocytic perivascular infiltration in tissues around contemporary metal-on-metal joint replacements. *J Bone Joint Surg Am* 2005;87:18-27.

53. Callaghan JJ, Dysart SH, Savory RF, Hopkinson WJ: Assessing the results of hip replacement: A comparison of five different rating systems. *J Bone Joint Surg Br* 1990;72:1008-1009.

54. Bryant MJ, Kernohan WG, Nixon JR, Mollan RA: A statistical analysis of hip scores. *J Bone Joint Surg Br* 1993;75:705-709.

55. Boardman DL, Dorey F, Thomas BJ, Lieberman JR: The accuracy of assessing total hip arthroplasty outcomes: A prospective correlation study of walking ability and 2 validated measuring devices. *J Arthroplasty* 2000;15:200-204.

56. Soderman P, Malchau H: Is the Harris Hip Score System useful to study the outcome of total hip replacement? *Clin Orthop Relat Res* 2001;384:189-197.

57. Majnoni d'Intignano JM: Articulations totalesen résine acryligne [Total articulations in acrylic resin]. *Rev Orthop Chir Appar Mot* 1950;36:535-537.

58. Walldius B: Arthroplasty of the knee joint employing an acrylic prosthesis. *Acta Orthop Scand* 1953;23:121-131.

59. Walldius B: Arthroplasty of the knee using an endoprosthesis. *Acta Orthop Scand* 1957;24(Suppl):1-112.

60. Shiers LGB: Arthroplasty of the knee: Preliminary report of new method. *J Bone Joint Surg Br* 1954;36:553-560.

61. MacAusland WR: Total replacement of the knee joint by a prosthesis. *Surg Gynecol Obstet* 1957;104:579-583.

62. Young HH: Use of a hinged vitallium prosthesis for arthroplasty of the knee: A preliminary report. *J Bone Joint Surg Am* 1963;45:1627-1642.

63. Witvoet J: GUEPAR total knee prosthesis. *Exerpta Med* 1973;298:28.

64. Matthews LS, Sonstegard DA, Kaufer H: The spherocentric knee. *Clin Orthop Relat Res* 1973;94:234-241.

65. Gunston FH: Polycentric knee arthroplasty: Prosthetic simulation of normal knee motion. Interim report. *Clin Orthop Relat Res* 1973;94:128-135.

66. Bryan RS, Peterson LFA, Combs JJ: Polycentric knee arthroplasty: A preliminary report of postoperative complications in 450 knees. *Clin Orthop Relat Res* 1973;94:148-152.

67. Coventry MB, Upshaw JE, Riley LH, Finerman GA, Turner RH: Geometric total knee arthroplasty: I. Conception, design, indications and surgical technique. *Clin Orthop Relat Res* 1973;94:171-176.

68. Coventry MB, Upshaw JE, Riley LH, Finerman GA, Turner RH: Geometric total knee arthroplasty: II. Patient data and complications. *Clin Orthop Relat Res* 1973;94:177-184.

69. Ranawat CS, Shine JJ: Duocondylar total knee arthroplasty. *Clin Orthop Relat Res* 1973;94:185-195.

70. Waugh TR, Smith CS, Orofino CF, et al: Total knee replacement: Operative technic and preliminary results. *Clin Orthop Relat Res* 1973;94:196-201.

71. Freeman MAR, Swanson SAV, Todd RC: Total replacement of the knee using the Freeman-Swanson prosthesis. *Clin Orthop Relat Res* 1973;94:153-170.

72. Insall J, Ranawat CS, Scott WN, Walker P: Total condylar knee replacement: Preliminary report. *Clin Orthop Relat Res* 1976;120:149-154.

73. Insall JN, Lachiewicz PF, Burstein AH: The posterior stabilized condylar prosthesis: A modification of the total condylar design. Two to four-year clinical experience. *J Bone Joint Surg Am* 1982;64:1317-1323.

74. Alicea J: Scoring systems and their validation for the arthritic knee, in Insall JN, Churchill SN (eds): *Surgery of the Knee*, ed 3. New York, NY, Churchill Livingstone, 2001, p 1507.

75. Insall JN, Dorr LD, Scott RD, Scott WN: Rationale of the Knee Society clinical rating system. *Clin Orthop Relat Res* 1989;248:13-14.

76. Heck DA, Robinson R, Partridge C, Lubitz RM, Freund DA: Patient outcomes after knee replacement. *Clin Orthop Relat Res* 1998;356:93-110.

77. Saleh KJ, Dykes DC, Tweedie RL, et al: Functional outcome after total knee arthroplasty revision revision: A meta-analysis. *J Arthroplasty* 2002;17:967-977.

78. Ewald FC, Jacobs MA, Miegel RE, Walker PS, Poss R, Sledge CB: Kinematic total knee replacement. *J Bone Joint Surg Am* 1984;66:1032-1040.

79. Hirsch HS, Lotke PA, Morrison LD: The posterior cruciate ligament in total knee surgery: Save, sacrifice, or substitute? *Clin Orthop Relat Res* 1994;309:64-68.

80. Cook SD, Barroch RI, Thomas KA, et al: Quantitative histologic analysis of tissue growth, into porous total knee components. *J Arthroplasty* 1989;4(suppl):33.

81. Branson PJ, Steege FW, Wixon RL, Lewis J, Stulberg SD: Rigidity of initial fixation with uncemented knee implants. *J Arthroplasty* 1989;4:21-26.

82. Buechel FF, Pappas MJ. New Jersey low contact stress knee replacement system. Ten-year evaluation of meniscal bearing. *Orthop Clin North Am* 1989;20:147-177.

83. Bhan S, Malhotra R, Kiran EK, Shukla S, Bijjawara MA: A comparison of fixed-bearing and mobile-bearing total knee arthroplasty at a minimum follow-up of 4.5 years. *J Bone Joint Surg Am* 2005;87:2290-2296.

84. Insall J, Aglietti P: A five to seven-year follow-up of unicondylar arthroplasty. *J Bone Joint Surg Am* 1980;62:1329-1337.

85. Laskin RS: Unicompartmental tibiofemoral resurfacing arthroplasty. *J Bone Joint Surg Am* 1978;60:182-185.

86. Mallory TH, Damfi J: Unicompartmental total knee arthroplasty: A five- to nine-year follow-up study of 42 procedures. *Clin Orthop Relat Res* 1983;175:135-138.

87. The Knee Society: Available at http://www.kneesociety.org. (Accessed March 20, 2007)

88. American Shoulder and Elbow Surgeons: Available at http://www.ases-assn.org. (Accessed March 20, 2007)

89. Harryman DT, Sidles JA, Harris SL, Lippitt SB, Matsen FA: The effect of articular conformity and the size of the humeral head component on laxity and motion after glenohumeral arthroplasty: A study in cadavera. *J Bone Joint Surg Am* 1995;77:555-563.

90. Wright TW, Cofield RH: Humeral fractures after shoulder arthroplasty. *J Bone Joint Surg Am* 1995;77:1340-1346.

91. Wirth MA, Rockwood CA: Current concepts review: Complications of total shoulder replacement arthroplasty. *J Bone Joint Surg Am* 1996;78:603-616.

92. Froimson AI, Silva JE, Richey D: Cutis arthroplasty of the elbow. *J Bone Joint Surg Am* 1976;58:863-865.

93. Gill DR, Morrey BF: The Coonrad-Morrey total elbow in patients who have rheumatoid arthritis: A ten to fifteen-year follow-up study. *J Bone Joint Surg Am* 1998;80:1327-1335.

94. Dee R: Total replacement of the elbow joint. *Orthop Clin North Am* 1973;4:415-433.

95. Newton SE III: An artificial ankle joint. *Clin Orthop Relat Res* 2004;424:3-5.

96. Saltzman CL: Total ankle arthroplasty: State of the art. *Instr Course Lect* 1999;48:263-268.

97. Cocharell JR, Guyton JL: Arthroplasty of the ankle and knee, in Canale ST (ed): *Campbell's Operative Orthopaedics*, ed 10. St Louis, MO, CV Mosby, 2003, p 245.

98. Cooke PH: Ankle and foot, in *Oxford Textbook of Orthopedics and Trauma*. Oxford, England, Oxford University Press, 2002, vol 2, p 1224.

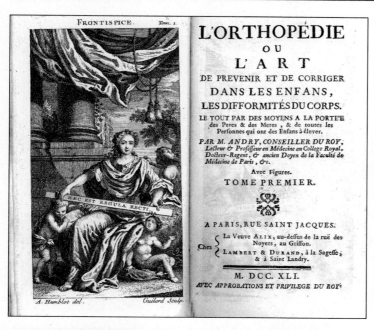

Figure 1 Frontispiece and title page of page of Nicholas Andry's book L'Orthopédie. The seated figure holds a ruler. Its Latin inscription translates as "This is the rule for straightness." (Reproduced from Andry de Boisregard N: *L'Orthopédie l'Art de Prevenir et de Corriger dans les Enfans les Difformités du Corps. Le Tout par des Moyens a la Porte'e des Peres et des Meres, et de toues les Personnes qui ont des Enfans à élever.* Paris, France, La Veuve Alix et Lambert et Levand, 1741.)

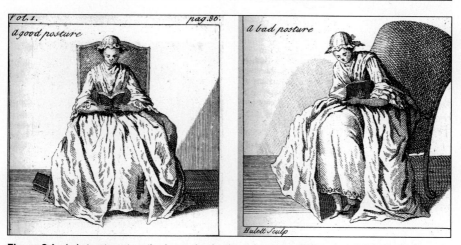

Figure 2 Andry's treatment methods emphasized good posture. (Reproduced from Andry de Boisregard N: *L'Orthopédie l'Art de Prevenir et de Corriger dans les Enfans les Difformités du Corps. Le Tout par des Moyens a la Porte'e des Peres et des Meres, et de toues les Personnes qui ont des Enfans à élever.* Paris, France, La Veuve Alix et Lambert et Levand, 1741.)

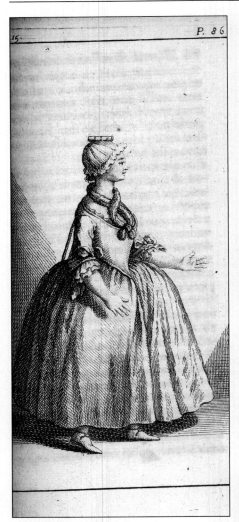

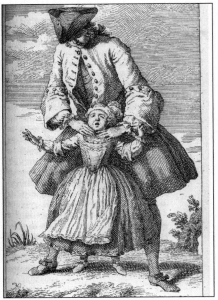

Figure 4 Andry advised against treating children roughly. (Reproduced from Andry de Boisregard N: *L'Orthopédie l'Art de Prevenir et de Corriger dans les Enfans les Difformités du Corps. Le Tout par des Moyens a la Porte'e des Peres et des Meres, et de toues les Personnes qui ont des Enfans à élever*. Paris, France, La Veuve Alix et Lambert et Levand, 1741.)

Figure 3 The girl is standing straight because she balances a book on her head. (Reproduced from Andry de Boisregard N: *L'Orthopédie l'Art de Prevenir et de Corriger dans les Enfans les Difformités du Corps. Le Tout par des Moyens a la Porte'e des Peres et des Meres, et de toues les Personnes qui ont des Enfans à élever*. Paris, France, La Veuve Alix et Lambert et Levand, 1741.)

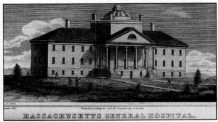

Figure 5 The Massachusetts General Hospital in the early 19th century. The large rectangular structure over the entrance was the operating theater. After the first documented use of anesthesia there in 1846, it became known as the "Ether Dome." (Reproduced from Snow CH: *A History of Boston: The Metropolis of Massachusetts From Its Origins to the Present Period*. Boston, MA, Abel Bowen, 1828.)

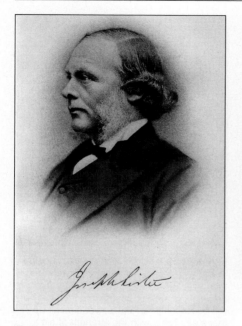

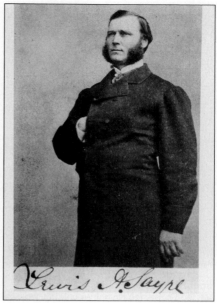

Figure 6 Sir Joseph Lister. After learning of Louis Pasteur's work on "germs," he developed antiseptic surgery and reduced the mortality from surgical infections to nearly zero. (Reproduced from Wrench GT: *Lord Lister: His Life and Work*. New York, NY, Frederick A. Stokes Company, 1913.)

Figure 7 Lewis A. Sayre, MD. When the Bellevue Hospital Medical College opened in 1861, Dr. Sayre was appointed Professor of Orthopaedic Surgery. The first person to hold this title in the United States, he has been called "the father of orthopaedics in America." (Photo courtesy of the Erhman Medical Library Archives, NYU School of Medicine.)

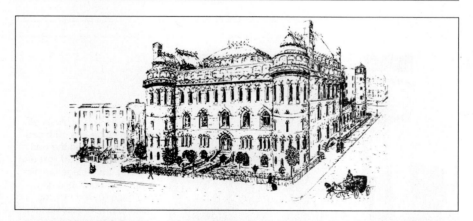

Figure 8 The Hospital for the Ruptured and Crippled, circa 1867. The first orthopaedic hospital in America, it is now known as The Hospital for Special Surgery. (Beekman F: A Historical Sketch on the Occasion of the Seventy-fifth Anniversary of the Hospital for the Ruptured and Crippled. New York, NY [printed privately].)

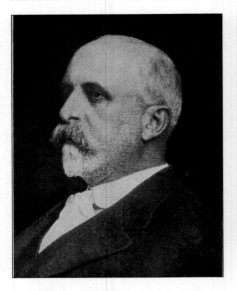

Figure 9 Virgil Gibney, MD. Gibney succeeded Dr. James Knight as chief at the
Hospital for the Ruptured and Crippled. A
pupil of Dr. Sayre's, he endorsed surgical
treatment of musculoskeletal deformities, a
controversial issue at that time.
(Reproduced with permission from Mayer L:
Orthopaedic surgery in the United States of
America. *J Bone Joint Surg Br* 1950;32:461-
569.)

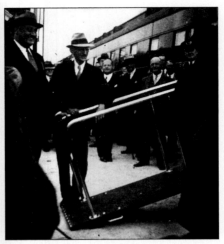

Figure 10 Dr. Michael Hoke about to help
Franklin D. Roosevelt ascend a ramp to the
train at Warm Springs, Georgia. The future
president is smiling despite the fact that he
will necessarily have to power himself up
that steep ramp with the strength of his
upper limbs. Dr. Hoke seems prepared to
swing in behind him should FDR fall over
backward. Roosevelt came to accept his
bilateral lower limb paralysis caused by polio
when Dr. Hoke became his physician.
During World War II, President Roosevelt
appointed an orthopaedic surgeon to the
post of Surgeon General of the Army.
(Reproduced with permission from the
March of Dimes Birth Defects Foundation,
White Plains, NY.)

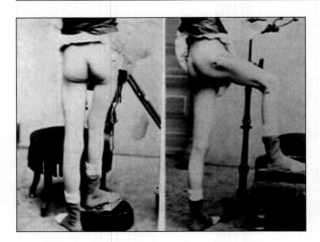

Figure 11 Tuberculosis of
the hip in the late 19th century. Treatment in the early
stages consisted of rest and
bracing. Late-stage hip disease with bone loss and
drainage (called morbus
coxarius) was occasionally
treated with "exsection."
(Courtesy of the New York
Academy of Medicine
Library, New York, NY.)

Figures

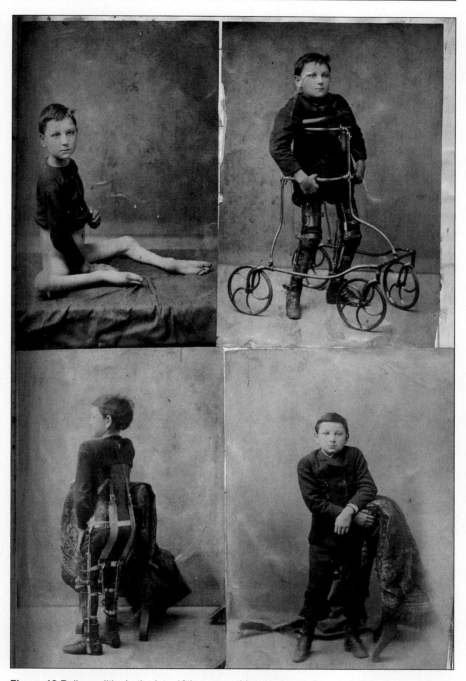

Figure 12 Poliomyelitis. In the late 19th century this was a rare disease. Ironically, as sanitation improved, the enteric polio virus disappeared from the water supply and humans lost their herd immunity to it. Massive epidemics of polio resulted in the 20th century. (Photo courtesy of the Ehrman Medical Library Archives, NYU School of Medicine.)

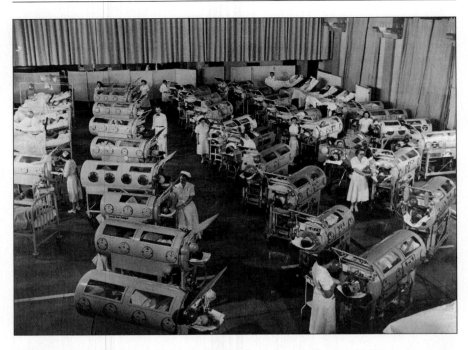

Figure 13 Iron lung ward of the Rancho Los Amigos in Downey, California, mid-20th century. (Reproduced with permission from the March of Dimes Birth Defects Foundation, White Plains, NY.)

Figures

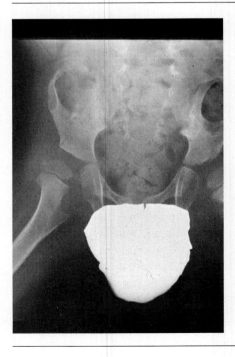

Figure 14 After the disappearance of tuberculosis and polio, improved neonatal care led to the survival of more babies with cerebral palsy and myelomeningocele. This radiograph of a child's pelvis reveals the large defects in the ilium through which the psoas muscles had been transferred in treatment of paralytic hip dislocation due to L4-5 myelomeningocele (the Sharrard procedure). (Reproduced from Poland J: *Traumatic Separation of the Epiphyses*. London, England, Smith & Elder, 1898.)

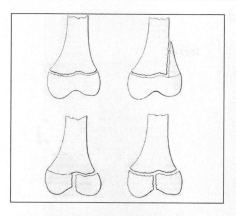

Figure 15 Dr. John Poland's 1898 classification of growth plate injuries in children. (Reproduced from Poland J: *Traumatic Separation of the Epiphyses*. London, England, Smith & Elder, 1898.)

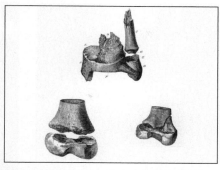

Figure 17 Poland studied amputation and autopsy specimens and patient outcomes and described them in a book nearly 1000 pages long. He compiled this information before radiographs became widely available. (Reproduced from Poland J: *Traumatic Separation of the Epiphyses*. London, England, Smith & Elder, 1898.)

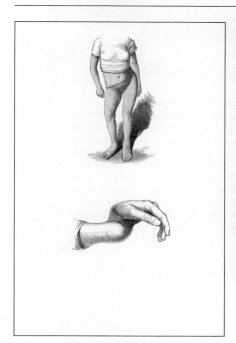

Figure 16 Deformities resulting from growth plate injuries. (Reproduced from Poland J: *Traumatic Separation of the Epiphyses*. London, England, Smith & Elder, 1898.).

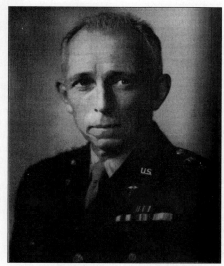

Figure 18 Major General Norman T. Kirk, MD. An orthopaedic surgeon and Surgeon General of the Army in World War II, Kirk was appointed by President Roosevelt over the objections of General George Marshall and Secretary of War Stimson. One of Kirk's first acts was to order that all fractures would be treated by orthopaedists. (Reproduced with permission from Major General Norman Thomas Kirk, 1888-1960. *J Bone Joint Surg Am* 1960;42:1450-1452.)

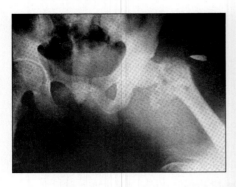

Figure 19 Radiograph of a soldier wounded in World War II. The German machine gun bullet that caused the fracture of the upper femur is clearly visible. (Reproduced from Coates JB, Mather C, McFetridge EM: Battle incurred compound fractures about the hip joint, in *Surgery in World War II: Orthopedic Surgery in the European Theatre of Operations.* Washington, DC, Office of the Surgeon General, 1956, p 229.)

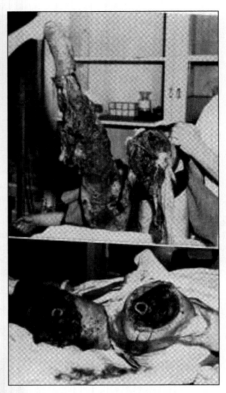

Figure 21 Massive wounds from a landmine explosion. Internal or external fixation for war injuries was prohibited. Débridement and open treatment, splinting, and traction were the mainstays of wound management. (Reproduced with permission from Coates JB, Cleveland M, McFetridge EM: *Surgery in World War II: Orthopedic Surgery in the Mediterranean Theatre of Operations.* Washington, DC, Office of the Surgeon General, 1957, p 248.)

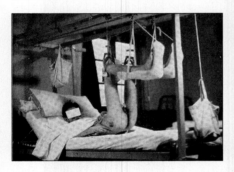

Figure 20 A wounded World War II soldier in skeletal traction. General Kirk required that treatment protocols be rigidly controlled. (Reproduced from Coates JB, Mather C, McFetridge EM: Battle incurred compound fractures about the hip joint, in *Surgery in World War II: Orthopedic Surgery in the European Theatre of Operations.* Washington, DC, Office of the Surgeon General, 1956, p 230.)

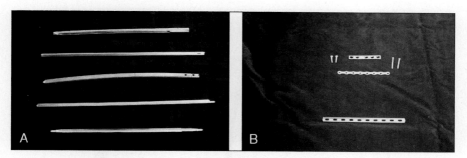

Figure 22 After World War II, open reduction and internal fixation with rods, plates, and screws came to dominate fracture care in civilian practice. A variety of femoral intramedullary rods (A) and various plates and screws (B) are shown here. Femoral rod designs have varied considerably: straight, bowed, solid, tubular, round, clover-leafed, diamond-shaped, with or without perforations for interlocking screws. The configurations of plates have also evolved. Thin beaded plates have lower profiles but lack the strength of other designs. Plates with slotted holes permit impaction of fracture fragments, but beveled screw holes and large hemispherical screw heads can actively produce compression at a fracture site. Locking screws (not shown) provide for the most rigid fixation. (Reproduced from the collection of the American Academy of Orthopaedic Surgeons.)

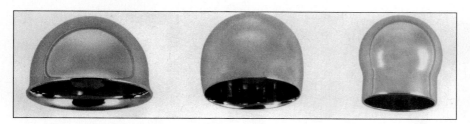

Figure 23 The Smith-Petersen cup arthroplasty was a standard operation for hip arthritis until the advent of hip prostheses. Smith-Petersen's first model (1926) was made of glass. (Reproduced with permission from Stryker Orthopaedics.)

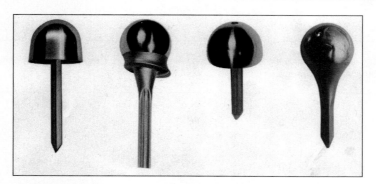

Figure 24 The Judet brothers developed femoral head replacements in the 1940s. Their first device was made of acrylic. (Reproduced with permission from Stryker Orthopaedics.)

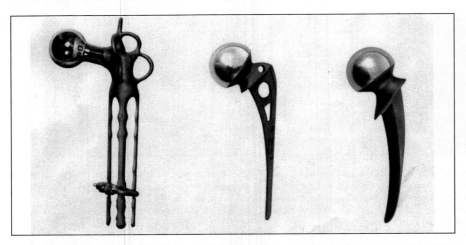

Figure 25 The Bohlman, Austin Moore, and Thompson prostheses (from left to right). Bohlman's hip prosthesis was devised for a patient with a large femoral giant cell tumor. It was probably the first hip prosthesis made from Vitallium. (Reproduced with permission from Stryker Orthopaedics.)

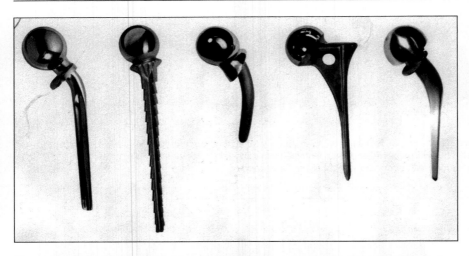

Figure 26 Many variations of the hip endoprosthesis were developed. (Reproduced with permission from Stryker Orthopaedics.)

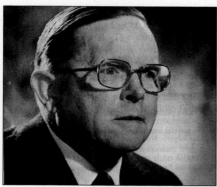

Figure 27 Sir John Charnley, a seminal figure in the development of total hip replacements. (Reproduced with permission from In Memoriam: John Charnley. *J Bone Joint Surg Br* 1983;65:84-86.)

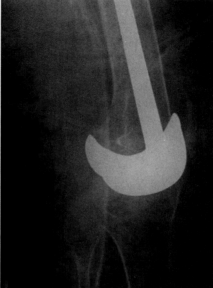

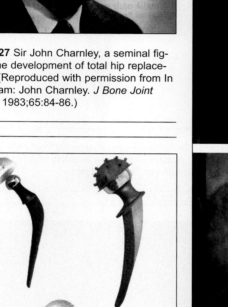

Figure 28 The Charnley, McKee-Farrar, and Charnley-Müller total hips (left to right) came to the market in America in the early 1970s.; The Charnley models featured metal-on-polyethylene bearing surfaces and the McKee-Farrar featured metal on metal. The components of all three were secured in place with methylmethacrylate. (Reproduced with permission from Stryker Orthopaedics.)

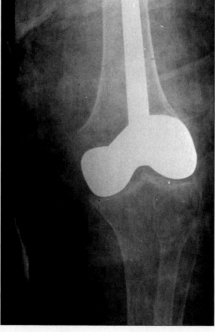

Figure 29 The MGH femoral condylar mold arthroplasty for arthritis of the knee. (Reproduced with permission from Stryker Orthopaedics.)

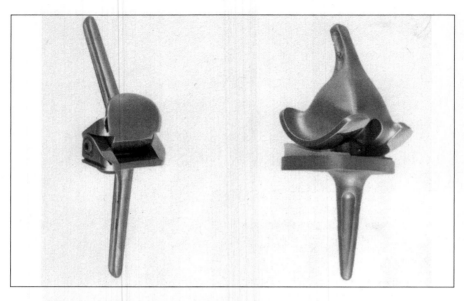

Figure 30 Fixed hinges worked poorly in the knee. The spherocentric knee prosthesis (on the right) was devised in an effort to permit motion in multiple planes. An example of a fixed hinge is on the left. (Reproduced with permission from Stryker Orthopaedics.)

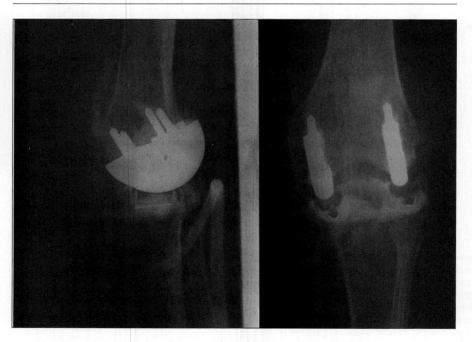

Figure 31 The Gunston prosthesis was one of the first to deal with the shifting center of rotation in the knee. (Reproduced with permission from Dr. John Gartland.)

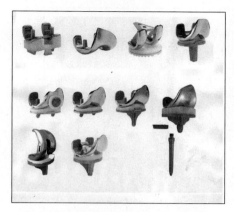

Figure 32 Later generations of the total knee. New models and designs appear regularly. (Reproduced with permission from Stryker Orthopaedics.)

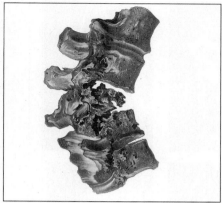

Figure 33 Pott's disease. The illustration is taken from Pott's book, published in the late 19th century. (Reproduced from Pott P: Remarks on the kind of palsy frequently found to accompany curvature of the spine. London, England, 1879.)

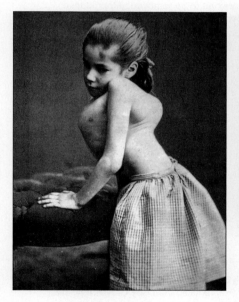

Figure 34 Clinical appearance of Pott's disease in a late 19th century child. The spinal fusions performed by Russell Hibbs and Fred Albee in the first decade of the 20th century were done to prevent this degree of deformity. (Photo courtesy of the Ehrman Medical Library Archives, NYU School of Medicine.)

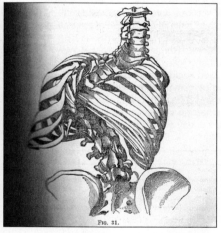

Figure 35 The rise of polio in the first half of the 20th century led to thousands of patients with severe paralytic scoliosis. This image is taken from Louis Bauer's book, published in the late 1860s. (Reproduced from Bauer L: *Lectures on Orthopedic Surgery Delivered at the Brooklyn Medical and Surgical Institute.* New York, NY, William Wood & Co., 1868, p 155.)

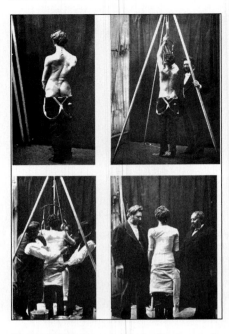

Figure 36 The Sayre method of treatment of scoliosis (circa 1880). Lewis A. Sayre's treatment of scoliosis consisted of longitudinal traction and manual application of translational forces. Correction was maintained by a plaster jacket. Removal of the jacket, however, resulted in loss of correction. Dr. Russell Hibbs used a variation of this method but ensured permanent correction of the deformity by performing a spinal fusion after the treatment of traction, manipulation, and casting. (Photo courtesy of the Ehrman Medical Library Archives, School of Medicine.)

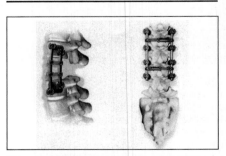

Figure 38 Examples of modern spinal fixation implants, which currently include rods, plates, screws, cages, and artificial disks. (Reproduced with permission from Stryker Orthopaedics.)

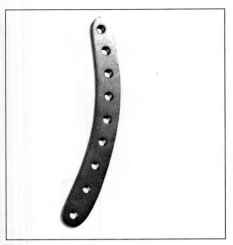

Figure 37 A Wilson plate. This device was curved to match the lordosis of the lumbar spine. The plate was secured to the spinous processess with screws in the sagittal plane. John F. Kennedy had a spinal fusion performed with this device in 1954. Infection complicated the recovery from surgery and the plate had to be removed. (Reproduced with permission from Stryker Orthopaedics.)

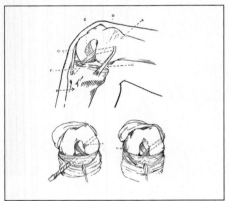

Figure 39 Hey Groves ACL reconstruction in 1919. (Reproduced from Hey Groves EW: The cruciate ligaments of the knee joint: Their function, rupture, and operative treatement of the same. *Br J Surg* 1920;7:505-515.)

Figures

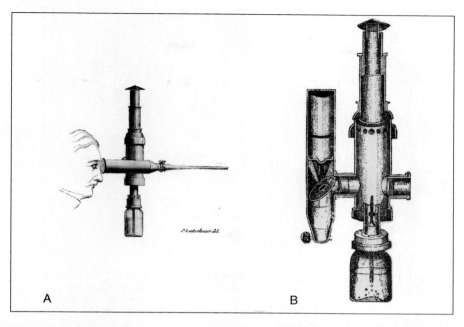

Figure 40 A, An early endoscope for use in joints. **B,** Interior view showing the light source for the scope—an oil lamp. (Reproduced with permission from Stryker Endoscopy.)

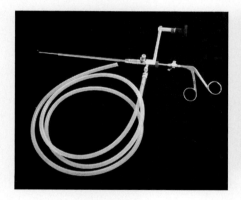

Figure 41 An operating arthroscope. The surgeon used the eyepiece to view the instrument, which was inserted through the cannula. Without video, only the surgeon could see inside the knee.

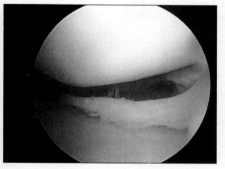

Figure 42 Video and triangulation have revolutionized arthroscopic surgery. This is the view of the interior of the knee, showing a tear of the medial meniscus. (Reproduced with permission from Stryker Endoscopy.)

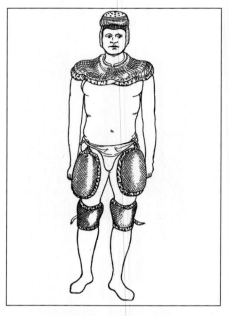

Figure 43 A 1909 drawing of a member of the Harvard football squad showing protective equipment required at the time. The knee supports were supposed to prevent injury but then, as now, they did not. (Reproduced from Nichols EH, Richardson FL: Football injuries of the Harvard squad for three years under the revised rules. *Boston Med Surg J* 1909;160: 33-37.)

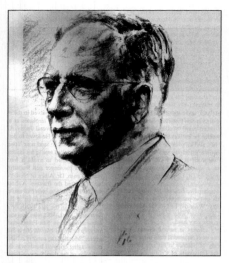

Figure 44 Sterling Bunnell, MD, the father of modern hand surgery. (Reproduced with permission from Newmeyer WL: The founding father. *J Hand Surg* 2003;28:161.)

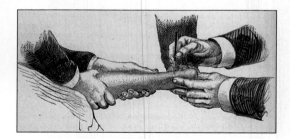

Figure 45 Tenotomy being performed for a foot deformity before the advent of antiseptic surgery. (Reproduced from Sayre LA: *A Practical Management of the Treatment of Club-Foot.* New York, NY, Appleton & Company, 1875.)

Figures

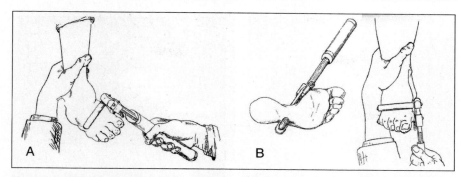

Figure 46 A, Correction of varus foot deformity without open surgery using the Thomas wrench. The Thomas wrench could also be used to correct adductus (B) and equinus (C). (Reproduced from Tubby AH: *Deformity Including Diseases of the Bones and Joints.* London, England, MacMillan & Co. Ltd., 1912, pp 281, 283.)

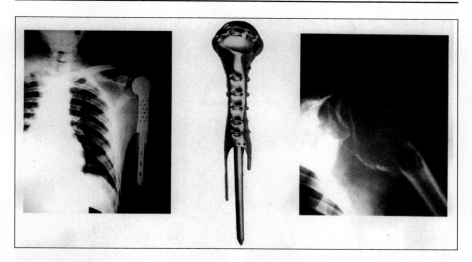

Figure 47 Modern chemotherapy, radiation therapy, and surgery based on staging of tumors have saved the lives and salvaged the limbs of many patients. The x-ray of a patient with a destructive tumor of the upper humerus is shown. His orthopaedic surgeon resected the lesion and replaced the lost bone with a custom made Vitallium prosthesis. The event took place in 1961 and is probably one of the earliest uses of a prosthetic implant in limb-salvage surgery. (Reproduced with permission from Stryker Orthopaedics.)

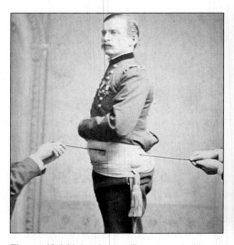

Figure 48 A Union Army officer wounded in 1862. His iliac osteomyelitis required surgical removal of most of his ilium. His wound drained for the rest of his life and required repeated removals and reinsertions of rubber drains. (Photo courtesy of the Ehrman Medical Library Archives, NYU School of Medicine.)

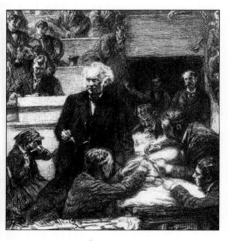

Figure 49 Portrayal of Dr. Samuel D. Gross performing a sequestrectomy in 1875. Surgical protocols based on staging classifications and antibiotics have changed the outlook for patients with bone infections since then. (Courtesy of the Athenaeum of Philadelphia.)

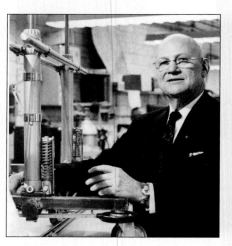

Figure 50 Dr. Homer Stryker, exemplar of the innovative and entrepreneurial individuals who created major corporations, engaged in the manufacture and marketing of orthopaedic products. Others included Revra DePuy, Joseph Zimmer, Dan Richards, Thomas Smith and his nephew, and many others. (Reproduced with permission from Stryker Orthopaedics.)

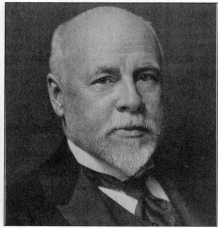

Figure 51 Dr. William Welch, the Dean of Johns Hopkins Medical College, was one of the creators of the modern system of medical education. (Reproduced from *Papers and Addresses by William Henry Welch: Volume 1. Pathology and Preventive Medicine*. Baltimore, MD, Johns Hopkins Press, 1920.)

Figures

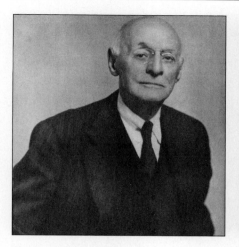

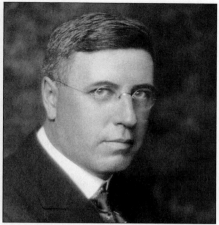

Figure 52 Abraham Flexner was recruited by Welch (and others) to make a national tour of inspection of all of the medical colleges. The Flexner report exposed the poor quality of medical education in 1911. (Reproduced with permission from Abraham Flexner: An Autobiography. New York, NY, Simon and Schuster, 1940.)

Figure 53 Dr. Melvin Henderson. A president of the AAOS, first chief of orthopaedics at the Mayo Clinic, and the first president of the ABOS in 1934. (Reproduced with permission from Mayo Historical Unit, Mayo Clinic, Rochester, MN.)

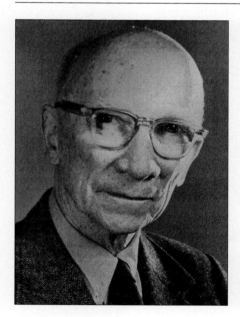

Figure 54 Dr. Alfred Shands Jr. founded the ORS and the OREF in 1954. (Reproduced with permission from Alfred Rives Shands, Jr., MD: 1899-1991. *J Bone Joint Surg Am* 1982;64:314-315.)

Figures

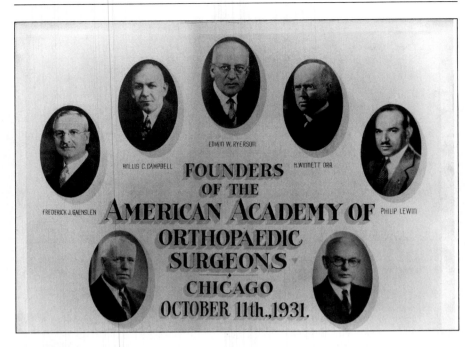

Figure 55 The founders of the AAOS.

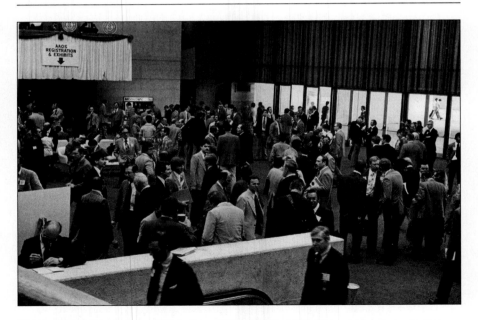

Figure 56 Activity at the Annual Meeting of the AAOS in 1978. Current attendance for the meeting exceeds 30,000.

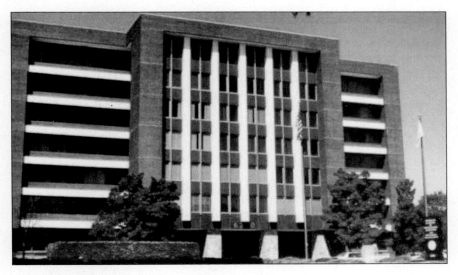

Figure 57 Headquarters of the AAOS in 2007.

CHAPTER 6
ORTHOPAEDIC SURGEONS AND THE SPINE

Tuberculosis and the Early Fusions

Orthopaedists could offer relatively little to patients with spinal diseases and injuries until the late 1890s. Many patients seemed to improve with bracing; external support with various devices was the mainstay of treatment during that period. The situation began to change in the late 19th and early 20th centuries. Several orthopaedic surgeons, having observed the apparent beneficial effects from fusing tuberculous hips or knees, postulated that surgically stabilizing infected spinal segments might produce the same positive outcome. Anesthesia and Listerism had made operations safe, paving the way for someone brave enough to attempt spinal fusion.

Berthold Ernest Hadra, a German immigrant orthopaedic surgeon practicing in Austin, Texas, read a paper at the 1891 meeting of the American Orthopaedic Association (AOA) describing how he had wired together the spinous processes of the sixth and seventh cervical vertebrae of a 30-year-old man. The patient had a C6-C7 fracture-dislocation, with painful instability and severe discomfort upon attempted motion. Hadra reported that the patient reported nearly complete pain relief after his operation. He also reported problems with drainage from the silver wire sutures he looped around the spinous processes. Nevertheless, the result of the operation had so encouraged him that he subsequently performed it on patients with spinal deformities caused by Pott's disease (Figure 33). He did not describe those patients' outcomes.

Another German orthopaedist, Fritz Lange of Munich, wrote a paper in 1910 for the *American Journal of Orthopaedic Surgery* describing the implantation of two long metal rods under the skin on the right and left side of the spinous processes in several children with Pott's disease. Lange observed that the metal bars used in braces held patients upright but were uncomfortable and often ineffective. He reasoned that placing the rods inside the body and suturing them securely to the spine would provide continuous and more efficient support than the awkward external spinal brace. Lange wrote that he experimented with various metals such as tin, steel, or silver, but in the end, the lack of a nonreactive material for use in the human body defeated him.

Two American orthopaedic surgeons made the essential breakthrough in 1911 when they performed spinal fusions using bone grafts in patients with Pott's disease (Figure 34). Russell Hibbs of the New York Orthopaedic Hospital described three patients upon whom he had performed spinal

fusion surgery in the *New York Medical Journal* of May 27, 1911. Fred
Albee of the Hospital for the Ruptured and Crippled described his spine
fusion surgery in the *American Journal of Orthopaedic Surgery* in the same
year. Albee also reported on only three patients, and both surgeons had
operated on patients with gibbus deformities resulting from Pott's disease.
Their techniques differed considerably. Hibbs exposed only the spinous
processes in the midline of the spine, cutting them off at their bases with a
small bone chisel. He then turned each spinous process at a right angle from
its normal upright position and used it to span the interlaminar space as a
fresh autogenous bone graft. Albee split the spinous processes longitudinally and wedged a long piece of the patient's tibial shaft into the defect created by the splitting of the spinous processes. Both Hibbs and Albee found
that the removal of the spinous process at the apex of the gibbus improved
the patient's appearance. More important, they found that the grafts caused
solid bridges of bone to form, fusing the involved vertebrae together. The
two articles by Hibbs and Albee, both surgeons from vigorously competitive New York hospitals, formed the basis of spine surgery as a modern surgical specialty. Over time, the Albee method declined in popularity. It
required the harvesting of a long tibial bone graft; in addition to the pain
inflicted on the patient, the technique imposed the risk of fracture at the
donor site when the patient resumed walking. Hibbs' method, supplemented with bone graft harvested locally, won out.

For the next 30 years, posterior spinal fusion served as the gold standard
for the treatment of Pott's disease. Orthopaedic surgeons performed thousands of these procedures worldwide. Spanning bone grafts across the back
of the spinal column, however, merely stabilized the spine to permit healing of the disease process, which involved the vertebral bodies. The fusion
was actually located some distance from the site of the disease. Most surgeons feared that a direct surgical attack on the locus of the infection might
cause the tuberculous infection to flare up. They could, however, use a cos-
totransversectomy to drain an expanding tuberculous abscess. By removing
the base of the rib and the transverse process of the thoracic vertebra, this
procedure permitted drainage from the site of an infected vertebral segment.
A direct frontal approach, though, seemed too risky.

In 1945, the advent of chemotherapy for tuberculosis changed the way
orthopaedic surgeons could treat Pott's disease. David Bosworth[1] of St.
Luke's Hospital in New York and the Seaview Tuberculosis Hospital on
Staten Island reported that streptomycin, isoniazid, and paraminosalicylic
acid prevented the dissemination of tuberculosis after surgery done directly
in an infected joint. Thereafter, Arthur Hodgson,[2] a British orthopaedic surgeon operating at the Royal Victoria Hospital in Hong Kong, began using
an anterior approach to achieve radical débridement of tuberculous foci in
the vertebral bodies of patients with Pott's disease. After removing the
tuberculous abscess with fragments of infected bone and fragments of intervertebral disks, he could place bone grafts directly into the infected areas
spanning diseased vertebral segments. These techniques provided immediate removal of the spinal disease with restoration of stability. Arthur

Hodgson's anterior surgical approach to the spine gave thousands of patients from mainland China the chance to be cured of spinal tuberculosis and also changed the way spine surgeons would routinely gain access to any portion of the spinal column. Subsequently, after the problems with resistance and hypersensitivity became known with regard to streptomycin and the other medications, new chemotherapeutic agents were developed as first-line drugs. These agents can control most spinal tuberculosis without surgery, and most patients can now expect to be cured by taking medication only. The era of spine surgery for tuberculosis has thus ended because the disease has essentially disappeared and the few patients afflicted with it respond so well to nonsurgical treatment. Nevertheless, attempting to cope with tuberculosis of the spine prompted orthopaedic surgeons to develop strategies and techniques for virtually all other diseases and deformities.

Pioneers of Spine Surgery

Russell Hibbs, chief at the New York Orthopaedic Hospital from 1899 to 1932, came from Birdsville, Kentucky. He was born in 1869 and educated at Vanderbilt University and the University of Louisville. After he received his medical degree, he started a general practice in Texas in 1890. His memorial, published in the *Journal of Bone and Joint Surgery* (*JBJS*) in 1933 a few months after his death, states that he came to New York in 1894 and became resident surgeon at the New York Orthopaedic Hospital and Dispensary, which at the time was "a small institution occupying a converted dwelling house." Because of their dissatisfaction with the current chief at the New York Orthopaedic Hospital, the trustees of the hospital offered the job to the young Hibbs. Hibbs took over the position at 30 years of age, serving in that capacity until his death 33 years later. He had numerous interests within orthopaedics, but he built his and the hospital's reputations primarily with his work in spine surgery.

Hibbs first reported on his original method in 1911, describing it simply as an osteotomy of the spinous processes with deflection of these to overlap the interlaminar spaces. His technique and indications continued to expand throughout the middle years of his career. He soon included decortication of the lamina and overlapping of bone from that source to cover the interlaminar spaces. Eventually, he also opened the facet joints and removed their articular cartilage to promote intervertebral fusion. In 1914, he began to perform his spinal fusion operation on children with scoliosis (Figure 35). Hibbs surmised that most of these scoliotic patients had paralytic deformities resulting from polio. In the first nine patients he did not attempt preoperative correction, but he soon decided that a better result could be achieved if he could correct the deformity before fusion. He tried several methods, settling on the "traction jacket" as the best (Figure 36). This technique had been described by Lewis A. Sayre nearly 20 years earlier. It consisted of longitudinal traction on the child's head and pelvis, coupled with lateral traction applied to the apex of the curvature on the convex side of the body. The patient was placed in a body jacket while the correction was applied. Hibbs repeated this process every two weeks until he had achieved what he considered to be maximum correction, at which point he removed the cast and performed the fusion. Two weeks after the fusion, he repeated the traction and body jacket, keeping the patient in the jacket for up to 12 months.

Hibbs had a profound effect on orthopaedics in the United States; his technique eventually became the standard operation for spine fusion. Orthopaedic surgeons from all over the country came to New York to learn about it. He also founded the New Jersey Orthopaedic Hospital in 1933 as an offshoot of the New York Orthopaedic Hospital and made sure that it functioned in the same manner as the New York Orthopaedic Hospital. A few years before his death, he founded an orthopaedic library at Columbia University in New York, now named after him. His name also survives in the Russell Hibbs Society and the Russell Hibbs Award presented annually by the Scoliosis Research Society.

Fred Albee, Hibbs' competitor in fusion surgery for spinal disorders, had a somewhat different background. He was a little younger than Hibbs, born in 1876 in Alana, Maine. He graduated from Bowdoin College in 1899 and from Harvard Medical School in 1903, spending most of his career as the Chief of Orthopaedics at the New York Postgraduate Medical School. After serving as an army colonel during World War I, he established a hospital in Colonia, New Jersey, where he cared for thousands of maimed veterans returning from France. Albee set up "curative workshops," based on the principles of rehabilitation established by Sir Robert Jones in Great Britain, to care for the veterans in Colonia. Albee's efforts led to the development of the New Jersey Rehabilitation Commission. One of Albee's residents, Henry Kessler, assumed the leadership role in this institution, which eventually became the well-known Kessler Rehabilitation Institute. Albee's spinal fusion techniques endured in some centers through the 1950s, but the large tibial onlay graft method has given way to the technique devised by Hibbs. Albee died in 1945 and was memorialized in the *Journal of the American Medical Association* as well as *JBJS*. He and Hibbs could not have been personally more different. Hibbs was moody and depressive, and apparently had actually dropped out at the beginning of his career to recover from depression. Albee was more jovial and outgoing. He had "an estate" in Florida, where he indulged his interest in horticulture. Albee lived a fuller life, but Hibbs had the more powerful legacy in orthopaedics.

Arthur Hodgson, whose efforts resulted in the now-routine use of anterior spinal surgery, received his medical education in Edinburgh and his orthopaedic training in Norwich with Brittain and McKee. He served in Burma, India, and Singapore during World War II and spent much of his working life thereafter in Hong Kong. His reports on the success of anterior spinal surgery with débridement and fusion of tuberculous lesions popularized this method and familiarized orthopaedic surgeons around the world with the possibilities of anterior spinal surgery. Hodgson did not originate the anterior approach, but he did publish several widely read papers that motivated his orthopaedic colleagues to give it consideration.

Scoliosis

In 1941, Hibbs published his last report on his treatment of progressive spinal deformities and nine years after his death, the AOA Research Committee reported at its annual meeting that it considered the findings of an "end result study of the treatment of idiopathic scoliosis."[3] The committee members, Alfred Shands Jr., as chairman, Joseph Barr, and Paul Colonna, with the assistance of Lawrence Noall, the research fellow at the Nemours Foundation, surveyed 16 orthopaedic clinics throughout the country. Although they collected some useless information such as the patients' nationalities and speculations of the clinics' chairmen or chiefs about the etiology of idiopathic scoliosis, the report presented a good deal of pertinent material. For example, it showed that Hibbs' evaluation of the deformities had not quantified the spinal curvatures adequately, and that the respondents in the study had switched to the method of John R. Cobb, which was described more thoroughly in 1948.[4] This technique consisted first of determining the extent of a given curve by defining the levels of the neutral vertebrae. The AOA report defined the various locations, degrees of severity, apices of the curve, ages of appearance, gender predilection, and various forms of treatment and outcomes.

In the late 1930s and early 1940s, the Risser turnbuckle cast became popular,[5] replacing Hibbs' body jacket with longitudinal and lateral traction, the fishnet horizontal suspension jacket, and various bent jackets employed by others. The Risser turnbuckle cast required application of a body cast extended over one hip to the knee and usually up to the occiput and mandible. Hinges and turnbuckles incorporated into the front and back of the cast facilitated gradual correction of the deformity. Results of the AOA survey of 1941 showed that when orthopaedists used these devices without following correction with a fusion, the deformity recurred 100 percent of the time, but with fusion, 67 percent of the patients achieved moderate to marked improvement.

During the war years, the cumulative index of *JBJS* recorded only five relatively minor papers under the general topic of scoliosis. In 1947, G. E. Thomas[6] of Liverpool published a paper on a new way to correct scoliotic deformities using longitudinal traction on a metal frame. Devices resembling house jacks mounted on the lateral bars of the frame could exert force on the apices of the curve and, if directed properly, could produce derotation of the deformed segments as well as lateral realignment. When the traction and jacks produced as much correction as possible, Thomas applied a body cast to his patients, as the corrective forces continued. Thomas reported that his localizer cast showed "encouraging improvement" over other methods.

In the 1950s, several important papers on the diagnosis and treatment of scoliosis appeared, encouraging other innovative clinical researchers to publish on this topic. For example, the paper by Ignacio Ponseti and Barry Friedman[7] of the University of Iowa reported on a review of 394 young patients with idiopathic scoliosis who had no treatment. Ponseti and Friedman identified five curve patterns: main lumbar, main thoracolumbar,

combined thoracic and lumbar, main thoracic, and main cervicothoracic.
They cross-referenced these curve patterns with four age groups (under 10
years, 10 to 12, 12 to 14, and over 14 years). They found that main lumbar,
thoracolumbar, and cervicothoracic curves generally had a good prognosis.
These curves did not progress rapidly and usually did not produce severe
deformity. Main thoracic curves progressed more rapidly than did other
curve patterns, and children younger than ten years of age progressed the
most rapidly. Thoracolumbar curves had a good prognosis in children older
than ten years of age but a poor prognosis in younger children. Some of the
deformities that had begun as minor curvatures with minimal rib humping
in young children eventually became severely disfiguring when untreated.

In 1958, *JBJS* presented a group of papers on scoliosis that summed up
the progress made after World War II. John R. Cobb,[8] the elder statesman
in the field at that time, wrote an editorial entitled "Scoliosis: Quo Vadis"
for the issue. Cobb sounded a mordant note, stating: "There has been great
enthusiasm for certain plaster casts, frames, body corsets, exercises, and
operations. Most of these have been discarded after arousing much hope in
some patients only to have it end in despair." After listing the many methods of treatment that had been discarded, he counseled conservatism, suggesting that surgeons did not yet have enough information about scoliosis
to choose surgical treatment in most cases. He pointed out that "many
spinal curves are mild, and few need any treatment" but "curvatures that
may progress until they seriously deform the child must be recognized and
they demand our best efforts."

The two articles by Blount and associates[9,10] that followed Cobb's somewhat acerbic remarks described Blount's results with a Milwaukee brace.
They described it as a "refinement of the distraction jacket and an improvement over the turnbuckle jacket." In these two articles, Blount and his colleagues described how the jacket should be fabricated, well molded over the
pelvic rim with two uprights in back and one in front. The uprights supported an occipital pad and a flat pad under the mandible, replacing the cup-
shaped arrangement for support of the chin that had previously resulted in
problems with an overbite. Strategically placed straps and pads produced
laterally directed forces at the apices of the curve. For nonsurgical treatment, Blount said that the brace was best used in three situations: in an
acceptable curve (20° or less) that has begun to progress rapidly, in convalescent polio patients with early structural scoliosis, and in chronic polio
patients with incipient pelvic obliquity.

Blount said that at the time he made this presentation in 1958, he had 12
years' experience with the brace. At that point, he concluded that the brace
could maintain alignment in rapidly developing curves in younger children
and delay or possibly eliminate the need for surgery. He cautioned that it
was necessary for patients to wear the brace most of the time; thus ortho-
tists needed to make them difficult to remove.

Parenthetically, Walter Bobechko[11] and others in the late 1970s and early
1980s also proposed a conservative treatment program for slowing the progression of scoliotic curves. They advocated using continuous electric

stimulation of the muscles on the convex side of the deformity. Children either wore electric pads or had them implanted internally to produce the muscle stimulation. This method failed to achieve reliable correction of the deformity, however, and most children did not like the sensation of the mild electrical shock. The technique is no longer in use.

The next article in the 1958 *JBJS* was by John Moe,[12] entitled, "A Critical Analysis of Methods of Fusion for Scoliosis: An Evaluation in Two Hundred and Sixty-Six Patients." Moe originally believed that the best preoperative correction of scoliotic deformity resulted from the use of the turnbuckle cast as described by Risser. Later, however, he switched to Risser's localizer cast, which was much like that described by G. E. Thomas. Moe employed several variations of the Hibbs fusion method and found that Cobb's modification of Hibbs's technique failed only 7 percent of the time.

Also in the 1958 *JBJS*, Joseph Risser[13] of Pasadena, California, described his various methods of preoperative correction with turnbuckle casts and localizer casts and said that he used Hibbs' fusion method exclusively. He suggested that surgeons should thoroughly investigate why a patient loses correction after fusion. This meant that one had to (1) act vigorously to detect and treat pseudarthroses, (2) extend fusions to adjacent levels, or (3) keep patients in postoperative body jackets for longer periods.

Risser contributed another insight in describing the importance of the ossification of the iliac crest as an important indicator of skeletal growth and maturation.[14] He observed that the radiographic appearance of the iliac crest apophysis coincides with the cessation of vertebral growth.

The final paper in the series of scoliosis articles published in *JBJS* in 1958 probably gave Cobb reason to remark:

> Today there are enthusiastic supporters of mechanical appliances of metal introduced at open operation for the interval correction of scoliosis. It is obvious that metal fastened to bone may hold bones or parts of bones in a certain position for a time. Certainly one cannot expect osteogenetic properties in them. Ultimately, unless something is done to stabilize the vertebral segments in an unsegmented form, there will be bone erosion or the device will slip or break if intervertebral motion is allowed to persist. One wonders if these devices will stand the test of time.[13]

Dr. Cobb appeared to be speaking about the work of Adam Gruca,[15] who presented a paper on scoliosis at the 1957 American Academy of Orthopaedic Surgeons (AAOS) annual meeting. Gruca based his thesis on "chronaximetric, myomechanical, and histological examination of the lower spinal muscles." These had a "dystonia" from asymmetric innervation or from reflex spasm introduced by inflammatory lesions in the spine, lungs, or mediastinum. The scoliosis thus could be cured by transferring muscles of the scapula to muscles on the convexity of the curves and denervating the hyperactive muscles on the concavity. The weakened muscles on the convexity, according to Gruca, would also need the support of compression springs and the hyperactive muscles would need distraction of a screw-spring device. In cases of lateral shifting of the trunk, muscle transfers of the latissimus, serratus anterior, trapezius, tensor fascia lata, and abdominal muscles should be performed. The radiographs the author used to illustrate his points showed springs attached to the ribs on the convexities of the curve, with distractors hooked to the ribs or the transverse processes on the concavities of the curves. Gruca's muscle releases, muscle transplants, and denervations failed to gain popular acceptance, but the springs and distraction presaged what came next in the treatment of scoliosis.

In 1960 and in1962, after Gruca had published his paper, Paul Harrington[16,17] published his own seminal articles on spinal instrumentation. Harrington, of Houston, Texas, had adopted orthopaedics as his life's work after seeing the effect of polio on thousands of children. Harrington strongly believed that internal stabilization was needed to treat collapsing paralytic spinal curvatures and began working on instrumentation for this in 1949. In his original 1962 paper, he described his numerous modifications and admitted that "many problems were encountered." By the time he was ready to present his first publication on the subject, he decided to use SMO 18-8 stainless steel to fabricate a distraction rod for use on the concavity of the curve. The rods were 3 to 15 inches long and ¼ inch in diameter. The lower end of the rod would fit into a hole in a curved hook that was placed over a lamina. The upper part of the rod had a series of circumferential notches, and when the rod was passed through the superiorly directed hook, which in turn had been placed under a superior facet, a special instrument would distract the vertebrae on the rod. He also developed a compression system for the convex side of the curvature. This consisted of a threaded semiflexible stainless steel rod that could be threaded through hooks over the transverse processes on the convex side of the curve. Small stainless steel nuts could pull the hooks together on the threaded rod to correct the deformity. Harrington reported that he used these instruments in the treatment of 129 patients. He encountered several complications but persevered, undaunted. Rod breakage, rod dislocation, vertebral erosion, pseudarthrosis of his attempted fusions, and two deaths did not forestall his efforts. He believed a child younger than ten years of age with a rapidly progressing curve could be treated with a rod only, avoiding a fusion. He believed, however, that older children would require a fusion. He also believed that his results in 129 patients treated over a period of eight years justified continuing with the development of correction and internal fixation of spinal deformities.

Paul Harrington's influence on spine surgery did not quite reach the same level of importance as that of Sir John Charnley's on hip surgery, but his work did have far-reaching consequences. The surgeons treating scoliotic deformities now had a potent (though admittedly imperfect) weapon for correcting and stabilizing deformed spines. It would permit them to bypass the unpleasant turnbuckles, localizers, and suspended fishnet techniques in many cases in favor of an operation at the outset. Although some patients would need preoperative traction, many, if not most, would not.

Paul Harrington[18] was born in Kansas City, Kansas, in 1911 and attended its public education system from grade school through the University of Kansas School of Medicine. He played basketball in high school and college and was captain of a college team that made it to three Big Eight championships. He completed an orthopaedic residency at St. Luke's Hospital in Kansas City in 1942, and then served in the U.S. Army until 1945. Instead of returning to Kansas City, however, he settled in Houston, where he spent the rest of his life. He died in 1980.

John Hall[19] of Boston Children's Hospital, who presented the annual Paul Harrington Oration at the Scoliosis Research Society meeting in 1988, recounted his visit with Harrington in 1958. Hall found that he alone was to assist Harrington with his surgery as "the residents from the Baylor program were not allowed to work with him because he was considered to be a madman." Hall went on to say that Harrington's instrumentation "yielded the lowest complication rate of any system I have used." His willingness to adopt a method as far removed from the standard way of doing things as Harrington's exemplifies Hall's own imaginative approach to the treatment of spinal deformities in children.

In 1964, two years after Harrington's original presentation, several surgeons interested in scoliosis decided that it was time to start a society. It began with 12 people as the Scoliosis Club at the AOA annual meeting in the Palmer House in Chicago and was convened by Bernard Levine. In 1966, the society held its first full meeting in Minneapolis. Evidently almost all of those invited regarded the project favorably, as most attended the function. Those in attendance elected John Moe president. He served in that capacity for two years.

John Hall, Dean MacEwen, Paul Harrington, and Robert Winter succeeded Moe and set the standard for those who followed. The Scoliosis Research Society (SRS) has maintained strict requirements for admission and continued membership. It requires regular submission of members' procedures, results, and complications, and members must submit papers for presentation at given intervals. In addition, the SRS strongly recommends that members devote their practice largely to scoliosis surgery. The stringency of these requirements reflects the opinion that only total commitment to scoliosis surgery will suffice. In his 1974 SRS presidential address, Robert Winter[20] questioned whether the "stupidity, laziness, and unawareness" of nonmembers had led to delays in referrals for surgical treatment and slowness in acquiring the necessary knowledge to care for scoliosis patients.

While the aforementioned scoliosis surgeons considered the ramifications of Harrington's inventions, Alan Dwyer, together with N. C. Newton and A. A. Sherwood of the Mater Misericordia Hospital in Sydney, Australia, published their results of anterior fusion.[21] After visiting Arthur Hodgson in Hong Kong, Dwyer devised a screw and cable system that could compress the convex side of a scoliotic deformity from the front. He found that anterior surgery was easier in a patient with scoliosis than in a patient whose spine had become deformed in the coronal plane by tuberculosis. In scoliosis patients whose spinal columns had shifted well to one side or the other, the spine was easily approached from the side of the convexity of the curve. In addition, the aorta and vena cava shifted into the concavity of the curve, and they could be retracted out of harm's way with little difficulty. Using his screw and cable system with tensioners and crimpers supplemented with multilevel diskectomies and interbody fusions, Dwyer successfully treated eight patients with scoliosis. In the words of John Hall, "Alan Dwyer did for anterior instrumentation what Paul Harrington had done for posterior." Dwyer's invention needed modification and reassessment, but the basic concept added a powerful new modality to scoliosis surgery.

When other orthopaedic surgeons began to perform Dwyer's anterior operation, they found that shortening the front of the spinal column resulted in lengthening the back of the spine. This did not cause much of a problem in the thorax, where the spine normally had that configuration; furthermore, scoliotic patients usually have a reversal of the normal thoracic alignment. Therefore, a system that corrected thoracic lordosis while correcting scoliosis provided a double benefit. In the lumbar spine, however, the tendency of the Dwyer system to produce kyphosis had adverse consequences. The lumbar spine must have a lordotic configuration for humans to maintain an upright bipedal posture. A reversal of lumbar lordosis forces a person to stand or sit like a quadruped. The Dwyer system tended to flatten the lumbar spine or even reverse the normal lordotic alignment, which traded the correction of the deformity in one plane for a deformity in another. With greater usage, the surgeons began to encounter problems with the cables and screws. They occasionally broke or dislodged, and the scarring and fibrosis resulting from the original anterior surgery obliterated the easily identifiable planes of the retroperitoneal space. Revision operations proved very difficult for that reason.

Manohar Panjabi and Augustus White[22] elevated spine surgery to a new level with the publication of their book *Clinical Biomechanics of the Spine* in 1978. Their text served as a benchmark for the application of physics and mechanical engineering to spinal deformities; subsequent efforts at treatment of scoliosis had to take into account the principles it discussed. The use of new systems intent on improving what Harrington and Dwyer had developed would require that inventors, manufacturers, and clinicians understand the mechanical principles of a new technique. In the early 1980s, Eduardo Luque[23] devised a system that corrected for several of the deficiencies of Harrington's original method. Harrington rods achieved correction of a spinal deformity primarily by exerting a traction force on the vertebrae at the upper and lower ends of a curve. Harrington's technique thus corrected a spinal curve as viewed in a front-to-back radiographic projection, but it did not take into account how the patient looked from the side (sagittally) or how much the vertebra had rotated in the axial plane. Harrington rods almost inevitably produced a "flat back" in the lumbar spine by straightening the patient's normal lumbar lordosis. In addition, Harrington rods worked well enough for severe curves, but less severe curves required transversely directed forces to achieve their best correction, not the powerful distraction of the Harrington system. Luque's methods seemed simple enough, indeed almost obvious. He passed flexible wires under each lamina and tied them to two metal rods, one on each side of the spinous processes. The rods also could be prebent to adjust to the level of correction deemed achievable. The Luque system thus did not use distraction, but depended on derotation and transverse forces to produce correction of the deformity, somewhat reminiscent of the method devised by Lange in 1910. The Luque method, however, required the surgeon to pass wires into and out of the spinal canal, a maneuver that placed the spinal cord at risk either by direct trauma or by the development of intraspinal hematomas. This occasionally resulted in paraplegia, and many surgeons expressed reluctance to use the Luque method for this reason. In fact, Denis Drummond,[24] then of the University of Wisconsin, modified the Luque concept by combining Harrington and Luque rods and tying the rods down to the spinous processes instead of directly to the lamina. The method produced distraction with some translation and derotation but not as powerfully as did the Luque sublaminar wire placement. However, it was safer.

In 1988, nearly 30 years after Harrington described his method of spinal deformity correction, three French surgeons—Cotrel, Dubousset, and Guillaumat—described a new technique.[25] Their system consisted of a series of pedicle and laminar hooks to insert into multiple levels on both the concave and convex sides of the curves. By using distraction on one side and compression on the other, their system straightened the deformity at multiple levels at once instead of at each end. By inserting blockers on the rod adjacent to the hooks, the correction could be maintained in the frontal plane, and by rotating the rod in the hooks, the rotational and sagittal misalignment also could be corrected. When the rods and hooks had finally been locked into place, a transverse loading device could connect the rods to create an extremely stable surgical construct. Cotrel, Dubousset, and others who used this system suggested that it provided such rigid support to the spine so that the patient would not need a brace postoperatively. The rigidity of the rods, hooks, and transverse loading would hold the spine solidly in place while a spinal fusion matured to maintain the correction permanently.

In the middle to late 1980s, a group of spine surgeons at the Texas Scottish Rite Hospital in Dallas developed a system that competed with the Cotrel-Dubousset assembly.[26-28] The Scottish Rite system featured different rod surfaces and offered different instrumentation, but it consisted essentially of the same segmental fixation on the concave and convex sides of the spinal deformity. Its early development was also different in that it incorporated the use of pedicle screws to achieve fixation of the spinal segment rather than relying solely on hooks and claws.

At the time that Luque, Cotrel, Dubousset, Ashman, and others worked on their modifications of the Harrington system, other surgeons did the same with Dwyer's anterior screw and cable system. A German surgeon, Klaus Zielke,[29] changed Dwyer's system by using a semiflexible rod instead of a cable and by using slotted screw heads instead of cannulated heads. These changes meant that a surgeon could prebend the rod slightly and drop it into the heads rather than thread it through the cannulations. In addition, Zielke's technique required posterior placement of the screws in the vertebral bodies to minimize the tendency to produce kyphosis in the lumbar spine. Most important, Zielke's technique provided for the application of an outrigger on each end of the rod and the use of derotation bars secured through the outrigger. By slowly twisting the derotator, the spine theoretically can be pulled into lordosis at the same time the deformity is corrected in the coronal plane. Both the Dwyer and Zielke systems included removal of the intervertebral disks and insertion of bone graft material into the disk spaces. Both of the surgeons also emphasized the importance of solid fusion and advocated using a brace until the fusion solidified.

The study of spinal deformity has included much more than devising ingenious ways to achieve correction of misaligned vertebrae with hooks and screws, rods, cables, braces, and electrical stimulation. In the past 50 years, many physicians and orthopaedic surgeons have also explored causation, natural history, prevention, early identification, and identification of spinal curves that will require surgical correction and fusion. Also, surgeons have sought ways to ensure intraoperative safety of children and adults with spinal cord monitoring or "wake-up tests" and have investigated methods for enhancing the rate of fusion by studying the biology of bone growth and repair.

In 1990, Gordon Robin, an orthopaedic surgeon from the Hadassah-Hebrew University Medical School in Jerusalem, published a 259-page book on the etiology of idiopathic scoliosis.[30] He stated that he had reviewed thousands of publications on the causation of spine curvatures in otherwise healthy children. He acknowledged the known causes such as polio, cerebral palsy, muscular dystrophy, myelomeningocele, congenital malformations, infections, tumors, and other recognizable entities. He also collated and summarized the available information regarding growth, genetics, neurology, biochemistry, and other disciplines, all without coming upon a single identifiable cause for the common "idiopathic" kinds of spinal curvature. In the book's conclusion, he favored "a functional abnormality in a neurologic content of posture, mainly related to the afferent side of the postural reflex system." The causes of spinal deformity in most children so afflicted therefore remain elusive.

Nevertheless, popular wisdom has dictated that physicians should recognize scoliosis in its earlier stages, presumably to start conservative treatment as soon as possible and to monitor young children who have early mild curves that might suddenly progress. The persuasive influence of motivated and articulate orthopaedic surgeons thus led to the organization of large-scale screening programs for school-aged children during the 1970s and 1980s.[31] School nurses, athletic trainers, pediatricians, family physicians, orthopaedic surgeons, and teachers have examined thousands of schoolchildren in many states and school districts. Typically, the examiners stood behind the upright child and looked at the bare back. The child then bent forward, and the examiner sighted along the bare back looking for rib humping or prominence of the paravertebral muscles on one side or the other. If a curvature was found, the examiner was supposed to report it to the child's pediatrician or an orthopaedic surgeon. School screening programs were often ineffective. Examiners tended to overdiagnose in fear of missing a problem, leading to many unnecessary referrals. A note from the child's school advising referral to an orthopaedic surgeon often needlessly alarmed parents, and unnecessary radiographs exposed children to radiation for no purpose. Furthermore, these efforts came at a time when the prevalence of scoliosis was declining. Many school districts questioned the expense and the cost-effectiveness of time-consuming programs that turned up so few affected individuals. Finally, the orthotic treatment of early curvatures has little appeal. Public health departments and school districts frequently decided that their scarce monetary resources would have a greater impact on public health if spent in other ways.

School screening did have the unintended benefit of providing an opportunity to study large numbers of children with scoliosis. John Lonstein and Martin Carlson[32] of St. Paul, Minnesota, reviewed 727 patients with idiopathic scoliosis in an effort to study the natural history of the condition and predict curve progression. They found that skeletal immaturity, curve location in the thoracic region, and curve severity correlated with rapid progression. Thus a young child with a tight, severe thoracic curve had a poor prognosis, which entailed significant progression of the curve. A physician should strongly consider prompt surgical treatment of such a child to prevent more severe deformity. Allowing a child to grow up with a severe thoracic deformity and permanent rib hump should bear heavily on the conscience of the child's physician, as this crooked appearance also correlates with progressively severe pulmonary disease. Individuals with rigid chest wall deformities have a diminished vital capacity and cannot take a deep breath. The compression of the lungs that these patients experience causes atelectasis, airway closure, hypoxemia, cor pulmonale, and reduced life span. Early surgical intervention can prevent the deformity and the chronic pulmonary disease. Indeed, in younger patients, the correction of the deformity can reverse it.

The question also arose as to what levels the surgeon should correct and fuse in treating the patient with a crooked spine. Howard King[33] of Seattle Children's Orthopaedic Hospital published a paper in *JBJS* that addressed this concern in 1983. His coauthors were John Moe, David Bradford, and Robert Winter of the Twin Cities Scoliosis Center. King defined five curve patterns that become the basis for making decisions regarding the selection of fusion levels. The curve patterns he and his coauthors described expanded on the classification system of Ponseti and Friedman of 1950 and an earlier system developed by John Moe. In King's classification, type 1 deformity consisted of an S-shaped curve in which both thoracic and lumbar curves crossed the midline and the lumbar curve was larger. Type 2 deformity also consisted of thoracic and lumbar curves that crossed the midline, but the thoracic curve was equal to or larger than the lumbar curve. Type 3 deformity consisted of the thoracic curve with a lumbar curve that did not cross the midline; type 4, a long thoracic curve; and type 5, a double thoracic curve. King and his associates analyzed the outcomes of 405 patients using this system, demonstrating that in type 2 curves, the surgeon can usually limit the fusion to the thoracic spine only, provided that the fusion ends in a neutral and stable vertebra. The other curve patterns require fusion of both curves, centering the lower level over the sacrum. Mild curves naturally do not require this level of surgical intervention.

Since the advent of Harrington's instrumentation procedures, scoliosis surgery has posed new risks for patients. The earlier Hibbs and Albee operations exposed patients to the hazards of preoperative correction such as pressure sores under the casts used to correct the deformity; children with respiratory insufficiency due to the thoracic deformity had additional chest wall restriction caused by the heavy body casts. Patients probably did not experience a great deal of blood loss with the earlier fusion methods when they were performed efficiently, and unless the surgeon made a terrible error intraoperatively, spinal cord injury or paraplegia were not major risk factors.

Harrington rods applied vigorous distraction to the spine and spinal cord. Also, heavy metal hooks passed over facet joints and laminae exposed the cord to greater risk of direct injury by the implants. Eduardo Luque's surgical method required that wires be passed under the laminae at multiple levels, and the Cotrel-Dubousset method and others like it exposed the cord to distraction and strong rotational forces. In an effort to forestall the potentially disastrous complications of postoperative paraplegia due to iatrogenic spinal cord injury, surgeons developed two strategies: the wake-up test and spinal cord monitoring. In his Harrington Lecture at the 1998 SRS annual meeting, John Hall gave the credit for the wake-up test to Pierre Stagnara. Stagnara was from Corsica but practiced in Lyon, France; Hall called him "the father of scoliosis treatment in France." In his book *Spinal Deformity*, Stagnara reported that 0.64 percent of patients who had corrective scoliosis surgery with Harrington rods before 1970 had severe spinal cord injury with paraplegia.[34] He autopsied one of those patients, finding complete necrosis of the upper thoracic and central necrosis of the lower spinal cord with thrombosis of the blood vessels in the affected segments. He wrote that intraoperatively he could not know if the distraction of the spine had injured the spinal cord, so he had to wait until the patient woke up. At that time, it was probably too late to do much about it. Later, while operating on another patient, Stagnara found that the anesthetist had not administered enough medication to keep the patient asleep; the patient began to move his hands and feet intraoperatively. Stagnara regarded this as a good indicator of continuing neural function of the spinal cord. He instructed the anesthetist to allow this to happen in subsequent cases, calling it the "wake-up test." He and others have acknowledged that rarely patients can self-extubate during surgery, but Stagnara regarded this as an acceptable risk. He said he could manage the problem by closing the incision quickly, turning the patient over, reintubating, returning the patient to a prone position, and continuing the operation. He felt that solid evidence of continuing spinal cord function was worth it.

Spinal cord monitoring with evoked potentials operates in one of two ways.[35-37] By using the somatosensory-evoked potentials (SSEPs), electroencephalographic responses in the brain are recorded through stimulation of sensory nerves in the upper and lower limbs. Motor-evoked potentials (MEPs) work the other way around. These require stimulation of the motor cortex of the brain with an electrical charge, and the recording of electromyographic activity in a muscle in the arm or leg. Both methods have gained general acceptance. SSEPs measure only dorsal column function and reveal little about possible motor function loss. Their sensitivity is fairly reliable, but false-positive results do occur. Thus, they have the potential to disrupt surgery frequently and unnecessarily. MEPs also have false-positive results about 20 percent of the time. They both require very light anesthesia, which may result in patient recall after the operation. Both SSEPs and MEPs diminish or disappear during periods of hypovolemia and hypotension intraoperatively. For these reasons, some surgeons have decided that they have less value than the wake-up test as devised by Stagnara in Lyon, but most scoliosis centers in the United States use spinal cord monitoring.

Bone Grafts and Bone Banks

Postoperatively, the patient and surgeon must work together to achieve successful healing and a solid bony fusion. The history of orthopaedics is replete with literature on bone fusions and how a surgeon can help facilitate them successfully. A solid fusion is the gold standard. Metal implants inevitably fatigue and break without it, causing the implants to loosen and then detach, which then leads to loss of correction of the deformity.

In attempting a spinal fusion, a surgeon uses sharp chisels, gouges, or osteotomes for elevating the involved cortical surfaces to expose the bleeding marrow beneath them. Usually the surgeon tries to overlap the fragments of bone generated by this process to bridge the gap between the vertebrae. Often this cannot be achieved without taking bone from another part of the body such as the iliac crest, ribs, or tibia. By cutting the bone into small fragments or by fashioning a large fragment into a spanning graft, the surgeon can create a large fusion mass of autogeneic bone, that is, bone derived from the patient and not another individual. Hibbs and Albee did their fusions this way, building on the experiences of earlier 19th-century surgeons and investigators such as Heine in 1836, Fluorens in 1842, Ollier in 1858, and others. P. von Walther performed the first free autogeneic bone graft in a human patient in 1820.

Subsequent laboratory and clinical investigations have established a biologic model of how the human body can transform a bed of bone chips into a massive sheet of rigid bone extending multiple spinal levels. Gary Friedlaender[38] of the Department of Orthopaedics and Rehabilitation at Yale University described this in a Current Concepts Review in *JBJS* in 1987. Apparently almost all of the bone cells in the graft die except for a few cells in the periosteum or very close to the surface of the graft that are kept alive from the hematoma about the fragments. The death of these cells initiates an inflammatory reaction, which in a few days results in the development of highly vascularized fibrous tissue as part of the healing process. This "fibrovascular stroma" carries newly formed blood vessels from the recipient bed to the bone fragments, bringing the necessary cells to the fragments to remove the dead bone and replace it with new bone. The graft itself has qualities that promote "osteoconduction" and "osteoinduction," two words that appear regularly in journal articles and on board examinations. Osteoconduction means that the graft provides a scaffold upon which new bone forms, and osteoinduction means that the bone actually induces the formation of new bone on the scaffold.

As the process continues, blood vessels rapidly invade the bone through the haversian canals in the graft fragments, bringing large cells with multiple nuclei (osteoclasts) to digest and remove the preexisting bone matrix and mineral crystals. The marrow of the donor supplies these cells from so-called hematopoietic stem cells precursors, that is, the same cells that give rise to blood-forming cells in the marrow.

As the osteoclasts digest and remove the bone fragments in the fusion bed, other primitive cells surrounding the invading blood vessels begin to differentiate into osteoblasts, which form new bone. The processes of removing old bone and depositing new bone overlap. During this time, the fusion mass has little structural strength, but as bone deposition accelerates, the mass of bone chips transforms itself into a homogeneous and increasingly solid sheet of bone. As time goes on, even over several years, the fusion remodels in response to the stresses placed upon it (Wolff's law). The soft bone mass develops surprising strength and structural integrity. The patient therefore no longer needs the metal support to maintain correction.

Many investigators studied the progression of this process over the years, but they did not develop a basic understanding of why these events occurred until fairly recently. Marshall Urist[39,40] conceived the idea of a bone morphogenetic protein (BMP) in the 1960s. He concluded that osteoinduction occurs in response to the production of proteins by cells genetically programmed to do so under certain conditions. When these conditions are right, undifferentiated cells will produce BMP, which is actually one of several growth factors necessary for the process to proceed successfully. Others subsequently described are transforming growth factor-β(TGF-β), which induces cells to synthesize collagen and proteoglycan, which in turn forms the organic matrix of bone. Other growth factors such as insulin growth factor-2 (IGF-2) control synthesis of collagen and cartilage matrix, and platelet-derived growth factor (PDGF) controls in part the initial inflammatory reaction about the bone graft.

Urist was born in Chicago in 1914. He earned degrees from the University of Michigan, University of Chicago, and Johns Hopkins. His residency training was at Hopkins for a short time and for a year at the Baltimore Children's Hospital before the doctors' draft sent him to England and Germany during World War II. After the war, he finished his residency at Massachusetts General Hospital under Smith-Petersen. Urist then moved to the West Coast and began research into bone formation at UCLA. He spent most of his working life on this. By the mid-1970s, he began work on the identification of the discrete protein within demineralized bone matrix, which he believed would act as an inducer of bone formation. He eventually identified the role of the protein (BMP) in the bone formation cascade in fracture healing and in bone graft incorporation into spinal fusion sites.

Surgeons often have trouble obtaining enough autogenous bone from patients who do not have enough in their vertebrae, pelvis, ribs, or tibia for a very large fusion mass. Sometimes long and severe spinal curves require both anterior and posterior fusions, thus calling for more bone than a patient can provide for an autograft. In these situations, the autogenous bone grafts may need to be supplemented with allografts (some surgeons use allografts only). The same general biologic responses follow the placement of allografts into a fusion as with autografts. An immediate inflammatory reaction precedes the elaboration of a highly vascular fibrous matrix around the allograft fragments. The surgeon hopes that the invasion of the allograft by the matrix will allow bone resorption and deposition to proceed uneventfully. The allograft, however, activates a host-donor inflammatory response through activation of the patient's histocompatibility genes. If the incompatibility is great enough, the patient's body may isolate the bone graft with elaboration of a dense fibrous tissue envelope about it or, alternatively, the graft may resorb and disappear. The initiation of the immunogenic response to the allograft depends not only on protein foreign to the host on the cell membranes but also in the collagen and proteoglycan of the bone. Therefore, even if all of the allograft cells are washed away, the graft retains its immunogenic properties as far as the host is concerned. Inevitably, allografts do not function as well as autografts and take longer to be incorporated into a fusion because of the host-donor inflammatory reaction. In addition, allografts in humans do not act osteoinductively. They serve only as a scaffold for the development of new bone made by the invading host cells into the allograft and function only as an osteoconductive trellis for the laying down of new host bone.

Despite the disadvantages, the use of allografts has expanded greatly. Obtaining, sterilizing, storing, and distributing human allografts has grown into an industry that serves not only scoliosis surgeons but also tumor specialists and surgeons who perform major total joint revisions.

There are now approximately 200 tissue banks in the United States, which supply about 250,000 allografts annually to surgeons for use in orthopaedic applications.

Spine surgeons now generally regard the use of allografts as quite safe, but several serious transmissions of donor disease occurred in the past. In 1954, Ned Shutkin[41] reported the transmission of hepatitis B to a Yale undergraduate who had received frozen tissue from a bone bank. In 1988, the Centers for Disease Control and Prevention[42] reported that a patient in New Jersey contracted the human immunodeficiency virus from bone taken from another patient who later died of acquired immunodeficiency syndrome. These and other episodes prompted regulations that require close supervision of procurement and storage.

Tissue donor programs have led to the development of teams available to harvest organs and tissues under sterile conditions in numerous hospitals around the country. In the case of bone tissue, removal of marrow and other cellular elements must precede final sterilization and storage.[43,44] Sterilization with gamma irradiation changes the physical properties of bone, making it unacceptably brittle; currently, most tissue banks use ethylene oxide instead. The bone banks store bone by either freezing or freeze-drying it. Freeze-drying makes it possible to use it at room temperature, an advantage when the surgeon needs allograft in a hurry. Otherwise, the operating room team has to thaw the bone before the surgeon can use it, and sometimes this lengthens the procedure by a fair amount of time.

Spine

In 1976, about 10 years after Moe and his associates convened the SRS, Harper and Row Publishers started a new journal called *Spine*. Henry LaRocca from New Orleans accepted the position of editor-in-chief. Spine has since had several editors-in-chief and a large editorial board. The SRS now recognizes *Spine* as its official journal. A review of this journal's contents during the past few years highlights the directions that scoliosis research and treatment have taken. *Spine*, is currently published by Lippincott Williams & Wilkins (a subsidiary of Wolters Kluwer, Amsterdam). James Weinstein is editor-in-chief, aided by 140 senior, deputy, and associate editors. A typical table of contents in recent years lists more than 100 entries under the heading of scoliosis. These reflect an extraordinary variety of interests that scoliosis researchers and clinicians have developed: video-assisted thoracoscopic surgery for anterior fusions of the dorsal spine, new classifications systems, meta-analyses of the literature on various issues related to scoliosis, new fixation technology, outcomes analyses, research into the causation of idiopathic scoliosis, and studies of scoliosis along with other diseases and conditions. In his presidential address before the SRS in 2002, Alvin Crawford discussed the future of the society. His remarks, later published in *Spine*, included a discussion of the numeric distribution of spine cases and the declining number of operations for correction of scoliosis. He reported that in 1999, there were 430,000 spinal fusions for disk degeneration worldwide and an additional 300,000 diskectomies without a fusion. He noted that 900 surgeons did more than 10 scoliotic fusions that year and that 1,500 surgeons did fewer than 10. Also, the most common CPT code used by the members of SRS was that of a laminectomy.

Disk Degeneration: Schmorl, Mixter, Barr, and Others

In 1925, Georg Schmorl[45] of Dresden embarked on a massive study of the human spine. He was a distinguished pathologist in the medical school there, with access to a remarkable volume of autopsy material. He removed entire spines in more than 12,000 postmortems, conducting detailed examinations. The project led to the publication of, *Die Gesunde und Kranke Wirbelsäule in Röntgenbild und Klinik* (*The Human Spine in Health and Disease*). Schmorl's research covered virtually every abnormality of the spinal column, including the study of intervertebral disks. After close scrutiny, he described the effect of aging on intervertebral disks, noting how the disk dehydrates, becomes fibrillar, and loses its resiliency. He recognized these findings as normal and part of the aging process. Schmorl also described how the degenerating disk prolapses, that is, how the material at the center of the disk finds its way into abnormal locations. His photographs and radiographs established the fact that the contents of the disk can and do break through the cartilage and bone of a vertebral end plate to herniate into the substance of vertebral bodies. These lesions are easily visible on a radiograph and today are called "Schmorl's nodes." He also noted that disk prolapses can occur in either forward or backward directions. When the disk prolapses anteriorly, it often produces a "marginal infraction," in which disk material pushes through the anterior or anterolateral edge of the rim of the vertebral body to lodge under the anterior longitudinal ligament. This produces a characteristic radiographic appearance, and Schmorl did not think a disk prolapse in this direction caused symptoms. Alternatively, the anterior anulus occasionally pulls away from the vertebral ring anteriorly, leading to increased distraction forces on the insertion of the anterior longitudinal ligament. The tension on the insertion of the ligament just above and below the level of the disk causes ossification and formation of bony spurs in these locations. Schmorl called this condition "spondylosis deformans."

Schmorl's chapter on disk degeneration and prolapse also described posterior herniation of disk material. Schmorl credited H. Luschka as the first to describe posterior prolapse of an intervertebral disk. Luschka reported on this condition in 1850.

Included in Schmorl's book are descriptions of posterior and posterolateral fissuring affecting the anulus. When fissuring has progressed sufficiently, it could permit prolapse of the contents of the disk back into the spinal canal, the recess, or the intervertebral foramen. Schmorl believed that this degree of disk prolapse could cause symptoms but stated that the symptoms most certainly resulted from aging, degeneration, and the stresses of everyday life. He did not think that the prolapses resulted from a specific injury.

Schmorl's work, complete with his extensive analysis of the autopsies of more than 12,000 human spines, gave the orthopaedic world an enormous amount of essential information. The problem for American orthopaedic surgeons, however, was that it was in German and no one had translated it. No one, that is, until Joseph Barr.

Barr began practicing orthopaedics in Boston around the beginning of the Great Depression. He was born in Ohio and attended that state's College of Worcester, but he came to Boston for a medical education. He graduated from Harvard with an MD and got his orthopaedic training at Boston Children's Hospital and Massachusetts General Hospital. He went into practice with Frank Ober, a well-known orthopaedic surgeon in Boston. Barr found that he had some time on his hands, however, and wanted to spend it reading Schmorl's book. Deterred by the German, he enrolled in a Berlitz course in order to understand Schmorl's work in its original language. At that time, Barr apparently also had become interested in the conundrum that certain spinal cord "tumors" contained no cells. He reviewed all of the slides of these cases on file in the pathology laboratories at Massachusetts General Hospital and found that they nearly all had the same characteristics as intervertebral disk tissue. Now armed with the experience of reading Schmorl's descriptions of posterior disk prolapses, Barr realized that the lesions removed in surgery were not chondromas or another other kind of tumor, but were, in fact, posteriorly prolapsed intervertebral disks.

Barr and his surgical associate, William J. Mixter, prepared a paper about the removal of disks from the spines of 19 patients. Mixter performed the surgery, but Barr reviewed and analyzed the slides. The Boston medical community expressed doubts about permitting a presentation, but eventually the New England Surgical Society relented. Mixter and Barr later published a paper in the *New England Journal of Medicine* in 1934,[46] acknowledging Schmorl's book and giving credit to Joel Goldthwait[47] of Boston as well as to G. S. Middleton and J. H. Teacher[48] of Glasgow. Barr and Mixter also cited Walter Dandy's article on "Loose Cartilage from Intervertebral Disk Simulating Tumor of the Spinal Cord," published in 1929. They definitively showed that disk herniations were not tumors and that removing them could relieve pain (in their series, 12 of 19 patients).

Barr went on to a distinguished career at Harvard. During World War II, he spent four years at Bethesda Naval Hospital, where he was Chief of Orthopaedics. Shortly after he returned to civilian life, he was appointed Chairman of Orthopaedics at Harvard, replacing the legendary Smith-Petersen. He served in that capacity for more than 15 years and died in 1964. His son, Joseph S. Barr, Jr., currently practices at Massachusetts General Hospital.

Most American orthopaedic surgeons regarded the Mixter and Barr paper of 1934 an essential breakthrough, a seminal contribution that established an entirely new field of surgery. Barr, however, was a relatively quiet and unassuming man; he might have difficulty comprehending the world of disk surgery today

In 1944, ten years after Mixter and Barr published their paper, Alan DeForest Smith of the New York Orthopaedic Hospital, together with Edwin Deery and George Hagman, published a review of 100 patients with herniation of the nucleus pulposus treated surgically.[49] Deery, a neurosurgeon, performed diskectomies in the lumbar spine in all 100 patients, and Smith performed fusions in 85 of them. Smith reported that all of the patients who underwent fusion had instability at the disk levels in question, basing this diagnosis on radiographic evidence of "asymmetrical lateral articulations, anterior or posterior displacement of the fifth lumbar vertebra, exaggeration of the lumbosacral angle, a thin intervertebral disk, and a transitional or partly sacralized lumbosacral vertebra." Smith reported that 83 percent of these patients had good to excellent results.

Smith's published paper was presented at a national meeting, and several members discussed it. One of these was Joseph S. Barr. He challenged the assertion of the radiographic diagnosis of instability and recalled a paper by Carl Badgley that had compared these "abnormalities" in asymptomatic and symptomatic patients. Badgley reported that the symptomatic and asymptomatic patients had the same incidence of these findings. Barr implied that he did not think fusion was necessary most of the time. He changed his mind, however, and stated in 1947: "The thesis that every patient should have a spine fusion done at the time of laminectomy is tenable."[50]

Clearly, eminent and authoritative surgeons disagreed on important aspects of the treatment of back pain. As interest in lumbar disk surgery increased after World War II, surgeons began to realize that they could not explain the variation in results of surgery. Some patients did very well, whereas others with similar diagnoses and similar kinds of treatment did not. These conflicting results stimulated investigations on several fronts. Carl Hirsch and Alf Nachemson of the Karolinska Institute in Stockholm, for example, conducted several studies on the mechanics of intervertebral disks. They found that normal disks respond differently to static and dynamic loads; that disk pressures vary with standing, sitting, and leaning forward; and that the normal disk behaves hydrostatically. Carl Hirsch and S. Friberg[51] conducted an analysis of 15,000 patients with back pain, correlating their findings with additional studies of hundreds of necropsy spines of the lumbosacral articulation. Their findings, published in a series of classic papers, indicated that disk degeneration begins early (in some individuals, in the second or third decade) and progresses inevitably with dehydration of the nucleus, fragmentation of the anulus, and prolapse of nuclear material into the anulus (often through it). Hirsch postulated that tears in the anulus produced inflammatory tissue which brought fine pain fibers into the outermost layers of the degenerating anulus. These mediated the pain response.[52-55]

Other investigators studied patient responses to pain stimuli and devised pain questionnaires and tests to classify them. As a result, a physician's assessment of the patient with back pain not only includes taking the history but also examining the patient's range of motion, reflexes, strength, circulation, sensation, and responses to sciatic nerve stretch tests. It also can include evaluation of the Waddell signs, Short Form-36, pain questionnaires, Oswestry Low Back Pain Disability Questionnaire, the McGill Pain Questionnaire, the Frymoyer multiattribute utility model, the Minnesota Multiphasic Personality Inventory, and others.[56-61]

In evaluating patients with back, neck, and extremity pain, physicians have increasingly relied on the imaging modalities such as plain radiographs, myelography, CT, and more recently MRI. Ernest Schmidt,[62] a radiologist from Denver, published one of the first articles on myelography in American literature in 1926, some eight years before Mixter and Barr's paper on diskectomy. In fact, myelography had achieved wide acceptance during that time, and Mixter and Barr used a myelogram to demonstrate that their patient did, in fact, have a herniated disk. Schmidt reported that Sicard and Forestier, two French radiologists, developed a technique of myelography by injecting an iodized oil into the cisterna magna or into the lumbar spine. The injected material, which they called lipiodal, had a high specific gravity and would pass rapidly from the cisterna down to the lumbar spine when the patient was placed in an upright position. Because of its high iodine content (40 percent by weight) it was radiopaque, and any mass in the spinal canal such as a tumor or herniated disk would create a defect in the column of dye visible on a radiograph. Schmidt acknowledged some reports of lipiodal toxicity and said that every patient developed at least a transient aseptic meningitis. It was therefore important for patients to remain in the sitting position in bed for a week after being injected. At the end of that time, local inflammation in the cauda equina would have fixed the lipiodal in that location, from which it would slowly resorb over a period of months. Occasionally, however, the mass of lipiodal in the low back caused considerable discomfort. Schmidt had to remove it from one patient by performing a laminectomy and draining it from the cauda equina under direct vision. Wayne Sharpe and Carl Peterson[63] of New York described a similar complication in *JBJS* in 1926. They found that a block in the middorsal spine in one of their patients had prevented lipiodal from running down into the cauda equina. The patient reported severe midback pain, and at a subsequent laminectomy, globules of encysted lipiodal were found enmeshed in "numerous newly formed adhesions." They advised against its use thereafter and recommended air myelograms instead.

Despite the problems encountered with myelography, orthopaedic surgeons and radiologists had few other imaging options for more than 40 years. Water-soluble contrast media replaced the oil-based media in the 1970s. Patients, however, still risked allergic reactions with their use; since the advent of MRI, myelography has less applicability in the diagnosis of spinal disorders. In the late 1980s and early 1990s, radiology texts touted CT myelography, but with improvements in MRI technology, invasive procedures such as myelography essentially have been abandoned. An axial view of the spine, created with CT, can show bony structures in great detail, but the spinal cord, nerve roots, and soft-tissue lesions in the spinal canal require contrast material to make them visible. In reviewing the history of spine imaging, CT and myelography appear to have been widely used only until MRI became widely available.

CT became commercially available in 1973 and was the best imaging modality available for about 10 years until MRI scanners came to the market. It is interesting that the technology, manufacturing, and marketing of CT scanners developed as rapidly as it did. CT's expeditious launch was made possible with backing from Electrical Musical Instrument, a British firm funded by the investments of John Lennon, Paul McCartney, George Harrison, and Ringo Starr.[64] The Beatles made a bet on the technology of computerized scans and profited greatly as a result.

Fifty years after William Conrad Roentgen discovered the x-ray, physicists at Harvard and Stanford, working independently, published papers on nuclear magnetic resonance.[65,66] Their discoveries, made almost simultaneously in 1946, earned a joint award of the Nobel Prize for physics in 1952. Felix Block of Stanford and Edward Purcell of Harvard demonstrated resonance absorption of radiofrequency energy by magnetic nuclei in the magnetic field. Their contribution to physics led to an application of nuclear magnetic resonance to investigation of the properties of matter in virtually all its forms and to the assessment of the parameters of magnetic fields in radiofrequencies that would elicit the nuclear resonance. By 1976, both Block and Purcell used nuclear magnetic resonance to evaluate magnetic resonance on parts of their own bodies (Block, a finger; and Purcell, his head). By the late 1970s, the science and technology of nuclear magnetic imaging had improved to an extraordinary degree, making it possible to generate images of remarkable resolution and tissue discrimination. During the mid-1980s, MRI scanners came into the market in very large numbers; thousands of hospitals in the United States acquired them by the early 1990s. The technology continues to advance: improved software, developments of new pulse sequences, and refined applications of MRI to molecular biology will eventually reduce the importance of radiographs, CT, and other imaging modalities. The manufacturers have claimed that MRI scanner obsolescence should be slow because software can be altered without changing the hardware. MRI enthusiasts claim the advantages of the technology are so great that Roentgen's x-ray may not be needed for diagnostic purposes in the future.

Diskectomies

Surgical intervention for a patient with degenerative disk disease should take place only after a serious effort with nonsurgical treatment. The classic article demonstrating the wisdom of this approach was written by Weber in 1983.[67] Weber reviewed the results of treating a large group of patients with both surgical and nonsurgical modalities over a ten-year period. He found that at the end of ten years there were no differences in the outcomes overall between surgical and nonsurgical therapies.

Furthermore, from the time of onset of symptoms, most patients recovered within a period of 6 weeks. Thus, most individuals get better without surgery, and ten years after the onset of symptoms the results are the same with or without an operation. Weber suggested that a surgical procedure would be successful if it shortened the time of disability and alleviated the patient's pain more quickly. Nevertheless, many patients whose symptoms related to disk degeneration did not improve with nonsurgical therapy; for those patients, Weber concluded that surgical treatment is a reasonable option. The problem then becomes what kind of operation to perform. The formal open procedure by Mixter was a laminectomy or hemilaminectomy with retraction of lumbar roots or cauda equina and removal of the herniated disk. Mixter also performed durotomies on some of his patients to gain access to disk fragments. This operation, as described by Barr, required aggressive subperiosteal stripping of the erector spinae and multifidus muscles, along with removing a large amount of bone.

Nearly 40 years ago, Lyman Smith began to treat patients who had painful degenerated lumbar disks with intradiskal injection of chymopapain.[68] He based the procedure on studies done by E. F. Jansen and A. K. Dowes, as well as by Louis D. Thomas. They found that a plant enzyme from papayas had a chondrolytic effect on animals; rabbits' ears, for example, droop after being injected with it. With bigger doses, joint cartilage and bronchial cartilages also dissolve. Smith thought that injecting the enzyme into disk spaces could facilitate removal of the disk and conducted a study in dogs that proved his theory. Smith performed the procedure on a patient for the first time in 1963. He called the operation "chemonucleolysis." The U.S. Food and Drug Administration (FDA) then required a multicenter trial before the procedure could be approved for general use; it took place in the mid-1970s. Complications such as anaphylaxis and spinal cord injuries plagued the use of chymopapain, however, and the FDA-supervised trials showed little effectiveness. The FDA withdrew its approval for the use of chymopapain, prompting American patients to travel to Canada for the procedure. In 1979, the manufacturers of chymopapain and physicians interested in using it tried again. They changed the formula and dose, renaming it chymodactin. A new randomized, double-blind FDA-approved study showed the drug to be safe and demonstrated a 93 percent success rate. In the early and mid-1980s, the AAOS and the American Association of Neurologic Surgeons sponsored courses that taught more than 6,000 orthopaedists and neurosurgeons how to use the drug. Despite the best efforts of the leaders of the two specialties, serious neurologic complications still occurred in 46 of 120,000 patients, and the drug was again modified.

Relatively few surgeons now use chymopapain in the treatment of patients with back and leg pain caused by lumbar disk degeneration. Even with scant use, members of the Intradiscal Therapy Society, organized by Smith, E. J. Nordby,[69] and others, still present papers on the subject.

Other physicians have investigated ways to remove disk material using various kinds of percutaneous probes. Jeffrey and Joel Saal,[70] specialists in physiatry and rehabilitation medicine, developed a procedure they called "intradiscal thermal annuloplasty" in the mid-1990s and labeled it the IDET procedure. They used a flexible radiofrequency catheter threaded through a cannula inserted into a degenerated disk. By careful fluoroscopic guidance, they manipulated the catheter into a position in which they could heat the degenerated tissue to approximately 80°C, well above that required to denature protein. Presumably, the fine thin pain fibers that mediated the pain response also would be denatured and become unable to function, thereby helping to relieve the patient's symptoms. Peter Ascher of Graz, Austria, and Daniel Choy,[71] a New York internist, tried the same kind of treatment using lasers of various wavelengths. The IDET procedure and laser disk decompression have not achieved wide acceptance, although the originators of these operations report reasonable results in large numbers of patients.

Intradiskal surgery with mechanical devices has produced similar outcomes. Parvis Kambin[72] of Philadelphia developed a technique for arthroscopic microdiskectomy in the mid-1970s. This required the placement of an endoscope percutaneously into the disk space under fluoroscopic control and resection of disk material, usually using a two-portal technique. Kambin's indications for this procedure did not include treating patients with sequestered disk fragments or spinal stenosis. About the same time, Gary Onik[73] and J. C. Maroon, both of Pittsburgh, began using a nuclear probe that consisted of a suction device with rotating blade at the tip of a probe inserted into the disk. As the blade rotated, it removed disk material and pulled it into the cannula so that a continuous in-and-out saline infusion would remove it from the disk space.

Each of the percutaneous procedures, chemonucleolysis, thermal annuloplasty, arthroscopic microdiskectomy, and automated percutaneous lumbar diskectomy, have either been abandoned or are used by relatively few surgeons. All of them are limited to use in patients with contained disks, that is, disks that have not ruptured through the posterior longitudinal ligament into the spinal canal. Thus, they are performed in those patients most likely to recover spontaneously without surgery, making the results of the procedure difficult to evaluate.

The extensive dissection and wide laminectomy described by Mixter and Barr are no longer applicable for most patients with disk herniations. Surgeons now routinely perform diskectomies using loupes or an operating microscope, which allows much smaller incisions. Robert W. Williams,[74] a neurosurgeon from Las Vegas, published one of the early papers on microdiskectomy in 1978. The technique he described permitted complete decompression of a lumbar nerve root through a midline incision one inch long. Using a 400-mm lens to magnify the dura, nerve root, and disk, he reported that he achieved "satisfactory results" in 91 percent of his patients. A microdiskectomy, however, is not applicable to patients with severe degenerative changes, spinal stenosis, or those who require fusions.

Fusions for Lumbar Disk Degeneration

The indications for spinal fusions in patients with degenerative disk disease remain elusive. Most orthopaedists accept isthmic spondylolisthesis with pars interarticularis defects as a suitable reason to stabilize the spine in symptomatic patients, but that condition does not really signify a problem with the disk itself. Leon Wiltse convincingly defined pars defects as fatigue fractures in 1975 in the paper he published in *JBJS* with E. H. Waddell and D. W. Jackson.[75] Patients with mild forward displacement of the L4 vertebra on L5 associated with proven disk degeneration at that level might also qualify for fusions, and patients who have had wide decompression with removal of the facet joints might subsequently slip at the affected levels unless the surgeon stabilizes the vertebra. However, further definition of instability remains difficult. Nevertheless, performing spinal fusion in patients who appear to have pain because of disk degeneration has become commonplace recently.

The surgeons performing these fusions have deviated considerably from the basic Hibbs decortication and overlapping of bone graft derived locally from the laminae. The modern surgeon who has decided on a fusion can select from a wide range of possible techniques. After World War II, most American orthopaedic surgeons continued to rely on some variation of the Hibbs technique. This came to include fusions between laminae, across the posterior facet joints, with the placing of bone grafts over the transverse processes. In the mid-1950s, surgeons of the Hospital for Special Surgery (HSS) in New York devised the Wilson plate as an adjunctive internal fixator for spinal fusions (Figure 37). It consisted of a flat Vitallium plate, shaped to conform to the lordosis of the lumbar or cervical spines, with screw holes placed to permit transfixion of the plate to the spinous processes. Spine surgeons at HSS used the Wilson plate to supplement the spinal fusion they performed on John F. Kennedy in 1954,[76] but a severe surgical wound infection complicated the procedure and necessitated removal of the plate. Plates and screws did not gain wide acceptance thereafter for about 30 years.

During his many years of practice, Ralph Cloward conceived of and developed several instruments, surgical approaches, and techniques for spine surgery, including posterior lumbar interbody fusion (PLIF). Cloward,[77-80] a neurosurgeon who subsequently became better known for his anterior cervical fusions, was one of the first American surgeons to attempt PLIF in the lumbar spine in 1946; his first published paper on the subject appeared in a symposium on PLIF in *Clinical Orthopaedics and Related Research* in 1985.[79] Cloward's technique consisted of a partial removal of the lamina, wide spreading of the remaining parts of the lamina with a distractor, retraction of the cauda equina, and aggressive and complete disk removal with impaction of a large piece of bone into the disk space. Cloward recommended that certain operations for symptoms related to disk degeneration should be eliminated and replaced by PLIF, including simple diskectomy, decompressive laminectomy, and chemonucleolysis.

Cloward was not an orthopaedic surgeon, but he had a profound effect on the orthopaedists who practiced spine surgery. He did his medical training, including his neurosurgical residency, in Chicago. He moved to Honolulu, where he remained for the rest of his life. Cloward developed a huge practice in Hawaii, devoted mostly to spine surgery. He and his family reportedly occupied a beachfront estate at the tip of Diamond Head, from which they watched the Japanese attack on Pearl Harbor on the morning of December 7, 1941.

Philadelphian Paul Lin, also a neurosurgeon, was one of the spine surgeons who adopted Cloward's PLIF methodology. In 1983, Lin and associates[81] reported that they had performed 465 of these procedures, stating that over a ten-year period they obtained satisfactory results in 82 percent of patients, with an 88 percent satisfactory fusion rate. PLIF, as defined by Cloward and Lin, carried a considerable risk of complications. Lin and others reported neurologic deficits, graft dislodgement, failures of fusion, excessive bleeding, and other problems with the procedure. Arthur Steffee,[82] an orthopaedic surgeon from Cleveland, proposed to minimize these complications by supplementing the PLIF with rigid internal fixation by placing plates across the PLIF and securing them to the vertebrae with screws through the plates and into the pedicles and vertebral bodies. In writing about this procedure, Steffee acknowledged the work of H. H. Boucher,[83] who had attempted to stabilize lumbar spine segments by placing screws across the facet joints and into the pedicles. Steffee modified Boucher's operation by putting the screws all the way through the pedicles and into the vertebral bodies to secure the plates to the vertebrae. Steffee's procedure had broad appeal for many spine surgeons, who started to use it during the late 1980s and early 1990s. Initially, Steffee suggested that the plates and screws had their best use in stabilizing PLIF, but in his later reports he did not imply that. Instead, the Steffee system could stand on its own to support unstable spine segments until the posterior fusion on the lamina and transverse processes had time enough to consolidate. The wide popularity of Steffee's plates and screws led to the formation of a corporation to manufacture and market them. The success of this effort led to modification of Steffee's system by others. His plates, for example, were replaced by rods. The companies that manufactured these devices competed over the shape of the screw heads, the design of the screws, the metallurgy of the rods, and many other features.

The Spine Societies

In 1974, a group of orthopaedic surgeons established a new society to investigate the lumbar spine.[84] Harold Farfan, a Canadian; Leon Wiltse of the United States; and Alan Dwyer of Australia were the prime movers of the organization they named the International Society for the Study of the Lumbar Spine (ISSLS). They convened the first formal meeting of ISSLS in Longueville, near Montreal, with 71 surgeons in attendance. Their group was open to a very limited membership, and its stated purpose was "to serve as a forum for an exchange of information of both investigative and clinical nature which relates to low back pain and disability." Henry LaRocca was a founding member and the first secretary. A year earlier, he had been instrumental in establishing *Spine*, a journal devoted to spine research, which has remained in publication ever since as the official journal of the ISSLS and several other spine societies. ISSLS also established the Volvo Award for excellence in spine research and published a book, *The Lumbar*

Spine, which has had three editors over several editions: Stuart Weinstein, Samuel Wiesel, and Harry Herkowitz.

ISSLS became so important to low back surgeons that many wanted to join. In 1978, David Selby, Charles Ray, William Kirkaldy-Willis, Charles Burton, and others met in Excelsior, Minnesota, to establish a committee that would invite the ISSLS to support a North American spine organization. However, the effort failed. Several years later, Selby, with Vert Mooney, Mark Brown, Charles Burton, Alan Dwyer, Kenneth Heithoff, William Kirkaldy-Willis, Casey Lee, John McCulloch, Robert Watkins, Arthur White, and Leon Wiltse, gathered at a meeting of the AAOS to found the North American Spine Association. This group held its first meeting in Vail, Colorado, in 1984; approximately 175 individuals attended. Meanwhile, another group, headed by Robert Morrow, was attempting to create another organization, which they called the American College of Spine Surgeons. Members of both groups realized the benefit of joining forces and in 1985 they formed the North American Spine Society (NASS). NASS has become a very large organization of more than 4,000 members and attracts thousands of registrants at its annual meeting. NASS, too, has started its own periodical, *Spine Journal*. Its meetings and publications provide forums for orthopaedic surgeons and others to present their research and clinical studies.

As the organization able to bring the largest number of spine surgeons together in one location, NASS has the privilege and obligation of serving as a conduit for important information regarding spine surgery. The proceedings of recent meetings indicate that the membership has studied and reported upon all of the matters discussed previously as well as several items that have not been mentioned. For example, a group of NASS members have for the past few years engaged in treating painful compression fractures in elderly and osteoporotic individuals with methacrylate or bioactive hydrogels injected into compressed vertebral bodies through the pedicle of the vertebra. This procedure, known as kyphoplasty and/or vertebroplasty, can restore vertebral height and provide remarkable pain relief. Heretofore, such patients could only take narcotics and lie in as much extension as possible during the time it took for the fracture to heal.[85-87] The recent proceedings of NASS meetings also include papers on minimal access surgery, spinal infection, bracing strategies, annular repairs, gene therapy of disk degeneration, use of BMP as an adjunct to fusion, and the use of electrical stimulation of bone formation in fusion surgery. These issues could assume great importance and become the basis for major new developments.

The Pedicle Screw Lawsuits

During the early years of these societies, AcroMed, Synthes, Sofamor Danek, and other manufacturers of spinal instruments and implants worked closely with orthopaedic surgeons to provide the highest quality care to their spine patients. Studies of the efficacy of the use of bone screws in the pedicle of the back, plates, rods, and the instruments used to insert them were reviewed at meetings of NASS, SRS, the American Association of Neurological Surgeons (AANS), AAOS, and other meetings, along with other cutting edge treatments. During these discussions, it was noted that the FDA had not yet cleared the use of bone screws in the pedicle for marketing, although many considered such use to be state of the art.

At the 1992 meeting of NASS, reporters and lawyers interviewed several attendees; shortly thereafter, a prime-time exposé was aired on the television program "60 Minutes." Disgruntled patients with unsatisfactory outcomes were interviewed on the show. Plaintiffs' lawyers solicited clients unhappy with their spine surgery who filed thousands of lawsuits against the 24 companies that manufactured pedicle screws, including AcroMed, Smith & Nephew, and SofomorDanek. In addition, in a unique twist of legal theory, the societies that had offered continuing medical education courses covering the techniques of pedicle screw use were also brought into the litigation. In all, the AAOS and the other medical socieities were named as defendants in over 500 cases around the country, which were then consolidated with 3500 other pedicle screw cases for handling by Judge Louis Bechtle of the U.S. Court for the Eastern District of Pennsylvania.

In 1994, the FDA reclassified hooks, rods, and other posterior fixation and anterior screw and cable fixation systems. The agency also granted a 510(k) medical device exemption to Sofamor Danek to evaluate the use of pedicle screw systems in several spondylolisthesis fusions.

In 1997, AcroMed announced that it had created a $100 million fund to resolve all claims against it, its distributors, and all the surgeons who used their system of pedicle screw and plate fixation. By 1998, most of the issues had wound their way through the courts with resolutions mostly favorable to the defendants. In 1999, Judge Bechtel dismissed virtually all of these complaints for lack of subject matter jurisdiction and all claims of conspiracy and fraud. AAOS spent more than $1.6 million defending itself against these claims, although in the end the Academy and the other medical societies were removed defendants in all of them.

In the pedicle screw litigation, the Plaintiffs' Legal Committee tried several interesting tactics in the suits: suing the manufacturers for securities fraud because they had not told shareholders that they were marketing "experimental products," suing the FDA for reclassifying the screws during the litigation, and demanding the names of all the surgeons who had participated in an FDA-authorized studies. These arguments by and large were unsuccessful. In addition, some plaintiff law firms were fined for soliciting disgruntled spine patients and for providing fraudulent experts.

Spine Cages

Since the mid-1990s, many inventors have tried to improve interbody fusion techniques by implanting metal cages filled with bone graft into intervertebral disk spaces (Figure 38). Cages are metal cylinders with walls that have been perforated multiple times. They are strong enough so they will not collapse or break, and theoretically the osteoinductive bone grafts they contain promote bone growth from vertebral body to vertebral body across the disk space. George Bagby[88] began studying cages in the late 1970s in the treatment of horses with wobbler syndrome (cervical myelopathy) caused by herniated disks. He and his associates developed the "Bagby basket" for this purpose. Subsequently, Bagby and Steven Kuslich[89] of Minneapolis refined the basket for use in humans. The Bagby-Kuslich device, marketed as the BAK cage, was approved for distribution by the FDA after an investigational device exemption (IDE) study protocol was completed in 1991.

Charles Ray[90] of Norfolk, Virginia, also designed a cage. His differed from the BAK model in several ways (number of perforations, thickness of the cage walls, degree of beveling, and threads on the outer aspect of the cage), but the concept was the same. The arguments for fusion with cages are that the fusion is located at the center of vertebral segment motion and that smaller amounts of bone are required because of the milieu in which the cage is placed between the vertebral bodies; the strong metal cage prevents collapse at the disk space while the fusion takes place. In addition, the cages can be inserted from the front or the back and surgeons can use them with minimally invasive techniques or with larger open surgical exposures.

The use of cages has subsided in the early years of the new millennium because of the advent of the artificial disk. In 1996, D. H. Chow of Hong Kong and his associates published a report on the experimental analysis of forces applied to disk levels adjacent to those that had been fused using interbody techniques.[91] Chow and associates noted the growing concern that because interbody fusions were stiffer than posterior fusions they might be a cause of accelerated degeneration in disk levels adjacent to the fusion. Because of this problem, spine surgeons have attempted to develop and use an artificial disk that would combine pain relief, stability, and motion.[92-94] Ulf Fernström[95] published the first paper on this subject in 1966, 30 years before the resurrection of artificial disk technology in the mid-1990s. Fernström inserted a total of 204 large stainless steel ball bearings in 191 lumbar disk spaces and 13 cervical disk spaces in 133 patients. He employed a posterior approach in the lumbar spine and an anterior approach in the cervical spine. He reported that fewer than 1 percent of his patients experienced the complication of displacement of the ball bearings and described excellent short-term results. His report stimulated little interest, however. By 2005, inventive individuals had patented, tested, and brought to market devices that have been reported to maintain motion while relieving pain.[96,97] The basic model for a disk replacement consists of metal plates secured to the superior and inferior end plates of the disk space, between which is placed an ellipsoid of high-density polyethylene. The geometry of the metal plates keeps the polyethylene component securely in its assigned location. The insertion of the prosthetic disk, which must be done anteriorly, requires a good deal of distraction of the space to get the components properly seated. Any defects in the posterior arches, such as a pars defect or severe osteoarthritic changes in the facet joints, contraindicate the procedure. In its early use, the artificial disk led to some severe complications such as loosening and displacement, with injury to the aorta, vena cava, ureter, and other abdominal structures. In addition, scarring and fibrosis of the retroperitoneal space makes access for a revision procedure very difficult.

The Cervical Spine Research Society

J. William Fielding became interested in the cervical spine several years after he finished his orthopaedic training. A Canadian by birth, he studied orthopaedics at St. Luke's Hospital in New York in the tradition of Mather Cleveland, David Bosworth, and Frederick R. Thompson. Fielding had an early interest in photography and in the mid-1950s began using cineradiography to study motion in the cervical spine. He presented a dramatic paper at the 1959 Annual Meeting of the AAOS demonstrating how nonunions of odontoid fractures subject the upper cervical spinal cord to repeated and potentially catastrophic compression. This paper attracted a good deal of attention, and encouraged him to expand his investigations into the mechanics of the upper cervical spine and to study how various traumatic, inflammatory, and congenital conditions can adversely affect that area.[98,99] He subsequently published several papers on the upper cervical spine in which he elucidated the pathomechanics of rotatory atlantoaxial subluxations and dislocations, transverse ligament tears of the atlas, odontoid process fractures (especially in children), and other conditions of the upper cervical spine. Obviously, he was not the first person interested in abnormalities of the occipitocervical and atlantoaxial articulations, but this complex anatomic area had received relatively little attention. Fielding sought to increase the focus on this region, inviting a small group of like-minded people to his suite at the 1973 AAOS meeting to consider forming a society to study the cervical spine. Those present agreed that it was a good idea, and Fielding scheduled the first meeting of the Cervical Spine Research Society (CSRS) at the Essex House in New York in December 1973. Besides Fielding, the founding members were Robert Bailey, Henry Bohlman, Edward Dunn, Alice Garrett, Ashby Grantham, Robert Hensinger, Mason Hohl, Bernard Jacobs, Henry LaRocca, Donlin Long, Ian Macnab, Wesley Park, Joseph Ransohoff, Lee Riley, Richard Rothman, Henry Sherk, Edward Simmons, Wayne Southwick, Shannon Stauffer, Augustus White, and Thomas Whitesides.

A review of the programs at CSRS annual meetings reveals the gradual evolution of basic science research, diagnostic methodology, and surgical techniques, all refined by intense peer review provided by questioning presenters from the floor. The CSRS has also published the definitive book on the cervical spine, *The Cervical Spine*, now in its fourth edition. Charles Clark of the Department of Orthopaedics at the University of Iowa is the current editor. The society has also published an atlas of surgical exposures and procedures; Harry Herkowitz of Royal Oak, Michigan, served as editor of the second edition.

In 1982, at its 10th annual meeting, the society decided to offer instructional courses on cervical spine surgery and research, as suggested by Joseph Epstein, a New York neurosurgeon. Henry LaRocca of Tulane accepted the position of course chairman, and the first course was held in Palm Beach, Florida, in December 1983. It unexpectedly attracted over 100 attendees. The success of this endeavor led to the current biannual presentation of such instructional courses.

CSRS meetings attracted numerous European and Japanese spine surgeons, many of whom became members. In fact, the German, Swiss, French, Italian, Greek, and Portuguese members established a European section of the organization. They also meet annually, although at a different time of year. North American and European members often attend both meetings. Japanese physicians and surgeons also have presented many outstanding papers at CSRS meetings on their areas of expertise, such as ossification of the posterior longitudinal ligament, myelopathy, spinal stenosis, and laminoplasty.

The society's international membership, broad diversity of professional backgrounds, books, published research, educational courses, and support from individuals and industry has provided the CSRS with enough resources to support several large research grants annually. More recently, it also organized and developed traveling fellowships for young cervical spine surgeons. The CSRS is an outstanding example of what a small, focused organization can achieve. Fielding, who conceived of it, fostered the society by acting selflessly, offering criticism and advice but never really taking any credit. He died in 1998.

Advances in Treatment of Cervical Spine Injuries and Disorders

Several of the founders of the CSRS developed an interest in the upper cervical spine. Their presentations at the first CSRS meeting and subsequent publications complemented what Fielding had already disclosed in other venues. Thomas Whitesides,[100] for example, developed a retropharyngeal approach to the atlantoaxial joint for treatment of fixed deformities that might require decompression of the cervical canal from the front. A previously reported technique consisting of a transoral decompression proved unsuccessful because of a very high infection rate. Whitesides' approach avoided going through the oral mucosa and risking the contamination of the surgical field with a bacterial flora of the mouth and pharynx. Riley and Macnab[101] also used a retropharyngeal approach to gain access to the atlas, axis, and skull base from the front, but their surgical approach consisted of a dissection anterior to the carotid sheath instead of behind it. The different opinions on how to perform surgery in this difficult area might not have received the same level of educated discussion but for the forum that Fielding convened.

At the same meeting, Edward Simmons[102] presented his work on osteotomy of the lower cervical spine for fixed flexion deformity caused by ankylosing spondylitis. Simmons accepted patients for treatment whose necks fused in 90° of flexion, a condition so severe that even when standing or sitting fully upright patients could only look at their own feet. When viewed from behind, they appeared to have been decapitated. Simmons performed a C7 laminectomy, forcibly extending the neck and cracking through the fused vertebral column anteriorly. This set of maneuvers brought the head up into normal alignment. He maintained the correction by immediately placing the patients in a halo cast and claimed to have avoided quadriplegia by performing the laminectomy under local anesthesia and osteoclasis using a brief general anesthetic. The fact that his patients could communicate with him during surgery made it possible for him to do a very controlled correction.

Robert Robinson, another founding member of the CSRS, published a paper with George Smith on anterior approaches to the cervical spine in 1955 in the *Bulletin of the Johns Hopkins Hospital*. They reported on the surgical treatment of eight patients with cervical disk degeneration, and how those patients fared postoperatively. The authors first worked out the details of the surgical approach on animals. They dissected along the anterior border of the sternocleidomastoid and between the carotid sheath and esophagus to reach the anterior aspect of the cervical vertebrae. They identified the appropriate level by radiographs and removed the disk tissue from between the vertebral bodies. They achieved fusion by inserting a small piece of bone from the iliac crest between the vertebrae. They reported that five patients had good to excellent results, two had poor results, and one had been operated on too recently to evaluate the outcome. Two of the patients in this series had recurrent laryngeal nerve injury with vocal cord paralysis.

In subsequent papers, Robinson and his associates and former residents discussed further details about the surgical approach. Eventually anterior cervical spine surgery became commonplace. Riley, Southwick, Dunn, and Bohlman all came from the Johns Hopkins tradition of anterior cervical spine surgery. Wayne Southwick went on to become the head of the Division of Orthopaedics at Yale. There, Augustus White, Manohar Panjabi, and many other orthopaedic surgeons who received their education at Yale and Johns Hopkins benefited from learning Robinson's procedure firsthand or from those who had. Donlin Long, also a founding member of the CSRS, was a neurosurgeon at Johns Hopkins and colleague of Smith's. He also participated in the development of anterior cervical spine surgery there.

It is not clear, however, whether Smith and Robinson were the first American surgeons to perform anterior cervical spine surgery. Robert Bailey of the University of Michigan stated in a 1960 *JBJS* article that he had been performing this operation since 1952.[103] He noted that LeRoy C. Abbott had suggested it to him after Abbott evaluated a patient with a destructive process involving two cervical vertebral bodies. Furthermore, Bailey wrote, "This paper recounts chronologically the development and application of an original procedure for anterior fusion of the cervical spine." Bailey's original 1952 patient had a giant cell tumor that had destroyed most of the C4 and C5 vertebral bodies. Bailey performed a Hibbs posterior fusion from C3 to C7 to bridge a limited laminotomy of C4 for a progressive quadriparesis. The patient's condition deteriorated, however, necessitating an anterior resection of C4 and C5 vertebral bodies about four weeks later. Massive bleeding ensued, but with packing and transfusions the patient survived and her quadriparesis even improved. A month after removal of the tumor and almost all of the bodies of C4 and C5, Dr. Bailey operated on the patient a third time. He reopened the neck anteriorly and inserted long autogenous iliac crest bone grafts from C3 to C6. The patient recovered completely neurologically but died a year later from a recurrence of the giant cell tumor.

Bailey reported that the "use of the approach and the achievement of stability" in his original patient led him to perform the same operation in 17 other patients for varying indications such as postlaminectomy instability, fracture-dislocations of the cervical spine, tuberculous destruction of cervical vertebrae, and tumors of cervical vertebrae. It is interesting that none of his original anterior cervical fusions were performed for disk degeneration. He claimed that his first patient was "of historical significance in that the patient had the first known fusion by this approach." Bailey and Badgley presented their paper at the 1959 Annual Meeting of the AAOS, and Robinson was asked to discuss it. Robinson concluded his remarks by stating that "the principles and practice of cervical spine surgery are gradually evolving. The work of Dr. Bailey and Dr. Badgley is a solid addition to this body of surgical knowledge."

The third claimant to setting the precedent for anterior cervical spine surgery was Ralph Cloward.[104] He submitted a paper to the *Journal of Neurosurgery* on September 3, 1957, that described his own anterior surgical approach to the cervical spine. He reported that he began work on devising an anterior approach at least two years earlier, first on cadavers and then on patients. By the time he submitted his report, he had operated on 61 patients. Cloward used exactly the same surgical route as Robinson and Bailey, but his actual fusion procedure differed considerably. He performed the operation only on patients who had symptoms related to disk degeneration and used cervical diskograms to select patients for the surgery. In fact, he decided on the anterior approach while devising an anterior route for cervical diskography. Cloward used a large drill to core out the disk and performed an extensive anterior decompression. He then removed a plug of bone graft in the shape of a dowel from the patient's iliac crest, tamping it into the site of the defect in the vertebral bodies and disk space. Cloward performed the operation under local anesthesia. One patient in his series "was considered worse," but all the others had done well despite various complications, some of which required additional surgery.

Cloward presented his paper before publication at a meeting of the Harvey Cushing Society. As is the custom, several members of the society were asked to discuss it. The program chairman apparently had difficulty finding members to discuss Cloward's paper. A reviewer who ultimately did so noted that he was substituting for Spurling and Mack, who declined the invitation. John Raff took a light note in discussing Cloward's paper, declaring: "I am a great admirer of Dr. Cloward's prodigious energy and abundance of ideas, but so far I have not been able to bring myself to do either diskograms or anterior cervical fusions. It is true that there are a number of very fine blind pianists, but I doubt that one can pound on the strings that make up the brachial plexus with the same abandon that one can pound on piano strings." He said that he thought most patients with pain caused by cervical disk degeneration improved with conservative treatment, thus the operation was probably not necessary in most cases.

William Scoville, the second society member to discuss Cloward's paper, objected to the operation because he had obtained results that were "extraordinarily good" with a posterior keyhole through the facets with "uncapping and unwalling of the involved root." He noted that the "simplicity and excellence of the results in the posterior keyhole" and the possibility that a fused cervical interspace would stress adjacent interspaces were both contraindications for Cloward's operation. Smith and Robinson and Bailey and Badgley clearly enjoyed a more enthusiastic response to their presentations from orthopaedists than Cloward received from his fellow neurosurgeons.

Robinson and Smith, Bailey and Badgley, and Cloward all seemed to have had the same idea around the same time. Bailey probably did the first anterior cervical fusion, but did not report it in the literature until five years after Robinson and Smith. Cloward's initial report on his approach and technique for anterior cervical diskectomy was made in 1957, two years after Robinson and Smith, although clearly Cloward performed his first operations in 1955 and 1956. In the final analysis, it can be said that anterior surgery for the cervical spine developed in three places simultaneously.

In the decades that have elapsed, anterior surgery has assumed a major role in the treatment of cervical spine disorders. By the mid-1980s, numerous variations of the original concept were considered and explored. Modifications of the grafting techniques, outcomes assessments for single- versus multiple-level fusions, and extension of the indications to treat the conditions affecting the cervical vertebrae (trauma, tumors, infections, degenerative conditions) all came under scrutiny.

Overall, surgical treatment of intractable symptoms caused by cervical disk degeneration proved itself successful. In 1984, for example, Donald Gore[105] of Sheboygan, Wisconsin, reported that he achieved complete pain relief in 78 percent of 146 patients with discogenic neck and arm pain, with only 4 percent of patients experiencing little or no pain relief. A total of 97 percent of the disk levels fused successfully. Gore retained the essential features of the previously described operations, altering his technique with the use of autogenous fibular bone grafts for multilevel fusions instead of iliac crest grafts. He used an anterior exposure, completely removed the disk(s) that he identified as symptomatic by radiography and myelography, and fused the disk levels by impacting autogenous bone into the disk spaces. The excellent outcomes in his series illustrated the effectiveness of the anterior diskectomy operation devised by Smith and Robinson, Bailey and Badgley, and Cloward 30 years before.

Although Bailey and Badgley[103] reported that they used anterior fusion methodology to treat fractures and dislocations of the cervical spine successfully, others did not have their positive experience. Stauffer and Kelly,[106] reporting from Rancho Los Amigos National Rehabilitation Center in Downey, California, in 1977, found that disruption of the posterior stabilizers in the neck precludes a successful use of anterior fusion with a bone graft either between adjacent bodies or to replace an entire vertebral body after a corpectomy. They reported that flexion deformity recurred and that the grafts dislodged. These complications led to the development of internal fixation of the cervical spine with anterior plates secured with multiple screws to provide internal stability. In one of the classic articles on the subject, Jorg Böhler[107] suggested that after performing an anterior procedure with a bone graft, "additional fixation is necessary" with a Minerva jacket or internally with posterior or anterior osteosynthesis. Böhler preferred anterior osteosynthesis using a metal plate because it could be performed simultaneously with the bone graft procedure. Böhler gave due regard to several earlier papers on this subject, but most other reports cite his 1980 paper in *Spine* as the beginning of anterior plating in the United States. The earlier plating systems required fixation with screws that engaged both the anterior and posterior cortices of the vertebral bodies, an issue that raised the question of risking the cervical cord. Later designs incorporated the use of expanding screw heads or locking screws so that a surgeon could use much shorter 14-mm screws to achieve fixation without the need to engage two cortices. The chance of spinal cord injury was thus much reduced.

In the years since Smith and Robinson, anterior plating went through the same intense investigation by surgeons in multiple centers. Plate designs were extensively modified to minimize the possibility of esophageal perforation. Locking screws to eliminate bicortical purchase have become standard features. Donor-site morbidity has been largely eliminated because of successful substitution of autograft by allograft, bone substitutes, and adjuncts such as BMP. Large series of such patients have now been reported whose outcomes appear comparable to those reported by Gore and others. Allografts, however, even when used with plates, have a tendency to collapse, subside, or absorb. Although this may not have an effect on the final outcome of the procedure or require revision surgery, it is cause for concern. In response to the issue of subsidence of intervertebral allografts with or without plating, several manufacturers now offer cervical spine cages. As when used in the lumbar spine, they provide support to prevent collapse of the disk space; because they are filled with osteoinductive bone or other material, they promote fusion with stability. The evaluation of cages in the cervical spine and whether their use should be supplemented by anterior plating has interested several investigators and has been the subject of many presentations and publications in CSRS meetings and elsewhere. In the history of cervical spine surgery, it is not entirely clear that these frequent changes in methodology have improved the outcomes or lessened the risk. However, recent data may indicate better outcomes with anterior cervical spine plating techniques.

William Scoville, who discussed Ralph Cloward's anterior cervical fusion operation at the 1959 meeting of the Harvey Cushing Society, said that the possibility of accelerated adjacent segment degeneration "militated" against Cloward's technique. Scoville was prescient in this regard. Several studies since then have suggested that levels adjacent to a fusion in the cervical spine may degenerate more rapidly. Although anterior diskectomy and fusion in the cervical spine has an excellent track record of providing long-term pain relief, the adjacent-level degeneration may well cause a recurrence of symptoms in some patients. In an effort to keep the benefits of pain relief provided by anterior diskectomy while avoiding adjacent-segment degeneration, some clinicians have suggested replacing the disk with a prosthesis. Artificial disk technology therefore has become the next consideration in the history of anterior cervical spine surgery. Frank Phillips and Steven Garfin[108] reviewed cervical disk replacement in 2005, reporting that at that time, the FDA had approved investigational device exemption studies of four models of disk prostheses; therefore, a surgeon could use these devices only under carefully supervised and controlled conditions. Early reports suggest that total disk replacement preserves motion at the index level and does not cause adjacent-level hypermobility. Theoretically, the preservation of normal kinematics in the adjacent levels will delay the onset of degeneration and maintain satisfactory function and pain relief, but this had not been proved. Prosthetic wear, survival of the implant, and problems with revision surgery are issues that the investigators continue to address.

Multiple-level surgical disk degeneration in patients with congenitally narrow spinal canals presents problems that differ somewhat from those described previously. The size of the spinal cord does not vary much from one person to another, but the spinal canal does. A wide and capacious spinal canal protects against cord compression when disks herniate or osteophytes develop, but a narrow spinal canal makes the possibility of neurocompression more likely. The resultant pressure on the spinal cord causes it to flatten and splay out laterally. Patients with this problem report symptoms and findings that range from very mild motor weakness and ataxia to almost complete quadriplegia. These issues have been examined extensively in meetings of the CSRS since its inception.

Several British neurologists, notably Nurick[109] and Brain and associates,[110] studied the relationship of a congenitally narrow cervical spinal canal with spondylosis and myelopathy during the mid-20th century. They differed somewhat on the ultimate cause of loss of spinal cord function. Nurick concluded that compression produced spinal cord injury, whereas Brain believed that ischemia had a more prominent effect. Recent studies suggest that Nurick was more likely correct. Nurick also made a useful contribution to the evaluation of patients with myelopathy by devising the Nurick grading system (in which 0 means no myelopathy, and 5 means chair/bound or bedridden). Most orthopaedic surgeons who treat and write about cervical spondylotic myelopathy (CSM) use this classification system to determine their surgical indications and results.

Despite a large body of published information, indications for operating on patients with CSM and the appropriate operation to perform still remain somewhat controversial. In 1972, Nurick[111] compared treatment with a supportive collar to laminectomy and surgical decompression. He concluded that surgical decompression "should be reserved for those whose disability is progressive, particularly for those more than 60 years old." L. Simon and T. Lavender, who were cited by Nurick, performed multilevel laminectomies with removal of inbuckled and thickened ligamentum flavum to achieve an improvement rate of 70 percent in their CSM patients. Multilevel laminectomy, however, removes the attachment of the stabilizing extensor muscles and ligaments. In addition, if the laminectomy is carried far enough laterally, the surgeon also destabilizes the cervical vertebrae further by removing part of the facet joints. Patients who undergo this surgery often have swan-neck deformities with multiple subluxations and recurrent symptoms. To avoid the effects of instability caused by laminectomies, Japanese surgeons developed the technique of laminoplasty. Kiyoshi Hirabayashi,[112] for example, described this procedure in several papers he presented at meetings of the CSRS in the 1970s and 1980s. He found that the development of the high-speed air drill made it possible to create deep grooves in the laminae bilaterally where the laminae merge into the facet joints. By cutting completely through the laminae on one side, he could crack the laminae on the other side to raise multiple laminae together, hinging them open like a door. He thus called the operation "the expansive open-door laminoplasty." Hirabayashi found that laminoplasty achieved decompression of the spinal cord and also maintained stability of the neck. Japanese surgeons also confronted a condition known as ossification of the posterior longitudinal ligament (OPLL), which occurs less commonly in North America. They developed strategies, including laminoplasty, to address the severe narrowing of the cervical spinal canal caused by OPLL. Laminoplasty techniques varied, but the basic procedure purportedly yielded better outcomes than laminectomy in the Japanese literature.

Laminoplasty, however, may produce postoperative neck pain and loss of motion. It was thus natural for the intellectual descendants of Robinson to consider decompression of the cervical spinal canal from the front. In 1988, Harry Herkowitz[113] of Royal Oak, Michigan, compared the outcomes of surgery in patients with multilevel spondylotic radiculopathy treated with one of three kinds of operations: laminectomy, laminoplasty, or multiple anterior diskectomies and fusions as done by Robinson. Herkowitz found that laminectomy alone produced the least satisfactory outcomes, and Robinson's fusions produced the best. He also found that laminoplasty was associated with limited neck motion postoperatively. Since Herkowitz published his paper on anterior cervical fusion for the treatment of cervical spondylotic radiculopathy, several other authors have weighed in on the subject. Sanford Emery and associates[114] of Case Western Reserve

University in Cleveland, for example, published an important paper on the subject in *JBJS* in 2005. Their indications for the operation began with mild weakness and the demonstration of withdrawal reflexes in patients with demonstrable cervical spinal stenosis on MRI. They felt that this combination of complaints and findings justified surgery because, as far as historical controls indicated, the CSM inevitably worsens, albeit unpredictably.

Trauma

The freedom of motion in the cervical spine and its exposed position predispose it to injury. White and Panjabi[22] described the six degrees of freedom of the cervical spine and showed how the vertebrae move about axes of motion in the sagittal, coronal, and axial planes. The anatomic configuration of the seven cervical vertebrae permit a good deal of mobility, but when the neck is subjected to forces beyond the capabilities of its ligamentous and muscular restraints, dislocation and fracture can occur. Thereafter, stresses that the spine could have tolerated before injury cause abnormally large displacements; the cervical spine in this state is by definition unstable. Instability of the cervical spine has very grave consequences because it surrounds and protects the cervical spinal cord. Injury to the cord, of course, can result in neurologic impairments such as complete, central cord, Brown-Séquard, or anterior cord lesions. The orthopaedic and neurosurgical literature of the past century has tackled the issue of cervical spine injury in hundreds of articles, also examining the issues related to the subject of spinal cord injury after fracture and dislocation in the cervical area.

For example, Jeffrey Jefferson published his paper on fractures of the first cervical vertebra in *Lancet* in 1927. He determined that the vertebral ring breaks apart centrifugally because of axially directly forces and found that even considerable displacement did not prevent uncomplicated healing with minimal neurologic impairment. Jefferson's fracture, therefore, is regarded by many as a stable injury that does not need aggressive surgical intervention.[115]

In contrast, fractures of the odontoid process of the axis vertebra have a much greater chance of causing neurologic deficits. Immobilization of this injury with a Minerva jacket cast or a halo brace fails to achieve healing of the fracture in up to 40 percent of adult patients. Charles Clark and Augustus White[116] reviewed a group of patients with this injury in 1985 in a multicenter study. Using the classification system devised by Anderson and D'Alonzo[117] of the Campbell Clinic in Memphis, they found that type 2 injuries at the base of the dens fail to heal in a halo in at least one third of the patients reviewed. Posterior fusion of C1 and C2, however, resulted in satisfactory union of type 2 dens fractures in 96 percent of the patients. They also stated that "[fusion] appears to be the treatment of choice." The fusion technique for C1-C2 instability, however, also has been the subject of scrutiny.[118] In 1910, Mixter and Osgood described a method in which they passed a suture under the posterior arch of the atlas and tied it down over the spinous process of C2. This method became the basis of the "Gallie fusion" described by W. E. Gallie of Toronto just before World War II in 1939.

Despite the use of a bone graft, Gallie fusions failed to unite so often that they prompted the development of the Brooks fusion. Arthur Brooks of Nashville and Irwin Jenkins of Decatur, Alabama, passed two wire sutures under the posterior arches of both C1 and C2, tying them down over an "H graft" in 15 patients. They reported that fusion failed in only one patient. The Gallie and Brooks fusions, however, could not be used in patients without a C1 posterior arch; besides that, they lacked the ability to immobilize C1 and C2 completely. F. Margerl of St. Gallen, Switzerland, published an alternative technique in 1987. His procedure consisted of passing threaded screws from the outer edges of the C2 lamina across the atlantoaxial facet joints, ending in the lateral mass of C1. The fixation of C1 and C2 in this way immobilized an odontoid fracture well enough to achieve nearly 100 percent healing of type 2 dens fractures. Any C1-C2 fusion technique, however, necessarily results in limited rotation of the head. To overcome this objectionable outcome, Japanese, Swiss, and German surgeons chose screw fixation of the odontoid process from the front. To achieve this, they passed one or two cannulated screws from the distal-most part of the axis vertebral body upward across the fracture in the dens, then up to the tip of the odontoid process. They reported solid healing of odontoid process fractures in nearly 100 percent of patients without loss of neck motion and without using prolonged external immobilization in a halo brace or Minerva jacket.[119,120]

Fractures through the base of the neural arches of the second cervical vertebrae cause a traumatic spondylolisthesis of the second vertebra. In the late 19th and early 20th centuries, dissections of people executed by hanging showed that many of them sustained this injury. Good hanging technique required that the executioner place the knot in a submental position beneath the chin and that the victim should drop far enough to produce sudden and extreme hyperextension of the head on the neck. The resultant combination of forces should break the axis at the base of the neural arches and cause enough injury to the spinal cord at that level to produce a quick and relatively painless death. Authors writing about the injury often referred to it as the hangman's fracture. In recent times, the sudden and extreme hyperextension of the head, which occurs in head-to-windshield crashes or in diving accidents, can replicate the hangman's lesion, although without enough force to cause upper spinal cord injury. Richard C. Schneider, a neurosurgeon at the University of Michigan Medical School, made the connection between the two mechanisms of injury in the *Journal of Neurosurgery* in 1965.[121] In persons with minimally displaced or nondisplaced fractures, support in a halo, or even in an external brace or cast, will be sufficient to let the fracture heal without surgery. Occasionally, however, patients need internal fixation. The fracture can be fixed internally with an anterior plate-and-screw construct or posterior wiring and bone graft from C1 to C3.

In the recent past, several reports have been published on cranial cervical dissociation, usually caused by a high-speed vehicular crash or by a vehicle striking a pedestrian. The alar ligaments, anterior and posterior longitudinal ligaments, tectorial membrane, and cruciate ligament must all rupture simultaneously for the head and neck to separate from one another; the presence of such injuries implies great forces that must act in different directions in extremely rapid sequence. Injury to the spinal cord at this level usually results in death, but if a patient does arrive alive in an emergency department with an occipital cervical dissociation, treating physicians might not recognize it if no fractures have occurred. Bucholz and Burkhead[122] and Traynelis and associates[123] suggest that the injury occurs in more than 1 percent of spinal trauma patients and therefore physicians tend to underdiagnosis it. Traction with a halo brace or even with a halter can pull the head further from the atlas and axis because their restraining ligaments no longer connect the head to the upper cervical spine. Those who have had experience with this injury suggest that an occipital cervical fusion should be performed as soon as a patient can tolerate that level of surgery. A surgeon can select one of several available methods, such as contoured plates and screws, bent rods, or bone grafts wired to the occiput and neural arches of C1 and C2, and plates secured to the occiput with short screws to the atlas, axis, and subjacent vertebra with pedicle screws. Anterior fusion using bone graft has caused infections in a high percentage of cases; because the posterior fusion is easier and carries less risk, most surgeons elect to fuse the occiput to the cervical spine using a dorsal approach.

In adults, subaxial cervical spine injuries occur much more often than atlantoaxial trauma. In children, the most common cervical spine injury, however, is a separation of the odontoid process from the body of the axis at the level of a synchondrosis in that location. Unrecognized and untreated, the fracture may not heal. Fielding and associates[124] proposed this sequence of events to explain the development of an os odontoideum, in which the odontoid remains separated and unattached to the body of the axis. An os odontoideum produces pronounced anterior and posterior instability of the atlantal ring on the axis with a potential for severe damage to the spinal cord in the upper cervical region. Prevention of an os odontoideum requires that treating physicians recognize the dens separation in young children and that they provide adequate treatment, including about six weeks of immobilization with the dens in the reduced position.

A milestone in the evaluation and treatment of cervical spine injuries was reached with the publication of Henry Bohlman's paper on acute fractures and dislocations of the cervical spine in *JBJS* in 1979.[125] Bohlman is the son of Harold Bohlman, who invented the hip replacement, which later became the Austin Moore prosthesis. Henry Bohlman, while a research fellow in Robert Robinson's department of orthopaedics at Johns Hopkins Hospital in Baltimore, began the study of cervical spine fractures and dislocations occurring from 1950 through 1972. In all, he collected records and radiographs of 300 patients seen in Baltimore hospitals during that time. His review of this large group revealed that one third (100 out of 300) did not have the diagnosis of cervical spine injury made in the emergency department. Head injuries, alcoholism, and multiple other injuries may have precluded the treating physicians from eliciting a history of neck pain, but subsequent to Bohlman's report virtually all trauma physicians now recognize the need for "screening" cervical spine radiographs for all emergency department patients admitted to a hospital. The number of radiographs, what views to take, and whether MRI is needed remain matters of discussion, but the need to determine possible damage to the cervical spine is acknowledged as a necessary part of trauma protocols.

Bohlman's study also confirmed the futility of laminectomy in treating patients with anterior cord syndromes or complete spinal cord lesions. "The concept that laminectomy is contraindicated in these patients is supported by the high mortality rate and frequent loss of motor function . . . after this procedure." The study also showed that patients with flexion injuries and disruption of the posterior tension band should undergo a stabilizing posterior fusion, whereas patients with hyperextension injuries with disruption of the anterior column through an intervertebral disk should undergo an anterior diskectomy and fusion if external support fails to maintain stability. He concluded that burst fractures or other compression injuries of the anterior column strongly justify anterior corpectomy and fusion with a bone graft. This procedure would replace the vertebral body after removal of bone and disk fragments from the spinal canal.

Techniques for posterior fusion surgery have evolved since Bohlman's paper was published. Exposure of the posterior aspect of the subaxial cervical vertebrae is not difficult, and once a facet dislocation has been reduced several techniques can be used. Through the mid-20th century, various posterior wiring and grafting constructs were used to restore the posterior tension band side of the cervical spine. In later years, however, Raymond Roy-Camille[126] of Paris and other European cervical spine surgeons devised plate-and-screw techniques for use in creating posterior stabilization. Once a surgeon has reduced the cervical spine fracture and/or dislocation, placing a narrow plate over the lateral masses of adjacent vertebrae and securing them with short screws is a relatively straightforward and easy operation. It becomes more difficult and far more hazardous when the surgeon decides to secure fixation with pedicle screws in the cervical spine. Fluoroscopic control is not always certain, a concern that has led to the development of computerized navigation systems over the past several years to increase the accuracy of pedicle screw insertion in this location. Albert and associates[127] at the Rothman Institute in Philadelphia have been working on refinements of this technology. Their enthusiastic reports regarding its use have not led to its adoption by most cervical spine surgeons at this writing, yet computerized navigation may well become the most reliable guidance modality in the future.

References

1. Bosworth DM, Morgan C: Transpleural rupture of a tuberculous spinal abscess treated successfully by streptomycin: Report of a case. *J Bone Joint Surg Am* 1946;28:864-868.

2. Hodgson AR, Stock FE: Anterior spinal fusion: The operative approach and pathologic findings in 412 patients with Pott's disease of the spine. *Br J Surg* 1960;48:172-178.

3. End result study of the treatment of idiopathic scoliosis: Report of the Research Committee of the American Orthopaedic Association. *J Bone Joint Surg Am* 1941;23:963-977.

4. Cobb JR: Outline for the study of scoliosis. *Instr Course Lect* 1948;5:261-275.

5. Risser JC, Lauder CH, Norquist DM, Craig WA: Three types of body casts. *Instr Course Lect* 1953;10:131-142.

6. Thomas GE: Idiopathic scoliosis: A method of correction. *J Bone Joint Surg Am* 1947;29:907-917.

7. Ponseti IV, Friedman B: Prognosis in idiopathic scoliosis. *J Bone Joint Surg Am* 1950;32:381-395.

8. Cobb JR: Scoliosis—Quo vadis? Ed. *J Bone Joint Surg Am* 1958;40:507-510.

9. Blount WP, Schmidt AC, Keener ED, Leonard ET: The Milwaukee brace in the operative treatment of scoliosis. *J Bone Joint Surg Am* 1958;40:511-525.

10. Blount WP, Schmidt AC, Bridwell RG: Making the Milwaukee brace. *J Bone Joint Surg Am* 1958;40:526-528.

11. Bobechko WP, Herbert MA, Friedman HG: Electrospinal instrumentation for scoliosis: Current status. *Orthop Clin North Am* 1979;10:927-941.

12. Moe JH: A critical analysis of methods of fusion for scoliosis: An evaluation in two hundred and sixty-six patients. *J Bone Joint Surg Am* 1958;40:529-697.

13. Risser JC, Norquist DM: A follow-up study of the treatment of scoliosis. *J Bone Joint Surg Am* 1958;40:555-569.

14. Risser J: The iliac apophysis: An invaluable sign in the management of scoliosis. *Clin Orthop Relat Res* 1958;11:111.

15. Gruca A: The pathogenesis and treatment of idiopathic scoliosis: A preliminary report. *J Bone Joint Surg Am* 1958;40:570-584.

16. Harrington PR: Surgical instrumentation for management of scoliosis. Proceedings: The American Orthopaedic Association. *J Bone Joint Surg Am* 1960;42:1448.

17. Harrington PR: Treatment of scoliosis: Correction and internal fixation by spinal instrumentation. *J Bone Joint Surg Am* 1962;44:591-610.

18. Paul Randall Harrington, MD, 1911-1980. *J Bone Joint Surg Am* 1981;63:857.

19. Hall JE: Spinal surgery before and after Paul Harrington. *Spine* 1998;23:1356-1361.

20. Winter RB: The third era: SRS presidential address. *Spine* 1976;1:44.

21. Dwyer AF, Newton NC, Sherwood AA: An anterior approach to scoliosis: A preliminary report. *Clin Orthop Relat Res* 1969;62:192-202.

22. White AA II, Panjabi MM: *Clinical Biomechanics of the Spine.* Philadelphia, PA, JB Lippincott, 1978.

23. Luque ER: Segmental spinal instrumentation for correction of scoliosis. *Clin Orthop Relat Res* 1982;163:192-198.

24. Drummond DS: Harrington instrumentation with spinous process wiring for idiopathic scoliosis. *Orthop Clin North Am* 1988;19:281-289.

25. Cotrel Y, Dubousset J, Guillaumat M: New universal instrumentation in spine surgery. *Clin Orthop Relat Res* 1988;227:10-23.

26. Ashman RB, Birch JG, Bone LB, et al: Mechanical testing of spinal instrumentation. *Clin Orthop Relat Res* 1988;227:113-125.

27. Camp JF, Caudle R, Ashman RD, Roach J: Immediate complications of Cotrel-Dubousset instrumentation to the sacro-pelvis: A clinical and biomechanical study. *Spine* 1990;15:932-941.

28. Roach JW, Ashman RB, Allard RR: The strength of a posterior element claw at one versus two spinal levels. *J Spinal Disord* 1990;3:259-261.

29. Zielke K, Stunket R, Beaujeau F: Ventrale Derotations Spondylodese. *Arch Orthop Unfallchir* 1976;85:257-277.

30. Robin GC: The Aetiology of Idiopathic Scoliosis: A Review of a Century of Research. Boca Raton, FL, CRC Press, Inc, 1990.

31. Lonstein JE, Bjorklund S, Wanninger MH, Nelson RP: Voluntary school screening for scoliosis in Minnesota. *J Bone Joint Surg Am* 1982;64:481-488.

32. Lonstein JE, Carlson JM: The prediction of curve progression in untreated idiopathic scoliosis during growth. *J Bone Joint Surg Am* 1984;66:1061-1071.

33. King HA, Moe JH, Bradford DS, Winter RB: The selection of fusion levels in thoracic idiopathic scoliosis. *J Bone Joint Surg Am* 1983;65:1302-1313.

34. Stagnara P: *Spinal Deformity*. London, United Kingdom, Butterworth, 1988.

35. Forbes HJ, Allen PW, Waller CS, et al: Spinal cord monitoring in scoliosis surgery: Experience with 1168 cases. *J Bone Joint Surg Br* 1991;73:487-491.

36. Goto T, Crosby G: Anesthesia and the spinal cord. *Anesth Clin North Am* 1992;10:493.

37. Haghighi SS, Oro JJ: Effects of hypovolemic hypotensive shock on somatosensory and motor evoked potentials. *Neurosurgery* 1989;24:246-252.

38. Friedlaender GE: Current Concepts Review: Bone grafts: The basic science rationale for clinical applications. *J Bone Joint Surg Am* 1987;69:786-790.

39. Urist MR: Bone: Formation by autoinduction. *Science* 1965;150:893-899.

40. Urist MR, Silverman BF, Buring K, Dubuc FL, Rosenberg JM: The bone induction principle. *Clin Orthop Relat Res* 1967;53:243-283.

41. Shutkin NM: Homologous-serum hepatitis following refrigerated bone-bank bone. *J Bone Joint Surg Am* 1954;36:160-162.

42. Centers for Disease Control (CDC): Transmission of HIV through bone transplantation: Case report and public health recommendations. *Morb Mortal Wkly Rep* 1988;37:597-599.

43. Tissue and Organ Transplantation Assessment Report. Bethesda, MD, National Institutes of Health, Public Health Service Work Group on Organ and Tissue Transplantation, July 18, 1991.

44. Eastland T: Infectious disease transmission through tissue transplantation: Reducing the risk by donor selection. *J Transpl Coord* 1991;1:23.

45. Schmorl G: *The Human Spine in Health and Disease*. New York, NY, Grune & Stratton, 1959, pp 130-185.

46. Mixter WJ, Barr JS: Rupture of the intervertebral disc with involvement of the spinal canal. *N Engl J Med* 1934;211:210.

47. Goldthwaite JE: The lumbosacral articulation: An explanation of many cases of lumbago, sciatica and paraplegia. *Boston Med Surg J* 1911;164:365.

48. Middleton GS, Teacher JH: Injury to the spinal cord due to rupture of an intervertebral disc during muscular effort. *Glasgow Med J* 1916;76:1.

49. Smith AD, Deery EM, Hagman GL: Herniation of nucleus pulposis: A study of one
hundred cases treated by operation. *J Bone Joint Surg Am* 1944;26:821.

50. Barr JS: Ruptured intervertebral disc and sciatic pain. *J Bone Joint Surg*
1947;29:429-437.

51. Friberg S, Hirsch C: Anatomical and clinical studies on lumbar disc degeneration.
Acta Orthop Scand 1949;19:222-242.

52. Hirsch C, Ingelmark BE, Miller M: The anatomical basis for low back pain: studies
on the presence of sensory nerve endings in ligamentous, capsular and intervertebral
disc structures in the human lumbar spine. *Acta Orthop Scand* 1963;33:1-17.

53. Hirsch C: Studies on the pathology of low back pain. *J Bone Joint Surg Br*
1959;41:237-243.

54. Hirsch C: The reaction of intervertebral discs to compression forces. *J Bone Joint
Surg Am* 1955;37:1188-1196.

55. Hirsch C, Nachemson A: New observations on the mechanical behavior of lumbar
discs. *Acta Orthop Scand* 1954;23:254-283.

56. Waddell G, Kummel EG, Lotto WN, Graham JD, Hall H, McCulloch JA: Failed lumbar disc surgery following industrial injuries. *J Bone Joint Surg Am* 1979;61:201-
207.

57. Waddell G, McCulloch JA, Kummel E, Venner RM: Nonorganic physical signs in
low-back pain. *Spine* 1980;5:117-125.

58. Waddell G, Somerville D, Henderson I, Newton M: Objective clinical evaluation of
physical impairment in chronic low back pain. *Spine* 1992;17:617-628.

59. Fairbank JC, Couper J, Davies JB, O'Brien JP: The Oswestry low back pain disability questionnaire. *Physiotherapy* 1981;66:271-273.

60. Melzack R: The McGill Pain Questionnaire: Major properties and scoring methods.
Pain 1975;1:277-299.

61. Pfeiffer BA, Wong DA: Outcomes assessment and guidelines of care, in Farden D,
Garfin S (eds): *Orthopaedic Knowledge Update: Spine 2*. Rosemont, IL, American
Academy of Orthopaedic Surgeons, 2002, p 140.

62. Schmidt EA: The use of iodized oil (Lipiodol and iodipin) in the roentgen-ray diagnosis of spinal lesions. *Am J Roentgenol Radium Ther Nucl Med* 1926;15:431.

63. Sharpe W, Peterson CA: The danger of the use of lipiodol in the diagnosis of
destructive lesions in the spinal canal. *J Bone Joint Surg Am* 1926;8:348.

64. Orient JM: Review of saving lives and saving money: Transforming health and
health and health care by Newt Gingrich. *JAMA* 2004;291:251.

65. Block F: Past, present, and future of nuclear magnetic resonance, in Partain CL,
Price RR, Patton JA, Kulkarni MV, James AE Jr (eds): *Magnetic Resonance
Imaging*, ed 2. Philadelphia, PA, WB Saunders, 1998, pp 3-9.

66. Oldendarf W, Oldendorf L: MRI Primer. New York, NY, Raven Press, 1991.

67. Weber H: Lumbar disc herniation: A controlled, prospective study with ten years of
observation. *Spine* 1983;8:131-140.

68. Smith L, Brown JE: Treatment of lumbar intervertebral disc lesions by direct injection of chymopapain. *J Bone Joint Surg Am* 1967;49:502-519.

69. Simmons JW, Nordby EJ: Chemonucleolysis, in White AA (ed): *Spine Care*. St. Louis, MO, Mosby, 1995, p 991.

70. Saal JA, Saal JS: Intradiscal electrothermal treatment for chronic discogenic low back pain: A prospective outcome study with minimum 1-year follow-up. *Spine* 2000;25:2622-2627.

71. Choy DS, Asher PW, Ranu HS, et al: Percutaneous laser decompression: A new therapeutic modality. *Spine* 1992;17:949-956.

72. Kambin P, Brager M: Percutaneous posterolateral discectomy: Anatomy and mechanism. *Clin Orthop Relat Res* 1987;223:145-154.

73. Onik GM, Helms CA: Automated percutaneous lumbar discectomy. *Am J Roentgenol Radium Ther Nucl Med* 1991;156:531.

74. Williams RW: Microlumbar discectomy: A conservative surgical approach to the virgin herniated lumbar disc. *Spine* 1978;3:175-182.

75. Wiltse LL, Widell EH Jr, Jackson DW: Fatigue fracture: The basic lesion in isthmic spondylolisthesis. *J Bone Joint Surg Am* 1975;57:17-22.

76. Hart RA: Failed spine surgery syndrome in the life and career of John Fitzgerald Kennedy. *J Bone Joint Surg Am* 2006;88:1141-1148.

77. Cloward RB: The treatment of ruptured lumbar discs by intervertebral body fusion: A report of 100 cases. Read at the Harvey Cushing Society, Hot Springs, Virginia, November 15, 1947.

78. Cloward RB: The treatment of ruptured lumbar discs by vertebral body fusion: I. Indications, operative technique, after care. *J Neurosurg* 1953;10:154-168.

79. Cloward RB: Posterior lumbar interbody fusion updated. *Clin Orthop Relat Res* 1985;193:16-19.

80. Lin PM, Ralph B: Cloward, M.D. (Biography). *Clin Orthop Relat Res* 1985;193:5.

81. Lin PM, Cantilli RA, Joyce MF: Posterior lumbar interbody fusion. *Clin Orthop Relat Res* 1983;180:154-168.

82. Steffee AD, Biscup RS, Sitkowski DJ: Segmental spine plates with pedicle screw fixation: A new internal fixation device for disorders of the lumbar and thoracolumbar spine. *Clin Orthop Relat Res* 1986;203:45-53.

83. Boucher HH: A method of spine fusion. *J Bone Joint Surg Br* 1959;41:248-259.

84. Fraser RD: Presidential address: The formation of ISSLS and its impact on lumbar spine research. *Spine* 2004;29:1059-1065.

85. Tohmeh AG, Mathis JM, Fenton DC, Levine AM, Belkoff SM: Biomechanical efficacy of unipedicular versus bipedicular vertebroplasty for the management of osteoporotic compression fractures. *Spine* 1999;24:1772.

86. Wong W, Reiley MA, Garfin S: Vertebroplasty/kyphoplasty. *J Women's Imaging* 2000;2:117.

87. Belkoff SM, Mathis JM, Jasper LE, Deramond H: The biomechanics of vertebroplasty: The effect of cement volume on mechanical behavior. *Spine* 2001;26:1537-1541.

88. Bagby GW: Arthrodesis by the distraction-compression method using a stainless steel implant. *Orthopedics* 1988;11:931-934.

89. Kuslich SD, Ulstrom CL, Griffith SL, Ahern JW, Dowdle JD: The Bagby and Kuslich method of lumbar interbody fusion: History, technique, and 2-year follow-up results of a United States prospective, multicenter trial. *Spine* 1998;23:1267-1279.

90. Ray CD: Threaded titanium cages for lumbar interbody fusions. *Spine* 1997;22:667-680.

91. Chow DH, Luk KD, Evans JH, Leong JC: Effects of short anterior lumbar interbody fusion on biomechanics of neighboring unfused segments. *Spine* 1996;21:549-555.

92. Quinnell RC, Stockdale HR: Some experimental observations of the influence of a simgle lumbar floating fusion on the remaining lumbar spine. *Spine* 1981;6:263-267.

93. Lee CK: Accelerated degeneration of the segment adjacent to a lumbar fusion. *Spine* 1988;13:375-377.

94. Hambly MF, Wiltse LL, Raghavan N, Schneiderman G, Koenig C: The transition zone above a lumbosacral fusion. *Spine* 1998;23:1785-1792.

95. Fernström U: Arthroplasty with intercorporal endoprosthesis in herniated disc and in painful disc. *Acta Chir Scand* 1966;357(Suppl):154-159.

96. Eijkelkamp MF, van Donkelaar CC, Veldhuizen AG, van Horn JR, Huyghe JM, Verkerke GJ: Requirements for an artificial intervertebral disc. *Int J Artif Organs* 2001;24:311-321.

97. Klara PM, Ray CD: Artificial nucleus replacement: Clinical experience. *Spine* 2002;27:1374-1377.

98. Fielding JW, Cochran GB, Lawsing JF, Hohl M: Tears of the transverse ligament of the axis: A clinical and biomechanical study. *J Bone Joint Surg Am* 1974;56:1683-1691.

99. Fielding JW, Hawkins RJ, Ratzan SA: Spine fusion for atlanto-axial instability. *J Bone Joint Surg Am* 1976;58:400-407.

100. Whitesides TE Jr, Kelly PP: Lateral approach to the upper cervical spine for anterior fusion. *South Med J* 1966;59:879-883.

101. de Andrade JR, Macnab I: Anterior occipito-cervical fusion using an extra-pharyngeal approach. *J Bone Joint Surg Am* 1969;51:1621-1626.

102. Simmons EH: The surgical correction of flexion deformity of the cervical spine in ankylosing spondylitis. *Clin Orthop Relat Res* 1972;86:132-143.

103. Bailey RW, Badgley CE: Stabilization of the cervical spine by anterior fusion. *J Bone Joint Surg Am* 1960;42:565-594.

104. Cloward RB: The anterior approach for removal of ruptured cervical disks. *J Neurosurg* 1958;15:602-617.

105. Gore DR, Sepic SB: Anterior cervical fusion for degenerated or protruded discs: A review of one hundred forty-six patients. *Spine* 1984;9:667-671.

106. Stauffer ES, Kelly EG: Fracture-dislocations of the cervical spine: Instability and recurrent deformity following treatment by anterior interbody fusion. *J Bone Joint Surg Am* 1977;59:45-48.

107. Böhler J, Gaudernak T: Anterior plate stabilization for fracture-dislocations of the lower cervical spine. *J Trauma* 1980;20:203-205.

108. Phillips FM, Garfin SR: Cervical disc replacement. *Spine* 2005;30(17 suppl):S27-S33.

109. Nurick S: The pathogenesis of the spinal cord disorder associated with cervical spondylosis. *Brain* 1972;95:87-100.

110. Brain WR, Northfield D, Wilkinson M: The neurological manifestations of cervical spondylosis. *Brain* 1952;75:187-225.

111. Nurick S: The natural history and the results of surgical treatment of the spinal cord disorder associated with cervical spondylosis. *Brain* 1972;95:101-108.

112. Hirabayashi K, Watanabe K, Wakano K, Suzuki N, Satomi K, Ishii Y: Expansive open-door laminoplasty for cervical spinal stenotic laminoplasty. *Spine* 1983;8:693-699.

113. Herkowitz HN: A comparison of anterior cervical fusion, cervical laminectomy, and cervical laminoplasty for the surgical management of multiple level spondylotic radiculopathy. *Spine* 1988;13:774-780.

114. Emery SE, Bohlman HH, Bolesta MJ, Jones PK: Anterior cervical decompression and arthrodesis for the treatment of cervical spondylotic myelopathy: Two to seventeen-year follow-up. *J Bone Joint Surg Am* 1998;80:941-951.

115. Pierce DS, Barr JS: Fractures and dislocations at the base of the skull and upper cervical spine, in *The Cervical Spine*, ed 2. Philadelphia, PA, JB Lippincott, 1989, pp 312-324.

116. Clark CR, White AA: Fractures of the dens: A multicenter study. *J Bone Joint Surg Am* 1985;67:1340-1348.

117. Anderson LD, D'Alonzo RT: Fractures of the odontoid process of the axis. *J Bone Joint Surg Am* 1974;56:1663-1674.

118. Rao G, Apfelbaum RI: Dens fractures, in Clark CR (ed): *The Cervical Spine*, ed 4. Philadelphia, PA, Lippincott Williams & Wilkins, 2005, p 614.

119. Jeanneret B, Magerl F: Primary posterior fusion of C1-2 in odontoid fractures: Indiccations, techniques, and results of transarticular screw fixation. *J Spinal Disord* 1992;5:464-475.

120. Apfelbaum RI, Lonser RR, Veres R, et al: Direct anterior screw fixation for recent and remote odontoid fractures. *J Neurosurg* 2000;93(suppl 2):227-236.

121. Schneider RC, Livingston KE, Cearse AJL: "Hangman's fracture" of the cervical spine. *J Neurosurg* 1965;22:141-154.

122. Bucholz RW, Burkhead WZ: The pathological anatomy of fatal atlanto-occipital dislocations. *J Bone Joint Surg Am* 1979;61:248-250.

123. Traynelis VC, Marano GD, Dunder RO, Kaufman HH: Traumatic atlanto-occipital dislocation: Case report. *J Neurosurg* 1986;65:863-870.

124. Fielding JW, Hensinger RR, Hawkins RJ: Os odontoideum. *J Bone Joint Surg Am* 1980;62:376-383.

125. Bohlman HH: Acute fractures and dislocations of the cervical spine: An analysis of three hundred hospitalized patients and review of the literature. *J Bone Joint Surg Am* 1979;61:1119-1142.

126. Roy-Camille R, Saillant G, Mayel C: Internal fixation of the unstable cervical spine by a posterior osteosynthesis with plates and screws, in *The Cervical Spine*, ed 2. Philadelphia, PA, JB Lippincott, 1989, p 390.

127. Albert TJ, Klein GR, Joffe D, Vaccaro AR: Use of cervicothoracic junction pedicle screws for reconstruction of complex cervical spine pathology. *Spine* 1998;23:1596-1599.

CHAPTER 7

ARTHROSCOPIC SURGERY AND SPORTS MEDICINE

Injuries of the Menisci

Arthroscopy has radically altered the practice of orthopaedic surgery. Patients and surgeons prefer the limited morbidity associated with arthroscopic surgery, and as older orthopaedists have retired, the use of open surgery for many orthopaedic conditions has dwindled. Unless a patient requires a total joint arthroplasty, most knee and shoulder operations can now be done arthroscopically.

Before the advent of the arthroscope, knee, shoulder, and other joint injuries and conditions were treated with open surgical techniques. A review of some of the open surgical solutions will provide an understanding of how prearthroscopic orthopaedists managed these conditions. It will also show how they provided the foundation for modern treatment of such problems as knee ligament and meniscal injuries, shoulder subluxations and rotator cuff tears, and early articular cartilage injuries.

American orthopaedic surgeons did not pay much attention to these conditions in the early years of the specialty. The table of contents of the first 10 years of the *Journal of Orthopaedic Surgery* (the predecessor of *The Journal of Bone and Joint Surgery*) did not even mention them. A British physician, William Hey, coined the term "internal derangement of the knee" in 1803.[1] Another British surgeon, John Reid,[2] described the pathology of a meniscal tear in 1834, but American orthopaedists were too preoccupied with tuberculosis, spinal deformity, and various congenital malformations to concern themselves with meniscal injuries. In 1885, 2 years before a group of New York physicians met in the Park Avenue office of Lewis A. Sayre to establish the American Orthopaedic Association (AOA), Scottish surgeon Thomas Annandale[3] described the first operation for a displaced semilunar cartilage, in which he sutured the torn meniscal attachments back "to the fascia and periosteum covering the margin of the tibia." He reported that his meniscal repair worked "splendidly" and that the patient recovered with "perfect movement in the joint and had never had the slightest effusion or locking of the joint" thereafter. His report in the British literature, however, did not appear to have interested American physicians; in fact, very few papers on knee injuries, including meniscal tears, found their way into the American orthopaedic literature during the first two decades of the 20th century. A review of the *American Journal of Orthopaedic Surgery* during those years reveals little interest in the subject.

By 1920, American orthopaedic surgeons were devoting more attention to the subject of meniscal injury. In 1919, the *Journal of Orthopaedic Surgery* published an abstract of Melvin Henderson's paper on the results of 98 meniscectomies done at the Mayo Clinic. Henderson suggested that a patient should be treated conservatively first, but if that failed, a meniscectomy was required.[4]

In the same volume, Lt. T. G. Charles Painter, U.S. Naval Reserve, reported on the meniscal injuries at the U.S. Naval Hospital in Chelsea, Massachusetts. He wrote that if the physicians there suspected a meniscal injury they performed an air arthrogram; if positive, they did a meniscectomy. In his words, "There is no treatment at all satisfactory except excision of the displaced meniscus."[5]

By the mid-1920s, Willis C. Campbell published his review of 167 knee operations for semilunar cartilage injuries, loose bodies in the knee, and various other conditions. In the *Southern Medical Journal* in the same year, he declared: "Dislocation or fracture of the internal semilunar cartilage is the most common cause of derangement of the knee joint."[6]

In 1935, *The Journal of Bone and Joint Surgery* published a lengthy analysis of meniscal surgery by W. Rowley Bristow,[7] a well-known London orthopaedist. Bristow reported that he had operated on 725 patients with meniscal injuries. He strongly espoused removal of the entire meniscus and recommended that if that goal was unattainable with a single anterior incision, the surgeon should make a second incision in the back of the knee and remove any remaining posterior meniscal fragments.

Bristow's recommendations were in line with those of other influential British orthopaedists such as Reginald Watson-Jones[8] and I. S. Smillie,[9] who through the mid-1940s strongly recommended complete meniscectomy. American orthopaedic surgeons, influenced by published opinions from the Campbell Clinic, the Mayo Clinic, and elsewhere in the United States, as well as by the advice of renowned British authorities, undertook large numbers of total meniscectomies during the 1940s and 1950s. During World War II, they did so many that the Surgeon General of the Army mandated that a surgeon could perform this operation only after a review of the case by the surgeon's superior officers (see Chapter 4).

Orthopaedic surgeons had no reliable method to accurately diagnose a medial semilunar cartilage injury during those years. The history and physical examination frequently were not helpful despite the development of various physical signs for making the diagnosis. The most significant of these was the McMurray sign, devised by Thomas P. McMurray of Liverpool, England,[10] who deduced that he could detect tears of the posterior horns of the menisci by flexing the knee fully and rotating the tibia on the femoral condyles.

The opinion that total meniscectomy offered the patient the best chance for long-term success remained dominant into the 1960s. In his book *Diseases of the Knee*,[11] Anthony DePalma of Jefferson Medical College in Philadelphia stated: "Excision of the entire meniscus is the procedure of choice." He and others based this opinion on the claim that "failure to do this predisposes the posterior segment to trappings between the condyles of the femur and the tibia. The remaining posterior segment becomes hyper-mobile and eventually will be caught between the articular surfaces of the femoral and tibial condyles." Don H. O'Donoghue,[12] who wrote the first book on sports medicine in 1962, corroborated that all of the meniscal attachments must be divided, "care being taken to get all of the meniscus." If the surgeon could not do this from the front, the back of the knee would need to be opened to remove the offending posterior horn.

These surgeons held these opinions in the face of mounting evidence to the contrary. In 1936, Ben King of the Stanford University School of Medicine wrote two papers published in *The Journal of Bone and Joint Surgery*[13,14] detailing his experiments on the functions of the knee menisci. He noted that the menisci protect the hyaline cartilage of the knee by absorbing shock, increase stability by deepening the tibial surfaces, pro-mote lubrication of the joint, relieve incongruities, and increase mobility between the meshing femoral and tibial surfaces. He performed partial and total meniscectomies in dogs and found that removal of even a small seg-ment of meniscus produced degeneration of the articular cartilage. He also found that experimental tears in the menisci would heal if he made them at or close to the periphery of the meniscus; otherwise, they would not heal. It appears that the orthopaedic surgeons of the time ignored these findings. T. J. Fairbank of London[15] made an even stronger case for preservation of the menisci in his paper published in the British volume of the *Journal of Bone and Joint Surgery* in 1948, 12 years later. He reviewed the pre- and postoperative knee radiographs of 107 patients who had total meniscec-tomies. He found that by five months after surgery, 66 percent of medial meniscectomy patients and 50 percent of lateral meniscectomy patients had radiographically demonstrable joint-space narrowing, condylar ridge for-mation, or flattening of the femoral condyles. He challenged the widely held opinion that meniscectomy was an innocuous procedure and said that in his opinion it would predispose a knee to early degenerative changes.

Cruciate Ligament Injuries

In January 1983, John Feagin of Jackson, Wyoming, served as the guest editor for a symposium on the cruciate-deficient knee, published in *Clinical Orthopaedics and Related Research*.[16] The symposium is of considerable interest because it was published during the period just before the addition of arthroscopic surgery to the armamentarium of orthopaedic surgeons who treated these injuries. George Snook presented a brief history of the subject in the symposium and cited W. H. Battle, S. Alwyn-Smith, H. Goetjes, Mayo Robson, Ivar Palmer, and Hey Groves as the pioneers in anterior cru-ciate ligament (ACL) surgery in the late 19th century and the first few decades of the 20th century. The early reports provided little information on the outcomes of the various methods used to treat anterior ACL injuries, but direct repair intra-articularly must not have worked very well. Hey Groves and Alwyn-Smith, for example, reported that their poor results with this method prompted them to attempt reconstructions of the ligaments by passing fascia lata or tendon grafts across the knee joint through tunnels in the tibial and femoral condyles (Figure 39). Hey Groves accompanied his 1917 descriptions with drawings that bear a strong resemblance to modern ACL reconstruction. He wrote, "While the frequency and importance of this injury is becoming more widely known, there have not been any corresponding advances in methods of treatment. A rigid plaster or leather cast to be worn for a year, followed by a hinged apparatus, represents the generally accepted method. It is impossible to regard intraarticular suture of the ligaments . . . as an effective procedure." Hey Groves described his reconstruction in detail, reporting subsequently in 1919 that he had done this operation on 15 patients overall.[17,18] Despite Hey Groves' apparently good outcomes, his methods did not gain wide acceptance, at least not in America. In his 1950 *JBJS* article on surgical treatment of injuries to the major ligaments of the knee joint,[19] as well as in his book on treatment of injuries to athletes, Don H. O'Donoghue of Oklahoma City recommended direct repair of a torn ACL. O'Donoghue, however, made a noteworthy contribution to orthopaedics by focusing on ligament repair and educating his contemporaries about the importance of the subject. Willis C. Campbell[20] also wrote about ACL injuries and coined the term "the terrible triad" in 1936. The triad consisted of tears of the medial collateral ligament, medial meniscus, and ACL. Later, O'Donoghue called the same three injuries the "unhappy triad." Campbell and O'Donoghue had different approaches to the treatment of these injuries. Campbell reconstructed the ACL with a tendon graft passed through bony tunnels, whereas O'Donoghue simply reattached the torn ligaments.

By 1983, the year of Feagin's symposium, the orthopaedic community had gained a sophisticated understanding of ACL injuries. For example, there was now nearly universal appreciation of the biomechanics of ACL failure. Important papers by Victor Frankel[21] (New York), Frank Noyes[22] (Cincinnati), and J. C. Kennedy[23] (Toronto) and their associates described the physical properties of the cruciate ligaments, how rates of load modified these properties, and what effect aging had on them. Frank Noyes and his associates[22] found that selected sectioning of the ACL showed that the anteromedial portion of the ligament tightens when the knee is flexed, and this quality prevents anterior displacement of the flexed tibia on the femoral condyles. The posterolateral part of the ligament, on the other hand, is loose in flexion but tightens in extension, thus stabilizing the extended tibia on the distal femur. Anatomical studies by Steven Arnoczky, DVM,[24] and his associates at the Hospital for Special Surgery in New York demonstrated the rich blood supply of the ligaments from the middle genicular artery and the innervation of the ligament with sensory nerve fibers. These findings have clinical significance in that acute rupture of the ligament could also tear apart the blood vessels that surround it. Clinical studies have shown that a patient with an immediate hemarthrosis after a twisting or hyperextension injury has a 70 percent likelihood of an ACL tear.[25] The importance of the discovery of sensory nerve fibers in the ACL

lies in the knowledge that patients with these tears lose at least some pro-
prioception and position sense during motion. Regardless of the quality of
surgical reconstruction, patients thus have a permanent impairment after
such an injury.

During the 1970s and 1980s, orthopaedic surgeons interested in knee
surgery in general and ACL tears in particular developed numerous diagnostic physical findings to establish the diagnosis of cruciate and collateral
ligament injuries. They based their work on earlier fundamental research. In
1944, LeRoy C. Abbott of San Francisco, together with John Saunders,
Frederick Bost, and Carl Anderson,[26] published a classic article on injuries
to the ligaments of the knee. Their work in the mid-1940s, loosely based on
the writings of Ivar Palmer of Sweden,[27] provided the blueprint for the diagnosis and treatment of soft-tissue injuries about the knee joint. Surgeons
who were interested in treating athletes and others who had these injuries
developed several diagnostic maneuvers in an effort to pinpoint the location
of the injury.

In 1976, Dr. Joseph Torg and associates[28] described an important physical sign. The patient would lie supine, and the examiner would flex the knee
to about 15°. While holding the distal femur firmly, the examiner would
grasp the proximal tibia and gently displace it anteriorly. If the examiner
observed no end point to the anterior excursion of the tibia on the femur, it
could be assumed that the patient had an ACL tear. All of the patients with
ACL injury tested under anesthesia had a positive sign, and 80 percent of
those tested without anesthesia had a positive sign. The accuracy of the sign
far exceeded that of the simple anterior drawer test, which yielded a positive result in only 50 percent of patients tested under anesthesia and 10 percent of those tested without it. Torg trained in orthopaedics at Temple
University in Philadelphia, where John Lachman was his mentor. Having
learned this physical finding from Lachman, Torg immortalized him by
calling the maneuver the Lachman sign. The maneuver has gone by that
name ever since.

In 1980, Galway and MacIntosh[29] described the lateral pivot-shift test
for the diagnosis of ACL tears associated with rotational instability of the
knee. Jack Hughston,[30,31] who established the Sports Medicine Center in
Columbus, Georgia, described the same test in reverse. Hughston called his
test the reverse pivot-shift, or "jerk," test.

Orthopaedic surgeons have devised and described several other signs
used in the physical diagnosis of an injured knee. These include the
Slocum[32] anterior drawer test, the quadriceps active test,[33] the external rotation recurvatum test,[34] and the reverse pivot-shift sign of Jakob, Hassler,
and Stäubli[35] for posterolateral knee instability caused by injury of the PCL
(as opposed to the ACL injury diagnosable with the anterior pivot-shift
sign).

While these signs give an orthopaedic surgeon useful information, they
actually depend on a subjective appraisal of motion, displacement, and
crepitus of one bone moving on another. More precise measurements could
come about only with instrumentation; Kennedy and Fowler[36] provided the

much-needed equipment. In 1971, they reported that they had built a machine to deliver precisely measured force at a controlled rate to the components of the knee. Kennedy's machine evolved into the KT-1000 arthrometer. The KT-1000 is now the standard for objective evaluation of knee surgery outcome. The KT-1000 and KT-2000 provide surgeons with a numeric assessment of pre- and postoperative laxity, but they do not quantify patients' functional recovery. In 1982, Jacob Lysholm of Linkoping, Sweden, devised a scoring system that addressed this issue to the satisfaction of most surgeons who tried to evaluate their surgical outcomes objectively.[37] Lysholm modified the 100-point scale used by Robert Larson of Eugene, Oregon, who placed greater emphasis on instability defined as "giving way" of the knee by a patient.[38] His changes to Larson's scale defined the lowest activity level needed to produce pain or giving way or swelling during walking, running, or jumping. Lysholm's scale is still used as a reproducible way to evaluate patients' responses to treatment, and it complements numeric measurements of laxity provided by the Kennedy devices.

In John Feagin's 1983 symposium on ACL injuries, only one of the 30 papers in the symposium discussed the clinical use of the arthroscope in the overall treatment of the ACL-deficient knee. That paper, written by Kenneth DeHaven[39] of the University of Rochester, proposed that a surgeon should use the arthroscope as a diagnostic and evaluative device before proceeding to the actual repair or reconstruction of the torn ligaments. DeHaven stated, "Arthroscopic examination can help to demonstrate the associated lesion, especially meniscal tears." Later in his paper, however, he suggested that one might perform a partial meniscectomy "using arthroscopic techniques if possible or, if not, as an open operation."

Feagin's symposium was published on the cusp of the revolution in the treatment of knee ligament injuries. Arthroscopy completely altered the way surgeons think about this problem, but they were not quite ready to change. The material in Feagin's symposium therefore provides interesting insight into what treatment an orthopaedist considered just before arthroscopy came to dominate the surgical scene. The paper by James Andrews and Richard Sanders of the Hughston Clinic in Columbus, Georgia, for example, discussed extra-articular techniques in the treatment of anterolateral rotatory instability associated with an ACL deficiency.[40] They stated that although some surgeons preferred intra-articular repairs and reconstructions, the difficulties associated with duplicating ACL strength and durability intra-articularly led them to perform extra-articular stabilizing operations. Of course, these were not original with Andrews and Sanders. Ellison,[41] MacIntosh,[42] Johnson,[43] Galway,[44] and others had developed operations that looped tendon or fascia around the lateral collateral ligament to tighten the lateral capsule enough to prevent its subluxation anteriorly (which occurred during the pivot-shift test). Andrews and Sanders devised a "mini-reconstruction operation" in which they sutured the distal part of the fascia lata to the underlying bone and soft tissues through a 10-cm lateral incision, hoping to snug up the soft tissues on the lateral side of the knee. The Andrews-Sanders mini-reconstruction required another incision of the medial side of the knee, through which the transosseous sutures were tied. Andrews and Sanders reported that they did this operation on 62 knees and that "the results have been gratifying."[40] Subsequently, extra-articular procedures for treatment of the ACL-deficient knee have been abandoned.

In the same 1983 symposium, John Kennedy of London, Ontario, presented a paper that summarized the status of prosthetic ACLs.[45] He described the three kinds of synthetic materials: stents of polyethylene, designed to function as a temporary split; degrading scaffold replacements of carbon fiber designed to induce fibrous ingrowth and replacement; and ligament augmentation devices of Dacron or polypropylene to be used with autogenous graft to stabilize the knee while the tissue graft matured. Kennedy admitted that 12 years of experimentation with synthetic grafts failed to produce any lasting satisfactory results and claimed that "the evolution of synthetic materials to aid in the repair of ACL instability is in the embryonic stage of development." Several subsequent studies did not support the use of artificial ligaments, and interest in them largely disappeared by the late 1990s.

Other authors in Feagin's symposium on the ACL-deficient knee described various aspects of intra-articular reconstruction versus primary direct repair. Although the authors intended that the surgeons use open and quite wide exposures, they were actually setting the stage for less invasive arthroscopic methods. Frank R. Noyes and Kenneth Lambert described vascularized patellar tendon grafts, and William Mott discussed the use of semitendinosis tendon. George Hewson described a set of drill guides "for improving accuracy in anterior cruciate ligament repair and reconstruction," and several other authors discussed the rationale for repairing or reconstructing deficient ACLs to prevent chronic instability and early-onset osteoarthritis.[16] These reports began a tidal wave of information about the ACL that has continued up to the present.

Arthroscopy

Virtually every advance in medicine and surgery came about through discoveries made by nonphysicians. Physicians did not invent ether, nitrous oxide, or chloroform, but they found ways to apply them to surgical practice; similarly, it took Louis Pasteur to inspire Lister's revolution of antiseptic surgery. The same is true for arthroscopy.

The early 19th century endoscopes were profoundly limited by a poor light source (Figure 40). Before Thomas Edison and electric light, there were only candles and oil lamps, followed by glowing metal filaments. Medical histories and texts such as *Surgical Arthroscopy* (edited by John McGinty),[46] the *Textbook of Arthroscopy* (edited by Mark Miller and Brian Cole),[47] and the *Manual of Arthroscopic Surgery* (edited by Michael Strobel)[48] all recount the same information about these early attempts to look into the human body through a narrow tube. They describe the Bozzini

Lichleiter endoscope of 1806, which used a candle to reflect light into the bladder; the 1853 Gasogene endoscope of Desormaux, which used a flame of burning turpentine and alcohol; and the electrically heated glowing platinum loop of Nitze of 1876. Use of these scopes was hampered by poor visualization and excessive heat generation, which could burn patient tissue. Thomas Edison's invention of the light bulb therefore became the turning point for endoscopically oriented physicians. Robert Jackson, in his discussion of the history of arthroscopy in McGinty's text, references a 1912 report on diagnostic arthroscopy by Severin Nordentoft. Nordentoft devised a "trochar endoscope" that he presented to the German society of surgeons in 1912, describing in his report how it enabled him to visualize the components of the anterior part of the knee, such as the patellofemoral joint and the anterior horns of the menisci. He thought his device would be useful in differentiating tuberculous synovitis from syphilitic inflammations of the synovium. According to Jackson, Nordentoft died of aplastic anemia resulting from excessive radiation exposure.

Despite Nordtentoft's 1912 venture into diagnostic arthroscopy, the European and American surgical communities ignored the subject until several Japanese investigators proved that it really worked. In 1918, Kenji Takaji of Tokyo University began attempting to visualize the interior of a knee joint by inserting a 7.3-mm cystoscope into a cadaveric knee. By 1920, he developed a narrower 3.5-mm-diameter endoscope for use in the knee joint. He also developed a system of trochars, cannulas, and punches for synovial biopsies and succeeded in taking intra-articular photographs by 1932. Takaji, like Nordentoft, had little impact on mainstream orthopaedics in Europe and America. War between China and Japan, then between Japan and the United States, absolutely precluded any contact between American orthopaedists and their Japanese counterparts until many years later. Several Western surgeons, however, attempted to apply arthroscopic techniques to knee surgery. In 1921, Eugen Bircher, a Swiss surgeon, performed "arthroendoscopy" of the knee using carbon monoxide to distend the joint. In 1925, Philip Kreuscher published a paper in the *Illinois Medical Journal* entitled "Semilumar Cartilage Disease: A Plea for Early Recognition by Means of the Arthroscope and Early Recognition of this Condition." Michael Burman of the Hospital for Joint Diseases in New York published several articles on arthroscopy in the 1930s, two of them in *The Journal of Bone and Joint Surgery*, and R. Sommer and E. Vaubel published papers on arthroscopy in the German literature in the late 1930s on the same subject. World War II delayed further development of arthroscopy in orthopaedics until the 1950s. By then, Takaji had relinquished his interest in the subject to Mosaki Watanabi. Watanabi continued Takaji's work with the development of narrower arthroscopes and better light sources and optics. His early models featured a light bulb at the end of the arthroscope, but fiber optics facilitated the removal of the light source from within the joint. Development of high-intensity xenon lighting and effective irrigation systems made it possible to place the

light source outside of the joint and deliver light into the joint via a
fiberoptic cable. Despite a single paper by E. Hurter in 1955, American
orthopaedic surgeons remained indifferent to arthroscopy and its possibilities until 1964. In that year, Robert Jackson went to Tokyo
University to study tissue culture techniques, but he became sidetracked
by Watanabi's work. This serendipitous occurrence changed his career.
When Jackson returned to Toronto, he employed arthroscopic techniques in large numbers of patients with his new Japanese associate Isao
Abe. By 1968, Jackson and Abe had enough information to present an
instructional course in arthroscopy at the Annual Meeting of the
American Academy of Orthopaedic Surgeons. By then they had
received visits from other American orthopaedists eager to investigate
arthroscopy (most notably John McGinty of Wellesley, Massachusetts,
and Ward Casscells of Wilmington, Delaware). Other orthopaedists,
including Richard O'Connor, visited Watanabi; many others took up
arthroscopy, improving the instrumentation and techniques and popular-
izing it worldwide. Lanny Johnson, John Joyce, Kenneth DeHaven,
Ralph Lidge, and Robert Metcalf were among the "pioneers." The col-
legiality and the competition inherent in being the innovators of a new
technology that would revolutionize orthopaedic surgery led them to
organize a society. In 1982, the year before Feagin was guest editor for
his ACL symposium, they formed the Arthroscopy Society and elected
Watanabi as their first president. Since then, arthroscopy and arthroscopic surgery have transformed orthopaedics.

Most of the papers produced in the 1970s and 1980s related to knee
arthroscopy techniques and what could be learned diagnostically from
the method. The arthroscopist initially performed only a few simple procedures. For example, Ward Casscells' 1971 review of 150 cases published in *The Journal of Bone and Joint Surgery*[49] (which he claimed
was the first report in the English-speaking literature since 1934) found
three main uses for the arthroscope: (1) diagnosis of meniscal lesions
and defects of the articular cartilage; (2) follow-up with patients who
had previous surgery; and (3) visualization of the patellofemoral relationship to determine surgical options for patellofemoral disorders.
Casscells said that he preferred arthroscopy to arthrography, which at
that time was the only diagnostic modality available other than a physical examination and plain radiograph.

In the following year, Robert Jackson published his analysis of 200 consecutive arthroscopic examinations in the British volume of *JBJS*.[50] The
arthroscopic procedure in these 200 patients was restricted to diagnosis
only; Jackson thought the operation was extremely useful because he could
avoid operations on patients who had no abnormalities but reported knee
pain.

Richard O'Connor of West Covena, California, published his first paper
on the subject in 1974.[51] He had examined arthroscopically 21 patients who
sustained acute knee injuries. Like Casscells and Jackson, O'Connor used
the Watanabi model No. 21 direct-view arthroscope. The scope enabled him

to identify a characteristic peripheral detachment tear of the meniscus and to accurately assess injuries of the ACL and capsular ligament.

Kenneth DeHaven and H. Roger Collins[52] weighed in a year later with their paper on the arthroscopic diagnosis of internal derangements of the knee using the Watanabi No. 21 arthroscope. They performed a prospective study of 100 patients, all of whom warranted surgical treatment, comparing the diagnoses obtained by physical examination with those made by double-contrast arthrography, arthroscopy, and finally by arthrotomy. They concluded that by using arthrography and arthroscopy together, the orthopaedic diagnostician should be able to make the correct diagnosis 100 percent of the time.

John McGinty and Peter Freedman[53] published a similar paper in *Clinical Orthopaedics and Related Research* in 1976, a year after DeHaven and Collins. They reviewed 220 consecutive endoscopic knee examinations done with either the Watanabi No. 21 arthroscope or the Storz 2.7-mm or 40-mm fiber optic arthroscopes. Many of their patients had been referred for diagnostic arthroscopy with the understanding that they would return to the referring orthopaedists for definitive surgery if anything abnormal turned up at the arthroscopic examination. A total of 110 patients in McGinty's early series had an arthroscopic procedure without a subsequent arthrotomy, and 32 of these had no abnormal findings on arthroscopic examination. McGinty suggested that arthroscopy had saved those patients from an unnecessary operation.

Surgical arthroscopy may have begun with Casscells' arthroscopic synovial biopsy in 1971, but Casscells did not provide details of his procedure. Almost certainly triangulation was not involved, nor did he consider using video monitoring or have it available. At that time, the surgeon had to bend down to the eyepiece of the arthroscope to see inside the joint. The eyepiece frequently came in contact with the arthroscopist's facial skin, adding a risk of infection. Within a few years, several energetic and persistent orthopaedic surgeons developed video-assisted arthroscopic surgery with motorized instruments using triangulating techniques, which eliminated this problem.

By 1982, Jackson had reported on arthroscopic release of synovial plicas;[54] DeHaven[55] elaborated on the principles of triangulation for arthroscopic surgery; and Gilchrist, Oretorp, Dandy, and others published their techniques for arthroscopic meniscectomy.[56-58] The technique was taking off and entering the mainstream.

Triangulation made it possible to avoid using a surgical arthroscope. This device had a 7.5-mm sheath through which the arthroscope and cutting instruments were inserted. The setup required the use of a narrow-diameter arthroscope that reduced the field of vision and which in turn could easily be obstructed. The cutting instruments also had to fit through the sheath of the arthroscope, and thus had to be quite narrow as well. The large sheath made navigation inside the joint difficult, and even with an offset eyepiece, many surgeons found the operating arthroscope difficult to use (Figure 41). With triangulation, a surgeon could use the standard-sized arthroscope with a larger diameter and field of vision, and could put the cutting instruments through a separate portal into the knee joint. Because the cutting instruments did not have to pass through the same sheath as the arthroscope, they could be made larger and more efficient. Triangulation meant that the surgeon had to learn a new set of hand-eye skills, but once acquired, these skills greatly facilitated the procedure (Figure 42).

The subsequent meniscectomy papers were of particular interest because they emphasized removal only of the torn or injured part of the meniscus, versus the previous techniques requiring the meniscus to be removed entirely if any part was torn or detached. Arthroscopy thus made it possible to define tear patterns and preserve as much meniscal tissue as possible. Lanny Johnson,[58] Robert Metcalf,[59] and others during the 1980s also instituted the use of video monitors. This crucial innovation did not catch on at first, and in 1982 James Mullhollan[60] wrote: "Television is not mandatory for this procedure (arthroscopic meniscectomy)." In the same year,[55] DeHaven said: "Television is widely used . . . but it is certainly possible to perform arthroscopic surgery without the use of television." He noted that "As the surgeon learns to work from the video monitor, he can assume a more comfortable body position." Even so, DeHaven at that time attached a television camera to the arthroscope with a beam splitter. This would enable him to bypass the television and use the eyepiece to look directly into the joint if he felt it was necessary.

On the other hand, by 1982 Lanny Johnson[61] had wholeheartedly embraced video monitoring for arthroscopy and arthroscopic surgery. Since the mid-1980s arthroscopists, in cooperation with manufacturers, have progressed from using bulky tube cameras to single- and double-chip cameras, to relying by the early 21st century primarily on triple-chip cameras with high resolution and excellent color reproduction. By the mid- to late 1980s, arthroscopic surgeons were abandoning open procedures and opting instead to perform most meniscectomy procedures and ACL repairs arthroscopically.

One of the pioneers in this effort, Richard O'Connor, made the pilgrimage to Japan in the mid-1960s and became convinced that arthroscopy was the future for orthopaedics. Upon his return to America, he first plunged into the development of diagnostic arthroscopy, then devised the first operating arthroscope and produced high-quality intra-articular photographs. Technical limitations of the available instrumentation made arthroscopy difficult for many orthopaedists, however. Collaboration of early pioneers with manufacturers such as Richard Wolf Medical Instruments, Dionics, and others led to refinements that made arthroscopic operations practical. O'Connor died of lung cancer in 1980 at the age of 47. He had only a little over a decade to devote to his life's work, but he clearly made the most of it.[62]

Despite the progress American orthopaedists made in arthroscopy, skeptics still questioned the value of the new modality. A 1976 editorial in *Lancet*[63] entitled "Unnecessary Meniscectomy," for example, claimed that orthopaedic surgeons did not have the technical ability to diagnose symptomatic meniscal tears adequately. The authors of the editorial further commented that many elderly individuals have meniscal tears that do not cause symptoms. They disagreed with Watson-Jones' dictum that a surgeon who has opened the knee for a suspected meniscal tear should remove the entire meniscus even when a tear is not found because the posterior horn might still be torn although hard to visualize behind the femoral condyles. They also cited the papers by King and Fairbanks containing documentation of early osteoarthritis that developed after total meniscectomy. The editorial acknowledged the great increase in diagnostic arthroscopy in North America but proclaimed the modality impractical in Great Britain at that time because economic considerations precluded providing orthopaedists with arthroscopes.

A reply to the editorial came several years later in the British volume of *The Journal of Bone and Joint Surgery*, which published a paper, "In Defence of the Meniscus," by Jay Nobel and E. Erat.[64] Drs. Nobel and Erat reviewed 250 patients who were scheduled for meniscus surgery. With patients often waiting quite a long time for surgery, 50 of them improved spontaneously and thus did not need the operation. Nobel and Erat had also observed that many patients, despite preoperative arthrograms, had an indefinitive diagnosis before surgery. Worse yet, diagnostic arthroscopy and even open surgery occasionally failed to establish a diagnosis or at the very least revealed no definite meniscal tear. During the mid-1980s, knee surgeons in the United States began experimenting with MRI in an effort to improve their preoperative diagnostic accuracy. Two back-to-back papers published in the American volume of *The Journal of Bone and Joint Surgery* in 1991 reviewed the outcomes of these investigations.[65,66] The overall accuracy for meniscal tears varied widely from one hospital center to another and ranged from 64 percent to 95 percent when MRI findings were compared to those seen at arthroscopy.

The experiences of knee surgeons over the past 25 years as arthroscopic surgical techniques evolved have greatly modified the treatment of meniscal injuries. O'Donoghue, DePalma, Watson-Jones, and Smillie, among others had low thresholds for performing arthrotomies for removal of suspected torn menisci. They strongly advocated removing the entire meniscus, often even if the surgeon could not locate an obvious meniscal tear. Now knee surgeons take a much more conservative approach. They evaluate the meniscus arthroscopically through a very small incision, and if they find tears they remove as little meniscal tissue as possible, trying to maintain a stable rim of fibrocartilage. In fact, it is now considered preferable to repair a torn meniscus if possible than to remove all or even part of it. I. S. Smillie commented in 1946 that "the torn meniscus is an aggressive agent of great power."[9] Few if any orthopaedists accept that statement today.

The chapter on arthroscopic meniscal repair by W. Dilworth Cannon[67] in Surgical Arthroscopy covers the subject succinctly. Suturing a displaced meniscus to the perimeniscal ligament is not new, but in the past surgeons performed this operation only as part of a major open procedure. According to Cannon, Hiroshi Ikeuchi did the first arthroscopic repair in Japan in 1969 and Charles Henning of Wichita, Kansas, did the first one in the United

States in 1980. Henning and others suggested that the long-term effects of partial meniscectomy were not apparent, and removal of even part of a meniscus could result in early degeneration and disabling knee pain. Meniscal repair might obviate these concerns. Arthroscopists have devised several techniques for this operation. In 1988, Henning reported on his intra-articular technique with arthroscopic visualization using a supplemental posterior incision to insert a protective retractor.[68] Several variations in the technique have been described, including the "outside-in method" of Warren, Morgan, Casscells, and others; the all-inside technique of Morgan; zone-specific techniques (Rosenberg); and the double-barrel techniques (Clancy and Graf).[69] In 1993, P. M. Albrecht-Olson and others introduced a biodegradable meniscal arrow made from polymers of polylactic acid or polyglycolic acid.[69]

Arthroscopic Reconstruction of the Cruciate Ligaments

Since the mid-1980s, open repair reconstructions of the cruciate ligaments have gone from the rule to the rare exception. Most of the older surgeons who operated through long incisions about the knee joint have either learned to do the repair arthroscopically or have stopped doing these cases. Younger surgeons and those who trained in the recent past are so comfortable with arthroscopy that they use no other techniques. Orthopaedic surgeons tend to differ over the nuances of treating cruciate ligament injuries, but the experiences of the past two decades have indicated that tunnel placement is the most important factor in ensuring a good outcome. Since the late 1990s, S. M. Howell, Douglas Jackson, Freddie Fu, and others[70-73] have attempted to standardize tunnel placement.

Arthroscopic reconstruction of the cruciate ligaments has greatly lessened postoperative morbidity for these patients. The use of open techniques required many days of hospitalization, followed by difficult recoveries. ACL reconstruction is now performed on an outpatient basis in most cases, with minimal patient morbidity and early functional recoveries. Despite the improvements in surgical technique, however, complications and problems do arise. Some authors note, for example, that patients often develop disabling degenerative changes despite having their cruciate successfully reconstructed arthroscopically. Others have suggested that these degenerative changes cannot be avoided because an injury severe enough to rupture a cruciate ligament might well also injure other structures. Numerous reports have documented a high prevalence of meniscal injury associated with ACL tears, and most surgeons who follow these patients have reported that meniscal tears and osteoarthritis occurred in many patients who have not had their torn ACLs reconstituted. Technical errors might account for the premature development of osteoarthritis in some of these patients, but the outcomes of arthroscopic ACL repairs are generally quite good. These procedures, when performed proficiently, have a high possibility of restoring knee stability. Nonetheless, it is impossible to reconstruct the ACL so that it would function as anything other than a checkrein.

Besides infection, construct failures, and technical errors, patients undergoing ACL reconstruction face the possible complications of arthrofibrosis. This condition has received a good deal of attention in recent years. It results in excessive scarring and fibrosis in the knee after injury or surgery, ultimately causing loss of motion that can occasionally be quite severe. Arthrofibrosis occurs far more often in patients who have had ACL reconstructions soon after injury; most arthroscopists delay operating on a torn ACL until the patient has regained good motion without pain and until the effusion and swelling associated with the injury have subsided. This usually takes at least four weeks and more often six weeks after injury. Following the ACL reconstruction, a Cyclops lesion, infrapatellar tendon fibrosis, adhesions in the suprapatellar bursa, and fibrosis elsewhere can produce loss of flexion or extension or both with limitation of patellar motion because of entrapment of the infrapatellar tendon. Frank Noyes and others[74-77] published several papers on the treatment of arthrofibrosis during the 1980s and 1990s. Their experience suggests that prednisone or nonsteroidal anti-inflammatory drugs might slow down the development of arthrofibrosis, but when drugs and active motion fail to control the progressive stiffness a surgeon should consider arthroscopic or even open release of contracted peripatellar and infrapatellar tissue.

Patellofemoral Pain and Instability

Joel E. Goldthwait[78] of Boston published one of the first American papers on patellofemoral surgery in the *Annals of Surgery* in 1899. The paper presented the case of a 30-year-old woman who came to him for treatment of bilateral fixed lateral patellar dislocations. At the age of ten, she had worked on a sewing machine, pedaling its footplates in a repetitive motion for many hours a day, causing the dislocations. After a lengthy evaluation, Goldthwait performed surgery on both knees. He made an 8-inch incision anterolaterally over each knee and cut longitudinally through "the outer part of the capsule for a distance of 3 inches." This maneuver allowed him to correct the dislocation, but when the knee was flexed, the patella immediately redislocated because the tibial tubercle remained so far lateral. On one side, Goldthwait detached the patellar tendon and transferred it to the sartorius attachment. These maneuvers produced marked laxity of the medial capsule, which he corrected by plication of the loose tissue with sutures. He then performed a partial release of the quadriceps tendon to take tension off of the transferred infrapatellar tendon. He mentioned in his article, almost as an aside, that he performed bilateral supracondylar osteotomies to "straighten the limbs," but he did not make clear how they were deformed or angulated. On the second knee, instead of cutting off the infrapatellar tendon and sewing it to the sartorius insertion, the "whole tubercle of the tibia was chiseled off and thus nailed to a depression which was made on the inner side of the bone." With a two-year follow-up, Goldthwait[79] could report a successful outcome. Goldthwait described 10 other patients with recurrent patellar dislocations in 1904.

Nearly 35 years later, in 1933 (the same year the Academy held its first meeting), Benjamin Franklin Buzby[80] of Camden, New Jersey, reported his results using the Goldthwait operation modified by the Albee osteotomy. Albee recognized that the patella often dislocated because of deficiencies of the trochlea with flattening of the lateral femoral condyle. Albee proposed to correct this abnormality by elevating the lateral femoral condyle with a chisel and keeping it in its corrected position by propping it up with a bone graft. Buzby reported that he attempted to use soft-tissue procedures only, but his patients had recurrence of the patellar dislocations using these techniques. He cited the Krogius operation, which was a lateral release with a medial plication, and the Gallie operation, which used fascia lata sutured to the medial side of the patella and "fastened under tension to the inner femoral condyle." Buzby also outlined the orthodox thinking about the causes of patellar instability as promulgated in the 1930s, such as (1) congenital, with rudimentary patellae that are upwardly displaced with an elongated infrapatellar tendon; (2) traumatic, resulting from an acute injury in an otherwise normal knee; and (3) structural, with a knock-knee deformity, flattened lateral femoral condyle, and deformed shallow trochlea. Buzby noted that the structural deformity often occurred as the result of rickets.

Emil Hauser[81] of the Department of Orthopaedics at Northwestern University published an essay on the "Slipping Patella" in the 1938 *Surgery, Gynecology and Obstetrics* journal. The article mentioned all of the operations then extant for treatment of recurrent dislocations. He claimed that he had given due regard to "each and every procedure that has been devised," and he would classify them according to what their originators attempted to accomplish. He divided the procedures into six groups: plication of relaxed medial capsule, fascial transplantations, muscle transfers, free fascial transplants, osteotomies, and transfers of portions of the infrapatellar tendon. Hauser's own operation consisted of an extensive lateral release to permit the patella to be reduced from its dislocated position, then an aggressive shortening of the medial capsule to keep it there, and finally a medial and distal transfer of the tibial tubercle to correct the angulation of the extensor mechanism, which he believed led to the patellar instability. The Hauser procedure was very popular during the 1950s and 1960s until it became apparent that the distal and medial transfer of the tibial tubercle also transferred the tubercle backward somewhat because of the slope of the proximal tibia. Overdoing this kind of realignment pulled the patella down and backward, causing the patella to press so vigorously into the trochlea of the distal femur that the patients who had the operation developed early and severe patellofemoral arthritis. Most surgeons, in fact, had difficulty in determining how far they moved the tibial tubercle and its attached patellar tendon. Jack Hughston and Michael Walsh[82] of Columbus, Georgia, acknowledged this in a 1979 article on proximal and distal reconstruction of the extension mechanism for patellar subluxation. Donald Chrisman, George Snook, and Thomas Wilson reviewed 47 knees in patients with patellar dislocations treated with the Hauser operation. Eight years after the surgery, 24 of the 47 had significant degenerative changes of the patellofemoral joint. Chrisman, Snook, and Wilson[83] compared their outcomes using Hauser's operation with the less aggressive Roux-Goldthwait procedure[84] and found that 90 percent of the Roux-Goldthwait patients had good long-term results. It would become apparent that the Hauser procedure, with its aggressive tibial tubercle transfer, would have to be abandoned.

In 1976, Paul Maquet[85] of Liege, Belgium, reported on his studies of the mechanics of the patellofemoral joint. He determined that anterior displacement of the tibial tubercle would reduce the patellofemoral joint reaction forces, preserving the articular cartilage on both sides of the joint.

Several publications on the radiographic analysis of patellofemoral instability have influenced the diagnosis and quantification of the relationship between the patella and distal femur. A 1971 paper by Insall and Salvati,[86] for example, established a simple way to define "patella alta," the term used to define a high riding patella that is likely to be unstable. Axial views of the flexed knee, as described by A. C. Merchant and associates[87] in 1974, as well as others, revealed the relationship of the patella to the trochlea, the depth of the trochear groove, and the height of the lateral femoral condyle. H. Brattstrom,[88] a Swedish orthopaedic surgeon, described the Q angle in 1970. The Q angle is not a radiographic finding; rather, it measures or describes the relationship of the infrapatellar tendon to the pull of the quadriceps.

An acute dislocation of the patella involves detachment of the vastus medialis from the medial retinaculum and at least the distal part of the quadriceps tendon. Rupture of the medial patellofemoral ligament occurs in nearly 90 percent of acute patellar dislocations, and treatment of the acute injury requires open repair of the medial patellofemoral ligament with reattachment to the femoral condyle. Reference to the medial patellofemoral ligament did not appear in the literature before 1979, when it was described in detail in a paper by L. F. Warren and J. L. Marshall.[89] In previous papers related to acute patellar dislocations, Rorabeck and Bobechko[90] observed avulsions of ligament and soft tissue from the area of the abductor tubercle. They also noted that reattaching that tissue to the abductor tubercle produced uniformly good results with no recurrence of the patellar dislocation. Conversely, failure to do so usually resulted in a recurrence. Since Warren and Marshall published their findings in 1979, most surgeons who treat this injury also report that an acute patellar dislocation should be treated surgically by open repair and reattachment of the medial patellofemoral ligament and reattachment of the vastus medialis to the retinaculum.

The Shoulder

Recurrent Dislocation

In 1849, the Sydenham Society commissioned a London surgeon named Francis Adams to translate the works of Hippocrates. Adams produced *The Genuine Works of Hippocrates* and included a passage on the treatment of recurrent dislocations of the shoulder. According to Adams' translation, Hippocrates described the impairment caused by instability of the shoulder joint as follows: "Many persons owing to this accident have been obliged to abandon gymnastic exercises, though otherwise well qualified for them, and from the same misfortune have become inadept in warlike practices and have thus perished." Hippocrates advised such people to submit to a procedure that consisted of passing a red-hot iron through the skin of the axilla from below, upward to the front of the humeral head. He suggested that the surgeon performing the procedure should not go much deeper with the iron than the skin because of its proximity to the large blood vessels and nerves. He also advised that the patient should keep his arm close to his side for months after the procedure to allow the body to form the dense eschar that would keep the humeral head secure in its socket. Hippocrates also criticized his competitors, noting that many of them inserted the hot iron too deep or in the wrong place, such as above or behind the humeral head instead of in front of it.

In his commentary on the more than 60 procedures available for treating recurrent shoulder dislocations in his 1946 book on fractures and joint injuries, Sir Reginald Watson-Jones[91] stated: "The technique seemed to be unimportant so long as the operation was sufficiently traumatic and sufficiently bloody . . . the fact is that the success of this multitude of operations depends upon scarring and contracture in front of the joint with limitation of backwards extension and external rotation movement, so that the humerus cannot gain the position required to slide the posterior excavation of the head over the injured anterior glenoid margin." In other words, according to Watson-Jones, modern surgeons with access to multiple surgical techniques had only achieved what Hippocrates had, namely fibrosis, scarring, and an eschar that would hold the humeral head in place.

The operations, varied as they were, addressed different aspects of shoulder instability. Bankart,[92] for example, described several patients in 1923 with recurrent shoulder dislocations in whom "the essential feature is the detachment of the capsule from the fibrocartilaginous glenoid ligament." Fifteen years later, Bankart published another paper indicating that his thinking had changed somewhat.[93,94] In a 1938 paper, he said that a single shoulder dislocation would become recurrent only if "in its passage forward the head shears off the fibrocartilaginous ligament from its attachment to the bone." He wrote that while the capsular tear might heal, the detached labrum could not spontaneously reattach and heal itself to the bone of the glenoid rim. Therefore, in his words, "The only rational treatment is to reattach the glenoid ligament to the bone." Bankart performed a major operation to achieve this goal. Orthopaedic surgeons referred to the detached labrum as the Bankart lesion. Bankart had little regard for other surgeons' operations for treatment of recurrent shoulder dislocation. In particular, he excoriated the Clairmont procedure, which consisted of transferring a strip of deltoid muscle below and around the humeral head to act as a restraining sling. Bankart declared that this procedure prevented recurrent dislocations only when the patient developed enough local scar tissue to stiffen the joint so much that it would not redislocate. He also had little regard for the numerous other operations described by shoulder surgeons, merely noting in passing "the crude and irrational methods . . . based on erroneous ideas of the pathology of recurrent dislocation of the shoulder."

When other surgeons tried to apply Bankart's operation to their own practices, however, they frequently found that the anterior capsule had very little substance after they reflected the overlying subscapularis tendon and that reattachment of the capsule to the labrum was often difficult, if not impossible. In addition, they found that Bankart had oversimplified the matter because other osseous and soft-tissue abnormalities coexisted with the Bankart lesion. For example, Frederick Bost and Verne Inman[95] of the University of California Medical School in San Francisco found that multiple anterior dislocations of the shoulder often resulted in flattening, with erosion or fracture of the anterior glenoid rim. They also confirmed the presence of a grooved defect in the back of the humeral head in these patients. Hill and Sachs[96] described this lesion in 1940 and suggested that when the humeral head went anteriorly out of the shallow glenoid socket, the back of the head would rest on the anterior glenoid. Harold Hill and Maurice Sachs, radiologists in the Department of Medicine at Stanford, published their classic papers in *Radiology*. They cited several references from the 19th and early 20th centuries, such as Malgaigne, Perthes, Flower, and others who described the grooved defect in the back of the humeral head now referred to as the Hill-Sachs lesion.

During the years just after World War II, inventive orthopaedic surgeons devised several operations for recurrent shoulder dislocations and tested older techniques described in the past. Anterior soft-tissue operations besides the Bankart procedure included the Magnuson-Stack transfer of the subscapularis tendon;[97] the Putti-Platt "pants-over-vest" reefing of the anterior capsule and subscapular tendon;[98] and Moseley's modification of the Bankart operation by amplifying the anterior glenoid with a Vitallium rim, a prosthesis that he used to increase the elevation of the glenoid rim when repeated dislocations flattened and deformed it.[99] Other surgeons attempted to increase the height of the anterior glenoid rim by performing bone block operations. The Bristow procedure, for example, was quite popular during the 1960s and 1970s. A. J. Helfet[100] reviewed Bristow's procedure and reported on his own results in 1958. Bristow's operation consisted of transferring the coracoid process to the anterior rim of the glenoid including reefing of the anterior capsule. Helfet subsequently reported a high percentage of serious complications, including injury to the musculocutaneous nerve with consequent paralysis of elbow flexion, recurrence of dislocation, and the failure of the transferred coracoid process to heal satisfactorily in its new location. Eden[101] and Hybinette,[102] German and French surgeons, independently designed an anterior bone block procedure that consisted of screwing an iliac crest bone graft into the anterior glenoid rim that had flattened out under the repeated stresses inherent in repeated anterior dislocations. Other techniques used for correcting the osseous deformities associated with recurrent shoulder dislocations consisted of an osteotomy of the glenoid to direct the saucer-shaped socket backward, or an osteotomy of the surgical neck of the humerus to direct the Hill-Sachs defect in the humeral head away from the anterior glenoid rim.[103] Neither of these procedures gained wide acceptance.

Suspension procedures, however, were accepted techniques for a while, especially those of Melvin Henderson[104] (Mayo Clinic) and Toufick Nicola[105,106] (Montclair, New Jersey). Nicola read a brief paper at the 1928 meeting of the alumni of the Hospital for the Ruptured and Crippled, describing a procedure that transformed the long head of the biceps tendon into a sort of ligamentum teres similar to that seen in the hip. He drilled a tunnel in the proximal humerus from the bicipital groove to the middle of the head of the humerus. He then divided the biceps tendon just below the bicipital groove and threaded the proximal portion through the tunnel. He published the technique description in 1934, and in 1953 presented a paper reporting on follow-up of 25 patients on whom he performed the operation. He reported in the 1953 paper that he had corrected whatever other abnormalities he found in these patients' shoulders, such as a Bankart lesion, glenoid deformity, or a deficient anterior capsule.

Henderson's tenosuspension operation[104] consisted of harvesting a peroneus longus tendon graft, then threading the graft through a tunnel drilled in the acromion and anchoring it through a tunnel in the greater tuberosity of the humerus.

In the late 1970s and the early 1980s, investigations into the functional anatomy of the soft-tissue stability of the shoulder grew much more sophisticated. Research into the subtleties of structure and function of the capsular ligaments resulted in reclassification of shoulder instabilities and changes in their treatment. Anatomic studies by O'Brien and associates[107,108] delineated the functions of the superior, middle, and inferior glenohumeral ligaments and which part of the ligamentous complex grew taut in varying positions in the shoulder. These authors and other investigators elucidated physical signs based on these anatomic studies, differentiating between unidirectional and multidirectional, traumatic versus atraumatic, and involuntary and voluntary shoulder dislocations.

Zarins and associates[109] for example, writing on the treatment of recurrent shoulder dislocations after an acute traumatic dislocation, found that such patients almost always have a Bankart lesion and/or a tear in the anterior capsule, and occasionally a fracture of the glenoid rim or a Hill-Sachs lesion. In addition, they frequently have a widening of the seam between the subscapularis and supraspinatus tendons. Patients under 20 years of age at their first acute traumatic dislocation of the shoulder have a 90 percent chance of recurrence of dislocation because of the laxity of the connective tissue of young adults. In young patients with an acute traumatic recurrent dislocation, however, correction of the specific anatomic defect has an excellent chance of restoring the shoulder to functional stability. Zarins and associates[109] found that repairing only the specific lesion would also avoid the problem of restricted motion and stiffness that complicates overly aggressive capsular plication or tightening of the subscapularis tendon.

Multidirectional instability is less clear-cut. Patients with this problem do not generally have a Bankart lesion and usually do not have a history of injury. In fact, some of the patients with multidirectional instability can voluntarily dislocate their shoulders; Rowe and associates,[110] Neer,[111] and others warn that surgeons should not select such patients for surgical repair. They have too great a risk of recurrence to justify the surgery. Charles Neer and C. R. Foster[112] published a classic article on the surgical treatment of patients with multidirectional instability of the shoulder. These patients did not have Bankart lesions, and the etiology of their instability appeared to be "inherent laxity of the shoulder capsule" from overuse of the shoulder joint in daily and recreational activities. Neer used an inferior capsular shift to tighten the inferior glenohumeral ligament in these patients, either from the front or back, but rarely from both directions. Only one patient of the 37 he reviewed in his 1980 paper on inferior capsular shift had a recurrence, and most of the patients had normal or close to normal mobility.

In the late 1980s and early 1990s, Frederick Matsen[113] popularized a simplified classification system for determining what treatment to use for recurrent shoulder instability. He recommended that surgeons use the acronyms TUBS and AMBRII in deciding which surgical treatment to employ for recurring shoulder dislocations. TUBS is an acronym for *t*raumatic, *u*nidirectional, *B*ankart *s*urgery; AMBRII stands for *a*traumatic, *m*ultidirectional, *b*ilateral, *r*ehabilitation, *i*nferior capsular shift, *i*nternal closure. In their 1980 article on the inferior capsular shift, Neer and Foster[112] mildly disagreed with the "atraumatic" in AMBRII because some of their patients started their history of recurrent subluxations and multidirectional instability with an acute traumatic dislocation.

The Rotator Cuff
Virtually all orthopaedic surgeons who developed ideas about shoulder surgery in the late 20th century had an able predecessor. E. Amory Codman, unknown to many present-day orthopaedists, probably thought up their "new" ideas over 70 years ago. He wrote lucid discourses on these concepts in his numerous papers on shoulder surgery and in his 1934 book, *The Shoulder: Rupture of the Supraspinatus Tendon and Other Lesions in or About the Subacromial Bursa.*[114]

Amory Codman came from one of the most privileged backgrounds in America.[115] In 1869, he was born into a wealthy Boston Brahmin family, which had emigrated from England in 1637 and achieved financial success in the United States. He went to an elite private school (St. Mark's), moving effortlessly on to Harvard College and then to Harvard Medical School. He succeeded academically without appearing to work very hard. His friend and classmate, Harvey Cushing, wrote in a letter than he was "grouchy because Codman learned so much faster than I . . . I wish I had his 14-hour-a-day energy and enthusiasm. I get woozy after about three."[116]

Codman and Cushing began their practices about the same time that Roentgen discovered x-rays, and Codman embraced the new technology with enthusiasm. Codman published one of the first papers on the use of x-rays to diagnose fractures of the distal radius (a study of the x-ray plates of 140 cases of fracture of the lower end of the radius in the *Boston Medical and Surgical Journal* in 1900).[117] In the paper, he described a classification system for Colles' fractures remarkably similar to those used today. He recognized earlier than most the hazards associated with x-rays and published an article on this subject. (In fact, Cushing died of a malignant melanoma, which could have developed because of his exposure to high doses of radiation during his research.) Several years before the outbreak of World War I, Codman began to develop an interest in musculoskeletal surgery, whereas Cushing began to specialize in neurosurgery. Cushing's early results were horrifying. His biographer, Jay Fulton, states, "The question was raised whether he was justified in proceeding."[116] In 1915, Cushing organized the elite corps of Harvard physicians and surgeons (including Marius Smith-Petersen and Philip Wilson) that went to France to help the Allies treat the huge numbers of casualties. Codman stayed behind and embarked on his quixotic quest to implement his "end result idea," which in more modern terms would be called "outcome studies." After much campaigning, Codman organized a summit meeting with the Massachusetts General Hospital trustees, senior staff, the mayor of Boston, and others to review his ideas for possible implementation. During his lengthy speech at the meeting, he displayed a large, insulting cartoon that accused the trustees, Boston politicians, the university president, and the physicians of unconscionable greed and disregard of the medical needs of the people of Boston. In doing so, he committed professional suicide. His fortunes rapidly waned as he lost friends, position, and income. He tried to maintain his practice of general surgery but orthopaedics dominated his thinking, leading to his 1934 book on the shoulder.[114] The book contained an idiosyncratic 44-page preface and an equally unusual 29-page epilogue in which he discussed his career, successes, failures, and general philosophies of life and medicine. He died in 1940. In his book on the shoulder, he described almost everything that orthopaedic shoulder surgeons now regard as new information. In his chapter on fractures of the proximal humerus, for example, he anticipated Neer's four-part fracture classification system. Although Neer reordered and refined it, he did acknowledge his debt to Codman. Codman also described the impingement syndrome and noted the relationship of the "hypertrophic changes at the acromial edge seen in cases of longstanding subacromial bursitis and ruptures of the supraspinatus." He wrote on the frozen shoulder syndrome and probably coined the term. He delineated pendulum exercises, Codman's tumor (chondroblastoma of the humeral head of epiphysis), and what today would be called a "mini-open" repair of the rotator cuff. He discussed brachial plexus injuries, as well as the diagnosis and treatment of tears of the glenoid labrum, which he called "rents in the labrum," today known as SLAP (superior labrum anterior and posterior) lesions. Codman reported that he had looked for Bankart lesions in cases of recurrent dislocations but found that the tear of the anterior labrum was not always present. In patients with atraumatic recurrent shoulder dislocations, he described a procedure that sounded like a capsular shift.

Codman had an almost obsessive interest in rotator cuff tears—how they occur, in whom, why, how they varied, and how to treat them. He described six subgroups of conditions that affect the shoulder in his 1934 book: "complete and incomplete tendon ruptures, rim rents, calcified deposits, tendonitis, and arthritis." He wrote a 60-page chapter on rotator cuff tears, based on his experience operating on "perhaps 1,000 cases." In the chapter on rotator cuff tears, he included the age groups in which they occur, complaints and physical findings, and the effect of rotator cuff tears on scapulohumeral and scapulothoracic motion. He described the "painful arc syndrome" and surgical treatment of rotator cuff tears through a 1 ½-inch incision.

Charles Neer has expanded on Codman's ideas and trained a multitude of residents and fellows in shoulder surgery—unlike Codman, who was a crusading loner. Neer popularized treatment of the impingement syndrome and the recognition that decompression of the subacromial space could relieve painful pressure on the rotator cuff from a hooked acromion or osteoarthritic spurs arising from the acromioclavicular joint. Bigliani and associates[118] refined his concept in a classic anatomic study delineating the "hooked" acromion process, which would be likely to project down into the tendons of the rotator cuff.

Although Codman thoroughly explained the entities of adhesive capsulitis and calcific tendinitis, modern orthopaedists naturally have more to say about these clinical entities. Harrison McLaughlin,[119] J. S. Neviaser,[120] and B. J. Lundberg[121] all investigated and reported on the frozen shoulder. This entity usually resolves spontaneously over 6 to 12 months as patients regain pain-free shoulder motion with minimal treatment.

Neer, McLaughlin, Hawkins, Post, Rockwood, Neviaser, Matsen, and others have discussed surgical repair of rotator cuff tears. The treatment of massive, complete rotator cuff tears, poses special problems that even Codman could not solve. He noted that in some of his patients "the tendon was retracted to such a degree that I could not even attempt a suture."

Shoulder Arthroscopy

By 1980, diagnostic arthroscopy and arthroscopic surgery of the knee began to supplant open surgery, and orthopaedists began to appreciate the potential of this new modality. Naturally, a few orthopaedists recognized that endoscopic surgery also had potential in treating other joints, such as the shoulder. Fifty years earlier, Michael Burman[122] had similar thoughts, publishing an article on the subject in *The Journal of Bone and Joint Surgery* in 1931. Burman described an arthroscope he invented while serving as the Henry W. Frauenthal traveling fellow of the Hospital for Joint Diseases (Frauenthal founded that institution in 1905). Burman's arthroscope consisted of a 3-mm telescope and a 4-mm trochar. The telescope contained a lamp at its tip and a lens system angled so that the lamp was just outside the field of vision. This arrangement provided illumination of the inside of the joint without requiring the operator to look directly into the light. The differences in the diameters of the trochar and telescope made it possible to distend or evacuate the joint with liquid or gas.

Burman discussed the visualization of the interior of 40 knees, 25 cadaveric shoulder joints, 20 hips, and 2 or 3 ankles and elbows. He reported that in the shoulder he used both anterior and posterior punctures, and that distention and traction permitted him to see virtually the entire shoulder—the glenoid and labrum, biceps tendon, articular surface of the humeral head, and the entire capsule. He found that the shoulder was the easiest joint to examine arthroscopically, stating: "In general, it may be said that the shoulder is the easiest and most consistent of all joints to visualize."[122] Burman's remarkable paper had virtually no impact on orthopaedics at the time of publication. His explicit descriptions of his arthroscope, analysis of how he performed the examination of the joints, and clear exposition on what he saw all failed to spark the interest of his orthopaedic contemporaries. Not even Amory Codman, in the process of writing his book *The Shoulder*, picked up on Burman's work. In 1980, Lanny Johnson of Michigan State University in Lansing published one of the first papers on arthroscopic shoulder surgery nearly 50 years after Burman's article appeared.[123] Johnson advised arthroscopists to adapt their skills to the shoulder because shoulder specialists had not given enough attention to the possibilities of arthroscopy. At that time, Johnson was using video monitors and motorized shavers to accomplish such limited tasks as joint débridement. Nevertheless, it was a start, and the number of shoulder arthroscopies done since then has increased dramatically. Virtually every aspect of shoulder arthroscopy has come under intense scrutiny, including such issues as how to best position the patient (lateral decubitus versus beach chair), how much traction to apply to the arm, and the nuances of preliminary diagnostic evaluation and portal placement. The number of publications covering these issues has increased enormously as more surgeons enter practice with skill and experience in arthroscopic surgery. They begin their careers equipped with knowledge and technical capabilities researched and developed by their immediate predecessors during the past two decades. These arthroscopic pioneers, in turn, had the benefit of learning from the experiences and mistakes of orthopaedic surgeons of multiple preceding generations. It is extraordinary how rapidly arthroscopic surgery has developed in the past 20 years and how skillfully the beneficiaries of these developments now apply the technique to orthopaedic conditions that previously required major open surgery. It is not surprising that at least one third of all orthopaedic operations involve the use of an arthroscope at this time.

Arthroscopy of the Ankle, Elbow, Hip, and Wrist

The Ankle

The horizons of arthroscopic surgery have naturally expanded beyond the treatment of the knee and shoulder. Michael Burman, who tested arthroscopy in various cadaveric joints in the 1930s, reported that endoscopic evaluation of the elbow, wrist, and hip revealed little. He asserted that the tightness of these joints precluded the insertion of arthroscopes and that surgeons in the future would probably restrict arthroscopic surgery to the knee and shoulder. Burman correctly pointed out that examination and treatment of joints other than the knee or shoulder posed difficulties and, in fact, it took many years for orthopaedic surgeons to perform arthroscopic surgery in these joints.

In 1989, for example, a group of orthopaedists from the Hughston Orthopaedic Clinic in Columbus, Georgia, reported that surgeons there began to perform ankle arthroscopy in 1983; it took them six years to collect meaningful data on 57 patients.[124] They reported that arthroscopic surgery proved useful in treating synovitis and transchondral articular defects, but they had a 15 percent complication rate with various conditions such as infection, hemarthrosis, and postoperative neurologic deficits. In 1992, Keith Feder of Manhattan Beach, California, and George Schonholtz of Silver Spring, Maryland,[125] coauthored a report describing their results in treating osteochondral fractures, adhesions, osteoarthritis, and various other conditions of the ankle in 40 patients. They cited ten papers in their bibliography, all but one of which was published after 1985. Since then, arthroscopists have expanded the indications for endoscopic ankle surgery, which has made several kinds of open surgery nearly obsolete. The indications for arthroscopy include débridement of osteochondral fractures, chondroplasty, lysis of scar and adhesions, and some ankle fusions.

The Hip

Arthroscopic surgery of the hip poses difficulties not shared by other joints. Many of the reports on hip arthroscopy have appeared in the past 10 years; the best indications, techniques, and assessments of outcomes continue to evolve. Arthroscopic surgery of the knee and shoulder has progressed through the developmental phases of patient positioning, portal placement, and use of the modality in diagnosis, then on to minor procedures such as limited débridements and releases. Only after mastering these basic challenges could surgeons advance to more complicated reconstructive operations. Hip arthroscopy in the early 21st century appears to be in its relatively early stages. James Glick of the University of California in San Francisco, Joseph McCarthy of New England Baptist Hospital in Boston, Thomas Byrd of Vanderbilt Hospital in Nashville, and others have pioneered these efforts.[126-128]

Chondral Lesions

The outcome of hyaline cartilage injury has interested physicians and surgeons for a long time. It is theorized that Aesculapius and Hippocrates treated patients with arthritis, but actual research recognizable as the study of arthritis began much more recently. Peter Redfern[129] and James Paget,[130] both members of the Royal Society in mid-19th century

England, politely disagreed over whether hyaline cartilage could heal. Redfern's experimental incision into the surfaces of dog femoral condyles appeared to coapt fairly well after 29 weeks, but Paget maintained that fibrous tissue produced an apparent union but not real healing. He maintained: "There are no instances in which a lost portion of the cartilage has been restored, or a wounded person repaired, with new and well formed cartilage of the human subject."[130]

In 1982, Henry Mankin[131] of Massachusetts General Hospital and chairman of orthopaedics at Harvard published a review article entitled "The Reaction of Articular Cartilage to Mechanical Injury." He concluded that injuries of the articular cartilage that do not involve subchondral bone will not heal, and that lacerations or other defects in hyaline cartilage will look the same months and years after they were sustained. On the other hand, injuries that involved the subchondral bone will heal with fibrocartilage, which does not have the same physical properties as normal hyaline cartilage. Over time, motion and weight bearing usually erode this material, which eventually results in exposure of the subchondral bony tissue and onset of degenerative arthritis.

Because full-thickness hyaline cartilage defects heal with poor-quality fibrocartilage that cannot function properly with motion and weight bearing, and because defects in hyaline cartilage contribute to abnormal joint mechanics, many orthopaedic surgeons have recently attempted to repair these defects using a variety of methods. The easiest and longest used (but probably the least effective), known as marrow-stimulating techniques, attempt to deliver pluripotential marrow stem cells to the articular surface defect. A surgeon can do this easily enough in the knee by drilling, curetting, puncturing, or otherwise penetrating subchondral bone to release blood and fat from the marrow spaces into the full-thickness defect in the hyaline cartilage. If the patient avoids full weight bearing for 3 months postoperatively, the defect does not exceed 2 cm^2, and any ligamentous and/or meniscal alignment issues have been corrected, the fibrocartilage that develops in the defect might serve for several years. Lanny Johnson[132] of the University of Michigan, Richard Steadman,[133] of Vail, Colorado, M. R. Baumgaertner[134] of San Francisco, and others described their experience with abrasion arthroplasty, microfracture, and drilling procedures in the knee joint for full-thickness defects. One might assume that stem cell research, tissue engineering with manipulation of chondrocyte metabolism, and the development of a matrix for cartilage repair will change the way surgeons treat hyaline cartilage defects in the future. Research and clinical use, however, have led to the application of three techniques to that problem in the past 25 to 30 years: autogenous osteochondral grafting, cartilage cell transplantation, and implantation of osteochondral allografts.

Osteochondral autograft transplantation has the disadvantage of being applicable only to patients with fairly small defects in the articular cartilage. North American orthopaedic surgeons began to report on their experiences with the procedure in the 1980s when, for example, A. R. Outerbridge shared his technique with members of his family, H. K. and A. R.

Outerbridge, in 1981.[135] Thereafter, H. K. and A. R. Outerbridge performed the procedure in 18 patients.

In 1987, a group of Swedish investigators[136] performed their first autologous chondrocyte transplantation combined with a periosteal graft into a patient with a femoral condylar defect. Since then, this operation has gained considerable popularity.

Published results by American orthopaedic surgeons using the chondrocyte cell transplantation method vary considerably. Tom Minas[137] of Boston reported in 2001 that he applied this procedure to 169 consecutive patients with clinical improvement in 87 percent.

When patients have hyaline cartilage defects too large for treatment with an OATS mosaicplasty or autologous chondrocyte implantation, the surgeon might consider using a fresh or frozen allograft. Erik Lexer of Freiburg, Germany, may have performed the first such procedure in 1908. His 1925 report, however, indicated that he had done mostly large bulk transfers of bone and cartilage for filling in bone defects from excision.[138] Orthopaedic surgeons in the United States and Great Britain shared considerable interest in the potential of allografts for the treatment of articular cartilage defects during the 1960s. During those years, Medawar[139] and others worked out the details of the allograft reaction. It appeared that articular cartilage might survive for long periods in recipients because of the Millipore filter effect of the cartilaginous matrix that presumably isolated the allograft chondrocytes from the host antibodies. Since the late 1980s, numerous reports on the use of cadaveric osteochondrografts in the treatment of defects in hyaline cartilage have been published. Marvin Meyers, Wayne Akeson, and Richard Convery[140] of the University of California in San Diego, for example, used fresh cadaveric allograft to replace defects in the knees of 58 patients. Their experience showed that the best results occurred in localized cartilaginous defects in the femoral condyles, patella, and tibial plateau. Patients with unicompartmental arthritis, however, had poor results. The failures occurred mostly in patients with osteoarthritis and not in those with localized defects of the joint surface. Similarly, Beaver and associates[141] at Mt. Sinai Hospital in Toronto reported a 75 percent success rate at five years postoperatively using fresh osteochondral allografts for posttraumatic defects in 92 knees. They found that good results took a long time to deteriorate; chondrocytes in fresh osteocartilaginous allografts could survive for years because in the matrix in the cartilage they are isolated from the histocompatibility antigens that lead to deaths of cells and other tissues.

Sports Medicine and Arthroscopy: The Societies and the Journals

The American Orthopaedic Society for Sports Medicine

Jack Hughston had served on the Sports Medicine Committee of the American Academy of Orthopaedic Surgeons for nearly 10 years when he and Don O'Donohue of the University of Oklahoma decided that a smaller group might better serve the singular interests of orthopaedists who specialized in sports medicine. They and a few other like-minded individuals convened the American Orthopaedic Society for Sports Medicine (AOSSM) in 1972. The AOSSM Website lists the 67 orthopaedic surgeons who attended the first meeting, many of whom are prominent physicians serving high-profile professional teams and players. The initial mission of the AOSSM was to provide a peer group to establish appropriate protocols for handling unique problems associated with treating top professional players and their teams. The society, however, attracted such large numbers of physicians to its meetings that it was decided that membership should be offered to an expanded audience. AOSSM now has more than 2,000 members.

Four years after its founding in 1972, the AOSSM began publishing its journal, the *American Journal of Sports Medicine*. Hughston served as the first editor-in-chief, a post that he held for 15 years. Since he has stepped down, the journal has had two other editors-in-chief: Robert Leach of Boston, who served for 11 years, and Bruce Reider of Chicago, who currently holds the position.

Hughston guided the *American Journal of Sports Medicine* through the years that arthroscopic surgery changed the orthopaedic landscape. The journal now has more than 9,000 subscribers and a very high impact.

In addition to publishing a journal, Hughston and the other founders of the AOSSM encouraged the development of fellowship programs in sports medicine. This initiative required the approval and oversight of the Accreditation Council for Graduate Medical Education (ACGME). The ACGME is the accrediting body for post-medical school training programs in the United States; a new specialty such as sports medicine to achieve recognition requires meeting the ACGME's daunting standards. It took the AOSSM several years, but there are now approximately 57 ACGME-approved fellowships in orthopaedic sports medicine in the United States.

The AOSSM also began in 1988 the process to create a Certificate of Special Qualification (CSQ) in Sports Medicine when it formed an ad hoc committee chaired by John Bergfeld of Cleveland. Bergfeld's committees filed countless applications, recommendations, resolutions, and surveys. By 1993, when he became AOSSM president, Bergfeld could announce that the society had formally petitioned the American Board of Orthopaedic Surgery (ABOS) to approve a Certificate of Added Qualification (CAQ) in Orthopaedic Sports Medicine.[142]

The AOSSM vigorously strives to advance the art and science of sports medicine: orthopaedic surgeons and others submit numerous excellent papers for consideration at the annual meeting; the society publishes an excellent journal; AOSSM offers 11 awards for excellence in research; and in 2001, it established the Sports Medicine Hall of Fame. The list of inductees that year included Fred Allman, Martin Blazina, Joseph Godfrey, Jack Hughston, Jack Kennedy, Robert Kerlan, Robert Larson, Don O'Donoghue, Donald Slocum, and Marcus Stewart. The society sponsors traveling fellowships and, with the Orthopaedic Research and Education Foundation, funds grants for research in sports medicine. It has also established cooperative relationships with other organizations, such as the

American Academy of Family Physicians, founded in 1947; the American College of Sports Medicine, founded in 1954; and the American Society for Sports Medicine. The members of these medical organizations (including physical therapists, athletic trainers, internists, and pediatricians) are also team physicians and sports medicine professionals.

The Arthroscopy Association of North America

For almost 10 years, the AOSSM was the only orthopaedic organization devoted to sports medicine. From 1972 to 1981, however, orthopaedic surgeons began to develop an interest in arthroscopy. At that time, the AOSSM generally recognized arthroscopy only as an adjunct to the methods used for obtaining diagnosis of sports injuries; thus, the physicians struggling to apply arthroscopy to surgical treatment of the knee, shoulder, and other joints had to present their work in other venues. The *American Journal of Sports Medicine* began publication in 1976 when arthroscopy was just gathering momentum in the United States. It published very few papers on the technique in its first 10 issues—never more than four; and in some years, none. Early pioneers in arthroscopic surgery of necessity formed their own group dedicated solely to the procedure and all of its parameters and possibilities "to promote, encourage, support, and foster . . . the dissemination of knowledge . . . of arthroscopic surgery in order to improve upon the diagnosis and treatment of diseases and injuries of the musculoskeletal system." The Web site of the Arthroscopy Association of North America (AANA), which posted that mission statement, notes that since its founding, arthroscopy has become involved in one third of all orthopaedic procedures, and claims that arthroscopy is now a "discipline" for which AANA will be a primary source of information, new techniques, and continuing medical education. It has grown from a small group of devotees to a large organization of thousands of members. AANA now publishes the journal *Arthroscopy*, with Gary Poehling, chairman of orthopaedics at Bowman Gray School of Medicine, serves as editor-in-chief. AANA also supports research grants, fellowship programs, and a spectacularly successful annual meeting. It has established, with the AAOS, an orthopaedic learning center in Rosemont, Illinois, where physicians receive expert instruction in arthroscopic techniques from AANA and AAOS members willing to share their skills in almost one-on-one educational sessions using cadaveric limbs.

The rapid emergence and success of AANA astounded even the individuals who founded it. David Caspari[143] of Richmond gave the presidential address at the 1991 AANA meeting, less than ten years after its founding, in which he quoted C. McAllister Evarts' remarks made at an AOA meeting about arthroscopy being one of the three great advances in orthopaedics in the 20th century, along with internal fixation of fractures and total joint arthroplasty. Caspari expressed alarm that arthroscopy had thus become mainstream, voicing concern that other larger, more established organizations might subsume arthroscopy as a surgical discipline in its own right and "assimilate it" into existing subspecialties such as reconstructive orthopaedics and sports medicine. Caspari also feared that AANA might lose the vitality and excitement that characterized it before Evarts made those remarks. He recalled that less than ten years earlier, arthroscopy had been considered "less than credible, not scientific, a flash in the pan" and was dismissed with the famous comment made by an anonymous critic: "Why look through the keyhole when you can open the door?" Dr. Caspari did not intend for his association to be co-opted, and urged members to maintain their independence and level of intensity. He must have struck a chord with them because interest in arthroscopy has exploded, paralleling endoscopic surgery in gynecology and otolaryngology, and laparoscopic colecystectomies, herniorrhaphies, and appendectomies in general surgery.

Rehabilitation and Bracing

The revolution in arthroscopic surgery attracted the attention of most orthopaedic surgeons, but many were not as cognizant of the changes in rehabilitative techniques occurring simultaneously. Arthur Steindler's 1955 book on the kinesiology of the human body presented his analysis of the musculoskeletal components of the body as a chain of overlapping segments connected by a series of joints.[144] He suggested that fixation of the distal segment of the chain, such as placing the foot on the ground during exercise, created a different set of circumstances from that which occurs during exercise with a distal segment not fixed. He referred to the situation as "closed kinetic chain versus open kinetic chain conditions." G. E. Lutz and his associates[145] at the Biomechanics Laboratory of the Mayo Clinic subsequently found that open-chain exercises of the knee produced high sheer forces at knee angles under 60°, forces large enough to disrupt a reconstructed ACL. With closed-chain exercises, on the other hand, the hamstring muscles co-contract with the quadriceps to stabilize the joint and decrease the stress on the ACL. Lutz and his associates also found that open kinetic chain exercises performed by a patient lying prone and flexing the knee against a weight would strengthen the hamstring muscles and protect the repaired ACL, but this type of open-chain exercise would correspondingly subject the PCL to excessive shear force. They concluded that surgeons should use closed kinetic chain exercises and not open kinetic chain techniques in rehabilitating patients after ACL surgery.

In addition to investigating and using closed versus open kinetic chain protocols, many orthopaedists have also studied muscle performance evaluation and isokinetics. During the polio decades, every junior orthopaedic resident could use the manual muscle testing technique and grade a patient's muscle weakness on the 0 through 5 scale (0 equaling no muscle contraction, progressing stepwise up to normal muscle contraction against resistance for a grade of 5). Since then, however, muscle testing has grown much more sophisticated, and the nuances of isometric versus isotonic versus isokinetic testing have been widely investigated.

Isotonic muscle testing (for example, lifting a free weight once or multiple times) subjects a muscle to a fixed amount of resistance and does not account for the fact that a muscle can generate different amounts of tension at different lengths. In addition, inertia forces can disguise the patient's real muscle strength, and strength without endurance can make testing with multiple lifts inaccurate. Isotonic muscle contraction, also called dynamic variable resistance weight lifting, served as the basis for the DeLorme progressive resistive exercises, which was a system of muscle strengthening that many orthopaedists and physical therapists used during the 1950s and 1960s. DeLorme[146,147] published a paper and a book on his methods in 1948 and 1951, respectively. Since then, basic scientists and others have aggressively investigated other muscle testing and strengthening techniques. In 1990, Alexander Sapega[148] of the University of Pennsylvania published the history of muscle testing, leading to the present and outlined current uses of isotonic, isometric, and isokinetic muscle testing and exercises. He noted the deficiencies of isotonic muscle testing and commented briefly on isometric muscle testing in which the patient contracts the muscle without moving the limb, thus maintaining the muscle at the same length throughout the time of contraction. Other means of muscle testing have been investigated. Isokinetic testing, which became available in the 1970s, now dominates muscle performance evaluation. Manufacturers such as Cybex International produce devices that measure the torque developed by muscle forces producing rotational movements about a joint. These isokinetic devices can help guide the rehabilitation of the patient recovering from knee or other joint surgeries. In the early 1980s, these devices relied on mechanical components, but since then, servo controls and microprocessors made the machines more user-friendly and capable of offering instant data in real time.

Bracing

Orthopaedics as a discipline distinct from general surgery began with bracing. The early European orthopaedists, including Nicolas Andry himself, did not even consider doing operations. In the United States, James Knight, who founded the Hospital for the Ruptured and Crippled (later to become the Hospital for Special Surgery), refused to allow surgery in his institution. Orthopaedics, however, has changed into a fellowship of surgeons who consider bracing as adjunctive.

The sports medicine community—team physicians and arthroscopists—debate issues on the role of bracing in their subspecialty. Prophylactic bracing has particular relevance for their discipline. Edward Nichols[149,150] addressed this issue in two papers published in 1906 and 1909. Violence on the football field had become so egregious in the late 19th and early 20th centuries that colleges had to revise the rules of the game under pressure from Congress and President Theodore Roosevelt. Nichols and his coauthors reported that in 1905, under the old rules, the Harvard squad of 70 men sustained 145 major injuries; in 1908, under the revised rules, they sustained 34. These included ten dislocations of the semilunar cartilage in 1905 and only two in 1908. Nichols and his associates attributed this reduction in knee injuries in part to the fact that "all men were absolutely compelled to wear proper protection," which included soft leather pads lined with heavy felting molded to fit the knees (Figure 43).

Eighty years later, Michael Sitler and his associates[151] won the O'Donoghue Award at the annual meeting of the AOSSM for their paper on the efficacy of prophylactic knee bracing to reduce knee injuries in football. They studied the knee injuries of 1,396 cadets at West Point, who had 21,570 athlete-exposures in intramural tackle football. They found that "the use of prophylactic knee braces significantly reduced the frequency of knee injuries" but noted that the effect was greater in defensive versus offensive players.

Carol Teitz and her associates[152] from the University of Washington in Seattle addressed the issue of prophylactic bracing in a 1987 paper just before the West Point study by Sitler and associates. Teitz and her associates reported, "Overall, players who wore braces on the knees had significantly more injuries to the knees than players who did not." They also said: "We could not recommend the use of these braces in an attempt to prevent injury to collegiate football players." They evaluated 2,389 braced players and 3,001 with no bracing. Those who wore braces used various devices made by manufacturers such as McDavid, Omni Scientific, Donjoy, and American Prosthesis Braces. No significant difference in injury rates was observed when players were grouped by the type of brace worn. Furthermore, these authors found that injury rates were actually higher in brace wearers, suggesting that braces were in fact harmful. This paper generated a great deal of interest, even prompting editorial comment by Harry Cowell, [153] then editor of *The Journal of Bone and Joint Surgery*. Cowell questioned why such devices had been used so extensively with so little data to support their use, advising physicians to harbor a healthy degree of skepticism when considering the use of a new device or procedure.

Although prophylactic knee bracing remains the subject of some controversy, functional and rehabilitative bracing does have a place in the armamentarium of orthopaedists and sports medicine specialists. A brace containing bilateral uprights with single or polycentric hinges and metal, fiberglass, metal, or plastic thigh and calf supports can provide stability to the knee of the patient with disabling ligamentous laxity. When a knee orthosis has a locking device as well, it can also control a moderate degree of muscle weakness. James Nicholas of New York (best known as the surgeon who cared for Joe Namath during his glory years with the New York Jets football team) designed the Lenox Hill brace to stabilize the knees of patients with anterolateral rotatory instability of the knee. George Bassett and Bryan Fleming[154] evaluated the Lenox Hill brace (named after Nicholas' hospital in New York) in its treatment of patients at Wright-Patterson Air Force Base in Ohio. They concluded that the brace worked as advertised under the low-force conditions of a physical examination of the knee in that it diminished anteromedial instability in the Lachman test.

They found that the brace should not be relied on to control anterolateral rotatory instability, however, unless the patient modified physical activities and pursued appropriate rehabilitative exercises.

Bracing can also provide stress protection to graft remodeling during rehabilitation of a cruciate ligament reconstruction. Basic science studies by Amiel and associates,[155] for example, show that graft remodeling goes through the stages of avascularity and necrosis, revascularization, cell repopulation, and finally structural remodeling over the course of a year. During this year-long process, a brace can prevent shearing and translational stresses that could disrupt the graft.

Finally, many patients with anterior knee pain related to poor patellar tracking and chondromalacia use supportive knee orthoses even without the advice of a physician. Drugstores and the purveyors of sporting equipment often display these prominently; patients do the right thing using these braces to alleviate discomfort.

A major component of the orthopaedic revolution has been the advent of arthroscopic surgery, a technique and way of thinking that entered the group consciousness of orthopaedic surgery in the early 1980s. A few interested individuals embraced it and worked through the early, somewhat awkward experimental phases, perfecting it as a diagnostic modality for internal derangements of the knee. Work on the operating arthroscope followed, but this device still required that the inside of a joint be viewed through an eyepiece. Video-assisted arthroscopy and surgery with triangulation came soon thereafter. These modalities led to an explosion in the popularity of arthroscopy, which has been adopted by a new generation of gifted specialists who can now offer major joint procedures done endoscopically. These techniques cause little morbidity compared with open surgery of the past, and patients require far less recovery time as a result. It is a tribute to these pioneers that arthroscopic surgery has progressed so far and become so widely adopted in so short a time frame.

Because arthroscopy is of greatest benefit to young, active adults, inevitably its practitioners have tended to apply this modality to injured athletes. Arthroscopy has thus become a major component of sports medicine. The specialty of sports medicine has a broad reach, however. It seeks to provide care to athletes of all ages, skill levels, and conditions. Sports medicine physicians thus concern themselves with such issues as exercise physiology, muscle strengthening, preparticipation evaluation, rehabilitation of injured athletes, the use of braces and orthoses, and the treatment and prevention of injuries in athletes. Arthroscopy is simply a treatment tool for an injured athlete and not the raison d'etre for sports medicine. Nevertheless, arthroscopic surgery has become one of the most important parts of orthopaedic surgery, a statement supported by the fact that one third of all of the operations performed by orthopaedists are done arthroscopically. As the skill and experience of the practitioners of arthroscopy increase, the percentage of surgical procedures performed arthroscopically will probably continue to grow.

References

1. Hey W: *Practical Observations in Surgery*. London, England, Capell, 1803.

2. Reid J: The healing of the semilunar cartilage of the knee joint. *Edinburgh Med J* 1834;42:377-378.

3. Annandale T: An operation for displaced semilunar cartilage. *BMJ* 1885;1:779.

4. Holt EZ: Abstract of Henderson MS: Derangements of semilunar cartilage of knee joint. Minnesota Medicine, April 1919. *J Orthop Surg* (Hong Kong) 1919;1:453.

5. Painter CF: Internal derangements of knee joints. *J Orthop Surg* (Hong Kong) 1919;1:416-422.

6. Campbell WC: Surgery of the knee joint. *South Med* 1924;17:82-87.

7. Bristow WR: Internal derangement of the knee joint. *J Bone Joint Surg Am* 1935;17:605-626.

8. Watson-Jones R: *Fractures and Joint Injuries*, ed 3. Edinburgh, Scotland, ES Livingstone, 1946, vol 2, pp 717-718.

9. Smillie IS: *Injuries of the Knee Joint*. Edinburgh, Scotland, ES Livingstone, 1946.

10. McMurray TP: *The Diagnosis of Internal Derangement of the Knee Joint*. Robert Jones Birthday Volume. London, England, Oxford University Press, 1928, p 305.

11. DePalma AF: *Diseases of the Knee*. Philadelphia, PA, JB Lippincott Company, 1954, p 169.

12. O'Donoghue DH: *Treatment of Injuries to Athletes*. Philadelphia, PA, WB Saunders, 1962, pp 494-502.

13. King D: The function of the semilunar cartilages. *J Bone Joint Surg Am* 1936;18:1069-1076.

14. King D: The healing of the semilunar cartilages. *J Bone Joint Surg Am* 1936;18:333-342.

15. Fairbank TF: Knee joint changes after meniscectomy. *J Bone Joint Surg Br* 1948;30:664.

16. Feagin JA Jr: Editorial: The cruciate deficient knee. *Clin Orthop Relat Res* 1983;172:2.

17. Hey Groves EW: The crucial ligaments of the knee joint: Their function, rupture, and the operative treatment of the same. *Br J Surg* 1919;7:505-515.

18. Hey Groves EW: Operation for the repair of the crucial ligaments. *Lancet* 1917;2:674-675.

19. O'Donoghue DH: Surgical treatment of fresh injuries to the major ligaments of the knee. *J Bone Joint Surg Am* 1950;32:721-738.

20. Campbell WC: Reconstruction of the ligaments of the knee. *Am J Surg* 1939;43:473-480.

21. Frankel VH, Burstein AH, Brooks DB: Biomechanics of internal derangement of the knee: Pathomechanics as determined by analysis of the instant centers of motion. *J Bone Joint Surg Am* 1971;53:945-962.

22. Noyes FR, DeLucas JL, Torvik PJ: Biomechanics of anterior cruciate ligament failure: An analysis of strain-rate sensitivity and mechanisms of failure in primates. *J Bone Joint Surg Am* 1974;56:236-253.

23. Kennedy JC, Hawkins RJ, Willis RB, Danylchuck KD: Tension studies of human knee ligaments: Yield points, ultimate failure, and disruption of the cruciate and tibial collateral ligaments. *J Bone Joint Surg Am* 1976;58:350-355.

24. Arnoczky SP, Rubin RM, Marshall JL: Microvasculature of the cruciate ligaments and its response to injury: An experimental study in dogs. *J Bone Joint Surg Am* 1979;61:1221-1229.

25. DeHaven KE: Diagnosis of acute knee injuries with hemarthrosis. *Am J Sports Med* 1980;8:9-14.

26. Abbott LC, Saunders JBM, Bost FC, Anderson CE: Injuries to the ligaments of the knee joint. *J Bone Joint Surg Am* 1944;26:503-521.

27. Palmer I: On the injuries to the ligaments of the knee joint. *Acta Chir Scand* 1938;81(suppl 53):3.

28. Torg JS, Conrad W, Kalen V: Clinical diagnosis of anterior cruciate ligament instability in the athlete. *Am J Sports Med* 1976;4:84-93.

29. Galway HR, MacIntosh DL: The lateral pivot shift: A symptom and sign of anterior cruciate ligament insufficiency. *Clin Orthop Relat Res* 1980;147:45-50.

30. Hughston JC: Knee ligament injuries in athletes. *J Med Assoc State Ala* 1966;36:1-9.

31. Hughston JC, Andrews JR, Cross MJ, Moschi A: Classification of knee ligament instabilities: Part II. The lateral compartment. *J Bone Joint Surg Am* 1976;58:173-179.

32. Slocum DB, Larson RL: Rotatory instability of the knee: Its pathogenesis and a clinical test to demonstrate its presence. *J Bone Joint Surg Am* 1968;50:211-225.

33. Daniels DM, Stone ML: Diagnosis of knee ligament injury: tests and measurements of joint laxity, in Feagin JA (ed): *The Crucial Ligaments.* New York, NY, Churchill-Livingstone, 1988, pp 287-300.

34. Larson RM: Clinical evaluation, in Larson RL, Granak WA (eds): *The Knee: Form, Function, Pathology, and Treatment.* Philadelphia, PA, WB Saunders, 1993, p 94.

35. Jakob RP, Hassler H, Staeubli HU: Observations on rotatory instability of the lateral compartment of the knee: Experimental studies on the functional anatomy and the pathomechanism of the true and reversed pivot shift sign. *Acta Orthop Scand Suppl* 1981;191:1-32.

36. Kennedy JC, Fowler PJ: Medial and anterior instability of the knee: An anatomical and clinical study using stress machines. *J Bone Joint Surg Am* 1971;53:1257-1270.

37. Lysholm J, Gillquist J: Evaluation of knee ligament injury results with special emphasis on use of a scoring scale. *Am J Sports Med* 1982;10:150-154.

38. Larson R: Rating sheet for knee function, 1972, in Smillie I (ed): *Diseases of the Knee Joint.* Edinburgh, Scotland, Churchill-Livingstone, 1974, pp 29-30.

39. DeHaven KE: Arthroscopy in the diagnosis and management of the anterior cruciate ligament deficient knee. *Clin Orthop Relat Res* 1983;172:52-56.

40. Andrews JR, Sanders R: A "mini-reconstruction" technique in treating anterolateral rotatory instability (ALRI). *Clin Orthop Relat Res* 1983;172:93-96.

41. Ellison AE: Distal iliotibial-band transfer for anterolateral rotatory instability of the knee. *J Bone Joint Surg Am* 1979;61:330-337.

42. MacIntosh DL, Darby TA: Lateral substitution reconstruction. *J Bone Joint Surg Br* 1976;58:142.

43. Johnson LL: Lateral capsular ligament complex: Anatomical and surgical considerations. *Am J Sports Med* 1979;7:156-160.

44. Galway R: Pivot shift syndrome. *J Bone Joint Surg Br* 1972;54:558.

45. Kennedy J, Willis RB: Synthetic cruciate ligaments: Preliminary report. *J Bone Joint Surg Br* 1976;58:142.

46. McGinty JB (ed): *Operative Arthroscopy*, ed 3. Philadelphia, PA, Lippincott Williams & Wilkins, 2003.

47. Miller MD, Cole BJ: *Textbook of Arthroscopy*. Philadelphia, PA, WB Saunders, 2004.

48. Strobel MJ: *Manual of Arthroscopic Surgery*. Berlin, Germany, Springer-Verlag, 1998. Translated by Terry C. Telger.

49. Casscells SW: Arthroscopy of the knee joint: A review of 150 cases. *J Bone Joint Surg Am* 1971;53:287-298.

50. Jackson RW, Abe I: The role of arthroscopy in the management of disorders of the knee: An analysis of 200 consecutive examinations. *J Bone Joint Surg Br* 1972;54:310-322.

51. O'Connor RL: Arthroscopy in the diagnosis and treatment of acute ligamentous injuries of the knee. *J Bone Joint Surg Am* 1974;56:333-337.

52. DeHaven KE, Collins HR: Diagnosis of internal derangements of the knee: The role of arthroscopy. *J Bone Joint Surg Am* 1975;57:802-810.

53. McGinty JB, Freedman PA: Arthroscopy of the knee. *Clin Orthop Relat Res* 1976;121:173-180.

54. Jackson RW: Memories of the early days of arthroscopy: 1965-1975. The formative years. *Arthroscopy* 1987;3:1-5.

55. DeHaven KE: Principles of triangulation for arthroscopic surgery. *Orthop Clin North Am* 1982;13:329-336.

56. Gillquist J, Oretorp N: The technique of endoscopic total meniscectomy. *Orthop Clin North Am* 1982;13:363-367.

57. Dandy DJ, O'Carroll PF: The removal of loose bodies from the knee under arthroscopic control. *J Bone Joint Surg Br* 1982;64:473-474.

58. Johnson LL: Impact of diagnostic arthroscopy on the clinical judgement of an experienced arthroscopist. *Clin Orthop Relat Res* 1982;167:75-83.

59. Metcalf RW: Operative arthroscopy of the knee, in *AAOS Instructional Course Lectures* 30. St. Louis, MO, CV Mosby, 1981, p 357.

60. Mulhollan JS: Swedish arthroscopic system. *Orthop Clin North Am* 1982;13:349-362.

61. Johnson LL: Creating proper environment for arthroscopic surgery. *Orthop Clin North Am* 1982;13:283-298.

62. Allen R, Shahriaree H: Richard O'Connor: A tribute. *J Bone Joint Surg Am* 1982;64:315.

63. Unnecessary meniscectomy. *Lancet* 1976;1:235-236.

64. Noble J, Erat K: In defence of the meniscus: A prospective study of 200 meniscectomy patients. *J Bone Joint Surg Br* 1980;62:7-11.

65. Raunest J, Oberle K, Loehnert J, Hoetzinger H: The clinical value of magnetic resonance imaging in the evaluation of meniscal disorders. *J Bone Joint Surg Am* 1991;73:11-16.

66. Fischer SP, Fox JM, Del Pizzo W, Friedman MJ, Snyder SJ, Ferkel RD: Accuracy of diagnosis from magnetic resonance imaging of the knee: A multi-center analysis of one thousand and fourteen patients. *J Bone Joint Surg Am* 1991;73:2-10.

67. Cannon WD: Arthroscopic meniscal repair, in McGinty JB (ed): *Operative Arthroscopy*, ed 3. Philadelphia, PA, Lippincott Williams & Wilkins, 2003, p 232.

68. Henning CE, Clark JR, Lynch MA, et al: Arthroscopic meniscus repair with a posterior incision. *Instr Course Lect* 1988;37:209-221.

69. Johnson DI: Meniscus repair with implantable devices, in McGinty JB, Burkhart SS, Jackson RW, Johnson DH, Richmond JC (eds): *Operative Arthroscopy*, ed 3. Philadelphia, PA, Lippincott Williams & Wilkins, 2003, pp 251-256.

70. Howell SM, Taylor MA: Failure of reconstruction of the anterior cruciate ligament due to impingement by the intercondylar roof. *J Bone Joint Surg Am* 1993;75:1044-1055.

71. Jackson DW, Gasser S: Tibial tunnel placement in ACL reconstruction. *Arthroscopy* 1994;10:124-131.

72. Fu FH, Bennett CH, Latterman C, Ma CB: Current trends in anterior cruciate ligament reconstruction: Part 1. Biology and biomechanics of reconstruction. *Am J Sports Med* 1999;27:821-830.

73. Cain EL, Gillogly SD, Andrews JR: Management of intraoperative complications associated with autogenous patellar tendon graft anterior cruciate ligament reconstruction. *Instr Course Lect* 2003;52:359-367.

74. Noyes FR, Wojtys EM, Marshall MT: The early diagnosis and treatment of developmental patella infera syndrome. *Clin Orthop Relat Res* 1991;265:241-252.

75. Noyes FR, Mangine RE, Barber S: Early knee motion after open and arthroscopic anterior cruciate ligament reconstruction. *Am J Sports Med* 1987;15:149-160.

76. Paulos LE, Rosenberg TD, Draubert J, Manning J, Abbott P: Infrapatellar contracture syndrome: An unrecognized cause of knee stiffness with patellar entrapment and patella infera. *Am J Sports Med* 1987;15:331-341.

77. Lindenfeld TN, Wojtys EM, Husain A: Surgical treatment of arthrofibrosis of the knee. *Instr Course Lect* 2000;49:211-221.

78. Goldthwait JE: Permanent dislocation of the patella. *Ann Surg* 1899;29:62.

79. Goldthwait JE: Slipping or recurrent dislocation of the patella with the report of 11 cases. *Boston Med Surg J* 1904;150:169-174.

80. Buzby BF: Recurring external dislocation of the patella. *Ann Surg* 1933;97:387.

81. Hauser ED: Total tendon transplant for slipping patella: New operation for recurrent dislocation of the patella. *Surg Gynecol Obstet* 1938;66:199.

82. Hughston JC, Walsh WM: Proximal and distal reconstruction of the extensor mechanism for patellar subluxation. *Clin Orthop Relat Res* 1979;144:36-42.

83. Chrisman OD, Snook GA, Wilson TC: A long-term prospective study of the Hauser and Roux-Goldthwait procedures for recurrent patellar dislocation. *Clin Orthop Relat Res* 1979;144:27-30.

84. Roux C: Luxation habituelle de la roule: Traitement operatoire. *Rev Chir Paris* 1888;8:682.

85. Maquet P: Advancement of the tibial tuberosity. *Clin Orthop Relat Res* 1976;115:225-230.

86. Insall J, Salvati E: Patella position in the normal knee joint. *Radiology* 1971;101:101-104.

87. Merchant AC, Mercer RL, Jacobsen RH, Cool CR: Roentgenographic analysis of patellofemoral congruence. *J Bone Joint Surg Am* 1974;56:1391-1396.

88. Brattstrom H: Patella alta in non-dislocating knee joints. *Acta Orthop Scand* 1970;41:578-588.

89. Warren LF, Marshall JL: The supporting structures and layers on the medial side of the knee: An anatomical analysis. *J Bone Joint Surg Am* 1979;61:56-62.

90. Rorabeck CH, Bobechko WP: Acute dislocation of the patella with osteochondral fracture: A review of eighteen cases. *J Bone Joint Surg Br* 1976;58:237-240.

91. Watson-Jones R: *Fractures and Joint Injuries*, ed 3. Baltimore, MD, Williams & Wilkins, 1946, pp 457-458.

92. Bankart ASB: Recurrent or habitual dislocation of the shoulder joint. *BMJ* 1923;2:1132.

93. Bankart ASB: The pathology and treatment of recurrent dislocations of the shoulder joint. *Br J Surg* 1938;26:23.

94. Bankart AS, Cantab MC: Recurrent or habitual dislocation of the shoulder-joint. 1923. *Clin Orthop Relat Res* 1993;291:3-6.

95. Bost FC, Inman VT: The pathological changes in current dislocations of the shoulder joint. *Br J Surg* 1938;26:23.

96. Hill HA, Sachs MD: The proved defect of the humeral head: A frequently unrecognized complication of dislocations of the shoulder joint. *Radiology* 1940;35:690.

97. Magnuson PB: Treatment of recurrent dislocation of the shoulder. *Surg Clin North Am* 1945;25:14.

98. Osmond-Clark H: Habitual dislocation of the shoulder: The Putti-Platt operation. *J Bone Joint Surg Br* 1948;30:19.

99. Moseley HF: *Recurrent Dislocation of the Shoulder*. Montreal, Canada, McGill University Press, 1961, pp 89-91.

100. Helfet AJ: Coracoid transplantation for recurring dislocation of the shoulder. *J Bone Joint Surg Br* 1958;40:198-202.

101. Eden R: Operation der habituellen schulterluxation. *Deutsch Chir* 1918;144:269.

102. Hybinette MK: De la transplantation d'un fragment osseux pour remedier aux luxations recidiantes de l'epanle. *Acta Chir Scand* 1932;71:411.

103. Chaudhuri GK, Sengupta A, Saha AK: Rotation osteotomy of the shaft of the humerus for recurrent dislocation of the shoulder: Anterior and posterior. *Acta Orthop Scand* 1974;45:193-198.

104. Henderson MS: Tenosuspension operation for recurrent or habitual dislocation of the shoulder. *Surg Clin North Am* 1949;29:997.

105. Nicola T: Recurrent dislocation of the shoulder. *J Bone Joint Surg Am* 1934;16:663-670.

106. Nicola T: Recurrent dislocation of the shoulder. *Am J Surg* 1953;86:85-91.

107. O'Brien SJ, Neves MC, Arnoczky SP, et al: The anatomy and histology of the interior glenohumeral ligament complex of the shoulder. *Am J Sports Med* 1990;18:449-456.

108. O'Brien SJ, Schwartz RS, Warren RF, Torzilli PA: Capsular restraints to anterior-posterior motion of the abducted shoulder: A biomechanical study. *J Shoulder Elbow Surg* 1995;4:298-308.

109. Zarins B, McMahon MS, Rowe CR: Diagnosis and treatment of traumatic anterior instability of the shoulder. *Clin Orthop Relat Res* 1993;291:75-84.

110. Rowe CR, Pierce DS, Clark JG: Voluntary dislocation of the shoulder: A preliminary report on a clinical, electromyographic, and psychiatric study of twenty-six patients. *J Bone Joint Surg Am* 1973;55:445-460.

111. Neer CS II: Involuntary inferior and multidirectional instability of the shoulder: Etiology, recognition, and treatment. *Instr Course Lect* 1985;34:232-238.

112. Neer CS II, Foster CR: Inferior capsular shift for involuntary inferior and multidirectional instability of the shoulder: A preliminary report. *J Bone Joint Surg Am* 1980;62:897-908.

113. Matsen FA, Thomas SC, Rockwood CA: Anterior glenohumeral instability, in Rockwood CA, Matsen FA (eds): *The Shoulder*. Philadelphia, PA, WB Saunders, 1990, pp 575-578.

114. Codman EA: *The Shoulder: Rupture of the Supraspinatus Tendon and Other Lesions In and About the Subacromial Bursa*. Boston, MA, Thomas Todd, 1934.

115. Mallon B: *Ernest Amory Codman: The End Result of a Life in Medicine*. Philadelphia, PA, WB Saunders, 2000.

116. Codman EA: A study of the x-ray plates of one hundred and forty cases of fracture of the lower end of the radius. *Boston Med Surg J* 1900;143:305-308.

117. Fulton JF: *Harvey Cushing: A Biography*. Springfield, IL, Charles C. Thomas, 1946, pp 87, 268.

118. Bigliani LU, Morrison D, April EW: The morphology of the acromion and its relationship to rotator cuff tears. *Orthop Trans* 1986;10:228.

119. McLaughlin HL: The "frozen shoulder." *Clin Orthop* 1961;20:126-131.

120. Neviaser JS: Adhesive capsulitis of the shoulder: A study of the pathological findings in periarthritis of the shoulder. *J Bone Joint Surg Am* 1945;27:211-222.

121. Lundberg BJ: The frozen shoulder: Clinical and radiographical observations. The effect of manipulation under general anesthesia. Structure and glycosaminoglycan content of the joint capsule. Local bone metabolism. *Acta Orthop Scand Suppl* 1969;119:1-59.

122. Burman MS: Arthroscopy on the direct visualization of joint: An experimental cadaver study. *J Bone Joint Surg Am* 1931;13:669.

123. Johnson LL: Arthroscopy of the shoulder. *Orthop Clin North Am* 1980;11:197-204.

124. Martin DF, Baker CL, Curl WW, Andrews JR, Robie DB, Haas AF: Operative ankle arthroscopy: Long-term followup. *Am J Sports Med* 1989;17:16-23.

125. Feder KS, Schonholtz GJ: Ankle arthroscopy: Review and long-term results. *Foot Ankle* 1992;13:382-385.

126. Glick JM, Sampson TG, Gordon RB, Behr JT, Schmidt E: Hip arthroscopy by the lateral approach. *Arthroscopy* 1987;3:4-12.

127. McCarthy JC, Busconi B: The role of hip arthroscopy in the diagnosis and treatment of hip disease. *Orthopedics* 1995;18:753-756.

128. Byrd JW, Jones KS: Prospective analysis of hip arthroscopy with 2-year follow-up. *Arthroscopy* 2000;16:578-587.

129. Redfern P: On the healing of wounds in articular cartilage, in Bick E (ed): *Classics of Orthopedics*. Philadelphia, PA, JB Lippincott, 1976, p 272.

130. Paget J: Healing of cartilage, in Bick E (ed): *Classics of Orthopedics*. Philadelphia, PA, JB Lippincott, 1976, p 276.

131. Mankin HJ: The reaction of articular cartilage to mechanical injury. *J Bone Joint Surg Am* 1982;64:460-466.

132. Johnson LL: Arthroscopic abrasion arthroplasty historical and pathologic perspective: Present status. *Arthroscopy* 1986;2:54-69.

133. Steadman JR, Rodkey WG, Rodrigo JJ: Microfracture: Surgical technique and rehabilitation to treat chondral defects. *Clin Orthop Relat Res* 2001;391(suppl):S362-S369.

134. Baumgaertner MR, Cannon WD, Vittori JM, Schmidt ES, Maurer RC: Arthroscopic debridement of the arthritic knee. *Clin Orthop Relat Res* 1990;253:197-202.

135. Outerbridge HK, Outerbridge AR, Outerbridge RE: The use of a lateral patellar autogenous graft for the repair of a large osteochondral defect in the knee. *J Bone Joint Surg Am* 1995;77:65-72.

136. Brittberg M, Tallheden T, Sjögren-Jannsen E, et al: Autologous chondrocytes used for articular cartilage repair: An update. *Clin Orthop Relat Res* 2001;391 Suppl:S337-S348.

137. Minas T: Autologous chondrocyte implantation for focal chondral defects of the knee. *Clin Orthop Relat Res* 2001;391(suppl):S349-S361.

138. Lexer E: Joint transplantations and arthroplasty. *Surg Gynecol Obstet* 1925;40:782-809.

139. Medawar PB: Biological problems of grafting: A symposium sponsored by the Commission Administrative du Patrimoine Universitoire de Liege and the Council for International Organizations for Medical Sciences. March 18, 1959.

140. Meyers MH, Akeson W, Convery FR: Resurfacing of the knee with fresh osteochondral allograft. *J Bone Joint Surg Am* 1989;71:704-713.

141. Beaver RJ, Mohamed M, Backstein D, Davis A, Zukor DJ, Gross AE: Fresh osteochondral allografts for post-traumatic defects in the knee: A survivorship analysis. *J Bone Joint Surg Br* 1992;74:105-110.

142. Bergfeld JA: Presidential address of the American Orthopaedic Society for Sports Medicine. *Am J Sports Med* 1993;21:770-772.

143. Caspari RB: Arthroscopy: An orthopedic surgical subspecialty or a technique: Presidential address. *Arthroscopy* 1991;7:390-393.

144. Steindler A: *Kinesiology of the Human Body Under Normal and Pathological Conditions*. Springfield, IL, Charles C. Thomas, 1955.

145. Lutz GE, Palmitier RA, An KN, Chao EY: Comparison of tibiofemoral joint forces during open-kinetic-chain and closed-kinetic-chain exercises. *J Bone Joint Surg Am* 1993;75:732-739.

146. DeLorme T, Watkins A: Techniques of progressive resistive exercise. *Arch Phys Med Rehabil* 1948;29:263.

147. DeLorme TL: *Progressive Resistive Exercise*. New York, NY, Appleton Century Crofts, 1951.

148. Sapega AA: Muscle performance evaluation in orthopaedic practice. *J Bone Joint Surg Am* 1990;72:1562-1574.

149. Nichols EH, Smith HB: The physician aspect of American football. *Boston Med Surg J* 1906;154:1.

150. Nichols EH, Richardson FL: Football injuries of the Harvard Square for three years under the revised rules. *Boston Med Surg J* 1909;160:33.

151. Sitler M, Ryan J, Hopkinson W, et al: The efficacy for a prophylactic knee brace to reduce knee injuries in football: A prospective, randomized study at West Point. *Am J Sports Med* 1990;18:310-315.

152. Teitz CC, Hermanson B, Kronmal RA, Diehr PH: Evaluation of the use of braces to prevent knee injury to the knee in collegiate football players. *J Bone Joint Surg Am* 1987;69:2-9.

153. Cowell HR: College football: To brace or not to brace. *J Bone Joint Surg Am* 1987;69:1.

154. Bassett GS, Fleming BW: The Lenox Hill brace in anterolateral rotatory instability. *Am J Sports Med* 1983;11:345-348.

155. Amiel D, Kleiner JB, Roux RD, Harwood FL, Akeson WH: The phenomenon of "ligamentization": Anterior cruciate ligament reconstruction with autogenous patellar tendon. *J Orthop Res* 1986;4:162-172.

CHAPTER 8

SPECIALIZATION IN ORTHOPAEDICS AND THE DEVELOPMENT OF SPECIALTY SOCIETIES

Orthopaedic specialty societies are generally founded by individuals with a special interest in a narrowly focused content area, such as an anatomic area (hip, knee, hand), a technique (arthroscopy, limb lengthening), a subset of patients (pediatrics, sports, trauma), or a disease (tumors, infections). Interests often overlap, such as does scoliosis with spine surgery and pediatrics, or trauma with microsurgery and rehabilitation and prosthetics. Belonging to more than one such organization, therefore, is a good way to keep current. This chapter focuses solely on those specialty societies not discussed in previous chapters.

The Hand Societies

A charismatic individual sometimes inspires the development of a specialty organization. The key stimulus for the founding of the American Society for Surgery of the Hand (ASSH) came in the person of Sterling Bunnell (Figure 44).[1,2]

Bunnell was born in San Francisco in 1882, operated a private practice of general surgery in San Francisco all his life, and died there in 1957. He attended the University of California as an undergraduate and for his medical degree.

Bunnell served in the U.S. Army in World War I with Norman T. Kirk, the head of the Letterman Army Hospital in San Francisco in the late 1930s and early 1940s and later the Surgeon General of the Army. Kirk admired Bunnell's prolific pre–World War II writings on hand surgery and appreciated Bunnell's ideas about restoring function and mobility to the injured, which mirrored his own philosophy that treatment of trauma should not end with the healing of the wound. As a consequence of their mutual interest, General Kirk ordered that patients with hand injuries receive special treatment in designated hand centers. He established nine centers in the United States and several others overseas. General Kirk insisted that the men in these units receive the best possible treatment, realizing the importance of salvaging injured hands. General Kirk apparently realized that the surgeons and other personnel in the hand centers would need training in orthopaedics, general surgery, plastic surgery, neurosurgery, and rehabilitation to provide total care for soldiers with hand injuries. Kirk had identified Bunnell as the one person who could change the thinking of army surgeons, who were recruited or drafted largely from civilian practices and relied on surgical principles derived from their own surgical specialties. Kirk made a unique offer to Bunnell, offering him the position of "civilian consultant for hand surgery to the Secretary of War" to oversee the treatment of the wounded in the hand centers. At about the same time, Bunnell began work on his definitive book, *Surgery of the Hand*. Although he was at the peak of his career, Bunnell nevertheless accepted Kirk's call and took on the monumental task of coordinating multidisciplinary treatment protocols for the army's network of hand centers.

Bunnell visited all of the nine centers at least once between 1944 and early 1947, staying in each for at least a month.[3] In all locations, he established an educational program consisting of lectures, demonstrations, case reviews, clinics, and surgery. He assisted the hand surgeons or performed the surgery himself with their assistance. Bunnell had a profoundly beneficial effect on the outcomes of treatment of the wounded. Beyond that, he influenced a new generation of surgeons whose careers reflected his own enlightened approach to the treatment of the hand, inspiring them to provide all aspects of care for these patients. Eventually, these surgeons became the nucleus for the beginnings of the American Society for Surgery of the Hand (ASSH), founded in 1947.[4] After the war, Bunnell returned to his practice in San Francisco and remained active there until his death. His legacy is his classic text on hand surgery and his multidisciplinary approach to the injured hand, passed down to subsequent generations of orthopaedic surgeons.

Bunnell's book went through three editions, and he personally wrote all but a few of the chapters. The definitive modern text, *Green's Operative Hand Surgery* (the fifth edition of which was published in 2005), now has four editors and 99 contributors. It contains so much material that it fills two volumes of 1,160 pages each. The third edition of Bunnell's book was a single volume of about 1,000 pages.

Inevitably, Bunnell's intellectual heirs modified or changed many of his principles and techniques. Comparing Bunnell's treatment of flexor tendon injuries to the technique presented in *Green's Operative Hand Surgery* perfectly illustrates the shift in operating philosophy. Bunnell regarded the restoration of normal function of the finger with a flexor tendon laceration as "one of the most baffling problems in surgery."[5] He wrote that his technically well-executed flexor tendon repairs in fingers worked very well for a few weeks, but gradually the tendons became "firmly embedded in scar tissue and united to the surrounding fingers in a solid mass." Adhesions inevitably followed repairs of the flexor tendons, particularly in that portion of the finger "between the distal crease of the palm and the middle flexion crease in the finger." He referred to this area as "no-man's-land," a direct reference to his World War I experience of the area between the German trenches and those of the Allies, so dangerous that troops used that term to describe it. Bunnell opined that "poor results the world over followed sutured flexor tendons" in that location and concluded that "when the problem of repairing a flexor tendon at that site is solved, the repair of all tendons will be comparatively easy."[5]

Approximately 50 years later, Martin Boyer, writing on flexor tendon injury in *Green's Operative Hand Surgery*, stated: "Major advances in the understanding of intrasynovial flexor tendon biology have made it possible to perform adhesion-free repairs in no-man's-land."[6] Thus, success in primary flexor tendon repair in this area depends on multistrand suture techniques that can provide a repair strong enough to permit vigorous postoperative rehabilitation protocols with preservation of motion.

In the 1960s, opinion began to shift away from Bunnell's proscription against performing primary flexor tendon repairs in no-man's-land. Boyer noted that Michael Mason of Chicago, Joseph Boyes of Los Angeles, William Littler of New York, and two European surgeons—Claude Verdan of Switzerland and R. G. Pulvertaft of the United Kingdom—performed studies suggesting that there was no need to close clean, fresh lacerations, wait three weeks for healing, and secondarily come back for a repair or reconstruction of the tendon. Verdan,[7] for example, excised the tendon sheath at the site of repair and repaired the tendon with multiple fine silk sutures. He protected the site of repair by transfixing the tendon above and below the repair site with needles.

In 1969, Isadore Kessler[8] of Tel Aviv reported his experimental and clinical findings using his "grasping suture" technique to reapproximate tendon ends. He claimed that Bunnell's figure-of-8 suture caused the tendons to split longitudinally and then separate. The Kessler suture, however, could maintain approximation of the tendon ends with sufficient strength to permit active and passive motion very soon after the repair. He reported that early motion prevented adhesions between the tendons and adjacent tissue and did not prevent end-to-end healing of the tendon laceration.

In the decades following these reports, many investigators became more aggressively involved in clinical and basic science research into flexor tendon physiology, kinesiology, and the biology of tendon healing. James Strickland[9] published a compendium on flexor tendon surgery in 2000 in the *Journal of Hand Surgery* in which he discussed these issues. He reviewed the controversy regarding intrinsic versus extrinsic tendon healing, noting that "continuing studies" by the numerous investigators he cited showed that tendons do, in fact, have an intrinsic capacity to heal, and healing does not depend entirely on extrinsic factors.

Frequently, of course, patients present with such severely mangled, contaminated injuries that a primary tendon repair cannot be performed. Bunnell discussed severe trauma at length in his book, suggesting various methods for preparing a suitable gliding surface for a tendon graft used for a secondary repair after coverage and healing occurred. He described techniques that employed stainless steel rods and celluloid tubes to construct artificial tendon sheaths. Presumably, placing such devices in the fingers through the pulleys in the bed of the flexor tendon would lead to the formation of a synovially lined sheath. Several weeks later, the surgeon could remove the rod and replace it with a tendon graft. In the mid-1960s, James Hunter[10] of Jefferson

Medical College in Philadelphia experimented with a silicone-Dacron reinforced rod for this purpose.

Bunnell apparently did not have as much interest in patients with crippling deformities caused by rheumatoid arthritis as he did in soldiers with war wounds. His clinics at the hand centers during World War II covered tendon transplants, tendon grafts and repairs, peripheral nerve repairs, skin resurfacing, transplantation of rays, treatment of nonunions and malunions, and almost anything else that thousands of young men would have endured during those years. Bunnell's text, however, devotes only a few pages to reconstruction of the rheumatic hand, and he devoted less than a page to the surgical treatment of hand deformities caused by rheumatoid arthritis. He suggested that surgery should be done "only on the burned out case" and advised fusion for wrist deformity, some finger joints, and both joints of the thumb. In just a few sentences, he went through tenotomy of the lateral bands for metacarpophalangeal joint contractures, and briefly acknowledged that patients with fixed deformities of the metacarpophalangeal joints might need resection arthroplasties with removal of the metacarpal heads. *Green's Operative Hand Surgery*, in contrast, devotes almost 90 pages to the subject, and the fifth edition of Adrian Flatt's book *The Care of the Arthritic Hand* runs to 454 pages.[11]

In 1961, Adrian Flatt[12] of Iowa City published a paper in the *Journal of Bone and Joint Surgery* on the use of metal prostheses to replace metacarpophalangeal and proximal interphalangeal joints in rheumatoid patients. The prostheses consisted of a hinged joint connecting two pronged stems, with fixation of the hinge provided by a transverse bolt. Flatt reported that he attempted to use the single-pronged model of E. W. Brannon as well as the single-pronged Richards model. Because these rotated within the medullary canals of the metacarpals and phalanges, he was forced to abandon them. Flatt's two-pronged prostheses had greater stability; he reported adequate outcomes in 12 patients with gross joint destruction, persistent swan-neck deformities, and ulnar drift deformities. Flatt followed these patients for about a year, but by then he had removed 6 of the 57 prostheses he had inserted.

About 10 years later, Alfred Swanson[13] of Grand Rapids, Michigan, in a paper published in the *Journal of Bone and Joint Surgery* described his results from correction of metacarpophalangeal and proximal interphalangeal deformities associated with rheumatoid arthritis using stemmed, heat-molded silicone rubber joint implants. He used Bunnell's resection arthroplasty techniques with their attendant capsular and tendon releases to correct rheumatoid hand deformities, but maintained correction by inserting semiflexible silicone implants into the canals of the metacarpals and phalanges. The procedure was not particularly difficult to perform. The prostheses in general held up well, and the Swanson prosthesis became the operation of choice for several years thereafter. Swanson published another classic paper in the same *JBJS* volume entitled "Disabling Arthritis at the Base of the Thumb: Treatment by Resection of the Trapezium and Flexible (Silicone) Implant Arthroplasty." That procedure involved resection of the trapezium and insertion of a spool-shaped silicone prosthesis mounted on an intramedullary silicone stem that fit into the shaft of the first metacarpal. Stability of the implant required reconstructing the capsular ligamentous structures of the first carpal metacarpal joint, often with the transfer of a slip of tendon taken from the flexor carpi radialis. Swanson reported that both techniques produced excellent results for over 5 years. Since 1972, improvements in the silicone elastomers have increased the strength of the prostheses. Joints implanted with all of the available prostheses (Flatt, Swanson, Niebauer, Schultz, Steffee) manifest deterioration in ranges of motion over a 10-year period, and replacement arthroplasty for the rheumatoid hand remains an intensely debated subject.[14]

In 2005, Nicholas Vedder and Douglas Hanel[15] of the University of Washington in Seattle wrote an excellent review of the issues related to salvaging the badly injured or mangled hand. They suggested that the advent of antibiotics in the 1950s, with control of life-threatening infections, has allowed surgeons to perform less aggressive débridements and make decisions biased toward preserving length rather than removing devitalized tissue. This policy led to an overreliance on antibiotics and to accepting the need for delayed closure and multiple débridements under anesthesia. The resultant multiple trips to the operating room and numerous operations of débridement, grafting, and wound revisions did not lead to better outcomes. By the 1980s, surgeons returned to Bunnell's principles for the treatment of mangling injuries, but added microsurgical free flaps to the surgical armamentarium. In addition, Bunnell's use of Kirschner wires and external splints has been supplanted by the application of "strong, low profile internal fixation devices." Rigid internal fixation of fractures, removal of all contaminated and dead tissue, and viable skin coverage have promoted the immediate repair of tendons and nerves in the same sitting. Immediate, concurrent repair of all damage is simply the application of Bunnell's principles with modern technology.

Bunnell's reconstruction methods for traumatic hand amputations have undergone a reappraisal, however. In the late 1940s and throughout the 1950s, patients who lost fingers or thumbs in accidents had few options. For thumb amputees, Bunnell described reconstructive procedures such as phalangization, pollicization with the index finger, and building a new thumb with a tubular pedicle graft and bone graft. In the 1956 edition of *Surgery of the Hand*, Bunnell described transferring toes to the hand to replace fingers or a thumb, but he had a low opinion of these surgical adventures. Bunnell described results that he personally observed to be aesthetically unacceptable and functionless.[5]

Reports of replantation of digits, hands, or even arms, however, appeared in the 1960s. Replantations have changed the outlook for many patients who suffered traumatic amputation of parts of an upper limb. These procedures came about because of the remarkable advances in microsurgery aided by operating microscopes and specialized microsurgical instruments capable of magnifications × 20. Richard Goldner and James Urbaniak of Duke University in Durham, North Carolina, wrote the chapter on replantation in the 2005 edition of *Green's Operative Hand Surgery* in which they outlined indications, contraindications, techniques, postoperative care, and possible outcomes.[16] Replantation procedures have important limitations—in particular, they apply largely only to patients with sharply amputated or moderately avulsed injuries and not to generally mangled and grossly contaminated war injuries like those Bunnell and his hand center surgeons saw. Replantation also requires a trained team of experienced surgeons and support staff. It also demands hospitals willing to pay for the acquisition and maintenance of specialized equipment, as even the most proficient surgeons could not perform the surgery successfully without it. Despite these limitations, Goldner, Urbaniak, and others have performed thousands of these procedures successfully, going beyond what Bunnell thought possible.

One could confidently assume that Bunnell would have supported the improvements made to his treatment methods by the hand surgeons who followed him. According to the accounts of those who knew him, he listened carefully to others' opinions and considered them in the light of his own experience. Furthermore, he accepted risks and took chances. He enjoyed aerobatics and flew World War I vintage airplanes as a hobby. He crashed on multiple occasions and limped because of a hip injury sustained in a crash that killed his passenger. This complex man surely knew that the future of his professional calling was not static; he took pleasure in founding the American Society for Surgery of the Hand (ASSH), an organization that would lead in the advancement of hand surgery. His presidential address at the 1947 meeting of the ASSH encapsulates what he thought about the subspecialty. He recalled the role of Norman Kirk, the orthopaedic surgeon who, as Surgeon General of the Army during World War II, called Bunnell to special service in hand surgery. Bunnell, although a general surgeon, declared hand surgery to fit within the specialty of orthopaedics. He said that hand surgeons needed to know how to perform skin grafts (including pedicle grafts) and nerve repairs but stated: "Hand surgery consists more of orthopaedic surgery than of plastic surgery or neurosurgery. It is the jewelry of orthopaedic surgery; the surgery of the extremities in miniature."[3] He looked forward to the advancement of hand surgery research and the development of new concepts and techniques. The ASSH kept Bunnell's dream alive and even surpassed it in creating a new surgical discipline with special training requirements and procedures to earn accreditation for programs and certification of trainees. George Omer[17] of the University of New Mexico in Albuquerque made the case in 1982 for the ASSH to achieve special status for accrediting and certifying programs and individuals in a newly created surgical discipline of surgery of the hand. He justified increased specialization as necessary to keep up with the rapid advances in biomedical science. He claimed that hand surgery "emerged as a subspecialty during World War II" and cataloged the achievements of the ASSH after the war. The ASSH had developed accredited continuing medical education programs; sponsored the *Journal of Hand Surgery*; set standards for fellowships; created the "annual bibliography of the hand"; published a book describing the 56 preceptorships or fellowships in hand surgery; and helped Omer establish the first Division of Hand Surgery in the United States. By 1971, the success in differentiating hand surgery as a distinct specialty led to formal discussions between the ASSH and the

American Board of Medical Specialties (ABMS) on establishing a conjoint (orthopaedics, plastic surgery, general surgery) Board of Hand Surgery, but a year later the ABMS rejected the idea, ruling that it had placed a moratorium on new boards of any kind. A year later, the ABMS agreed to certification of special competence if a "primary board," that is, one already in existence, went along with the idea. ASSH applied to the American Board of Orthopaedic Surgery (ABOS), the American Board of Plastic Surgery (ABPS), and the American Board of Surgery (ABS) for their approval in establishing certification of special competence in hand surgery, but all three primary boards refused.

In 1978, the ASSH went to the Liaison Committee for Graduate Medical Education for guidance, but received none. Two years later, ASSH tried again, petitioning the ABOS, ABPS, and ABS, as well as the ABMS, again to no avail. Omer and his committee of hand surgeons tenaciously reapplied in 1981, and by 1982 they could report that the three primary boards had agreed to establish a Joint Committee on Surgery of the Hand with representatives from orthopaedics, plastic surgery, and general surgery. By then the American Association for Hand Surgery (AAHS) had joined in the effort. This organization was founded in 1970 by a group of surgeons who trained under Joseph L. Posch in Detroit. It has grown to a society of over 1,100 members. Finally, by 1982, it looked as though a mechanism had been established for accreditation of hand fellowships and certification of individuals in hand surgery. The mechanism had not yet won complete approval, but as Omer stated in his address: "At long last the profession and the public may be provided with documented recognition of special competence in the well-defined surgical subspecialty."

In 1989, Omer, together with William Graham of Hershey, Pennsylvania, published an editorial in the *Journal of Hand Surgery* on the development of certification in hand surgery.[18] The 18-year quest for formal recognition of hand surgery as a distinct specialty had finally succeeded. Omer and Graham recounted the evolution of the accreditation and certification processes from 1920, when the Council of Medical Education first established committees to ensure "expertness" in various primary specialties. By 1982, Omer and fellow hand surgeons established the Joint Committee on Surgery of the Hand (JCSH), made up of representatives of the ABS, ABPS, ABOS, and the two hand societies (ASSH and AAHS). The JCSH worked with the three surgical boards to delineate requirements for accreditation of fellowships and to establish practice requirements and an examination for individuals who completed the approved fellowships. In 1986, the ABMS "in full assembly" approved the scheme.

American Orthopaedic Foot and Ankle
Society and *Foot and Ankle International*

The first issue of the *American Journal of Orthopaedic Surgery* was published in 1903. This forerunner of *The Journal of Bone and Joint Surgery* contained 34 articles, six of which referred to the foot and ankle. Thus, from the beginnings of orthopaedic surgery in America, physicians who concentrated on caring for the musculoskeletal system regarded the care of foot and ankle disorders of major importance.

The first published paper related to the foot in American orthopaedic literature was by Robert W. Lovett[19] concerning his observations on "painful affections of the feet among trained nurses." Lovett had examined 250 nurses and made "a series of 500 observations upon normal and disabled feet" in female nurses at a large general hospital in Boston. He reported that only a view of the sole of the foot in a mirror beneath a glass table on which the nurses stood had any prognostic significance. In his opinion, flat pronated feet more often caused trouble than feet "without breakdown of the arch." Lovett tried to mandate the use of a boot he designed that was "wide as the foot in front but [with a] straight inner edge and high arched, stiff shanked and constructed on a slightly curved line so as to hold the foot in its position of strength." The nurses rejected Lovett's design, saying that the shoes made to his specifications did not look good and made their feet hurt, but Lovett rejected their complaints. He said the nurses' feet hurt because they were working longer hours and claimed: "This outbreak of trouble was coincident with increased duty on account of the admission of soldiers returning from the Spanish War, and was probably due to that."

Lovett's subsequent comments have a comic quality. He described how he tried to modify his boot to placate the nurses and shoe dealers. Nothing he devised seemed to satisfy them, and he insisted: "If nurses were allowed to wear boots of their own selection, there would be much more trouble than there is now." He admitted that some of these women suffered foot pain severe enough to keep them from work; for these nurses, he prescribed a course of treatment of hot and cold soaks, felt pads, proper fitting metal plates, rest, and adhesive straps. In refractory situations he reported: "Strychnine in fairly large doses has been used in a number of cases in the hope of improving the muscular tone." Summing up his experience, Lovett said: "Although proof by figures is lacking, it is probable that the amount of trouble has been decidedly less than it would have been without the use of a proper boot."[19]

After such an inauspicious start, one would have hoped that subsequent reports on disorders of the foot would contain more science, but the article by Albert Freiberg and J. Henry Schroeder[20] of Cincinnati did not. In their paper, "A Note on the Foot of the American Negro," Freiberg and Schroeder examined the feet of 44 African Americans at the Cincinnati Hospital and took weight-bearing impressions by "the iron and tannic acid method." Freiberg and Schroeder said that they found a high percentage of flat feet and hallux valgus. In comparing those findings to those of 34 white patients at the same hospital, they found that white patients had a lower percentage of each condition. They were apologetic for the "homely observation and so incomplete an enquiry," and said that the whole matter needed more research. A third paper in the same volume entitled "The Abuse of Flat-Foot Supports" also borders on quackery. Wisner Townsend[21] published a three-and-a-half page lament that patients bought arch supports without consulting a physician, risking serious injury. He noted: "For the patient with a flat foot, who is his own surgeon or whose attention is called to the condition of his foot when purchasing shoes, there is but one kind of treatment—the application of the support sold at that store." He worried that lay people did not understand the principles involved. Joel Goldthwaite of Boston, among others, discussed the paper rationally, attempting to define which patients could benefit from arch supports and which would not. Goldthwaite described several patients with fixed valgus deformities of the foot that could not be improved with arch supports. He achieved corrections of deformity in these patients by excising the talonavicular joint and fusing it with the foot in the correct alignment. After the requisite several months in a cast, the correction of the deformity was maintained.

Royal Whitman, of the Hospital for the Ruptured and Crippled in New York, presented the most reasonable paper on foot surgery in a 1903 *American Journal of Orthopaedic Surgery*, describing "the importance of supplementary tendon transplantation in the treatment of paralytic talipes by other procedures designed to assure stability."[22] He had found that in treating paralytic foot deformities (probably resulting from polio), simply transplanting a tendon did not maintain correction. Thus, in treating a fixed inversion deformity, transferring the tibialis anterior laterally did not work as consistently on its own. He found that at least a limited bone resection and joint fusion were necessary before a tendon transfer could function effectively.

Whitman also described his operation for the treatment of foot malalignment associated with paralysis of the calf muscles. He observed that the foot developed a fixed dorsiflexion deformity when not supported by a brace or cast, and in 1903 one could assume that patients with such deformities had received little or no treatment until they found their way to Whitman. He reported, "I have found the most effective treatment to be an astragalectomy with backward displacement of the foot upon the leg." He also attempted a fusion between the tibia and heel, but found that "ankylosis is exceptional." Whitman thus found it necessary to shorten the heel cord and transfer the peroneal tendons to the insertion of the heel cord. Whitman's astragalectomy procedure found its way into the lexicon of orthopaedics for many years thereafter. Armitage Whitman, also of the Hospital for the Ruptured and Crippled in New York, published a paper on his father's results in volume 4 of the *Journal of Bone and Joint Surgery* in 1922. According to the younger Whitman, "In 65 cases the astragalectomy operation maintained good correction in all but a few patients, after a long period of time."[23]

The Whitman astragalectomy procedure with tibiocalcaneal fusion became the first of many eponymous foot operations that American orthopaedists presented in the ensuing decades. Michael Hoke, Naughton Dunn, E. W. Ryerson, Arthur Steindler, G. G. Davis, Paul Lapidus, C. L. Lambrinudi, Willis Campbell, A. B. Gill, and others described operations eventually named for them during the years following World War I, when polio epidemics ravaged the children of the United States and caused thousands of foot deformities needing their expertise. A review of the orthopaedic literature of the period shows the progress they made in devising techniques for correcting deformities and stabilizing instabilities of the hindfoot. In general, Whitman's radical astragalectomy operation lost out to more conservative osteotomies and tendon transfers, especially to Ryerson's triple arthrodesis procedure. Percutaneous tenotomies and forceful manipulation were the only usable techniques before the advent of these procedures (Figures 45 and 46).

Edwin W. Ryerson of Rush Medical College in Chicago, founder of the American Academy of Orthopaedic Surgeons (AAOS), published an article on arthrodesing operations in the foot in volume 5 of *The Journal of Bone and Joint Surgery* in 1923. He recalled how shoe modifications, forcible manipulations, and tenotomies failed to produce lasting correction of foot deformities. According to Ryerson, tendon transfers also failed to provide lasting correction. He found that Whitman's astragalectomy operation with an attempt at tibiocalcaneal fusion produced an ugly, painful foot, which too often rolled over into an inverted alignment. His report contrasted with the enthusiasm of Royal and Armitage Whitman. Ryerson concluded that none of these operations succeeded in giving patients pain-free walking and sourly suggested that patients with amputations had better gaits because their prosthetic feet worked only in flexion and extension with no lateral deformity to cause painful callosities or skin breakdown. Ryerson recommended fusion of multiple joints in the hindfoot to prevent lateral deformity. These joints might vary, according to Ryerson, but generally a surgeon should fuse the talocalcaneal, calcaneocuboid, talonavicular, and often the cuboid and fifth metatarsal joints. He described the techniques for these operations in detail, supporting his thesis with several pre- and postoperative photographs of his patients. Ryerson's hindfoot surgery techniques have withstood intensive analysis over many years, and today still serve as the basis for surgery of this area of the foot.

H. Augustus Wilson of Philadelphia published the first paper on forefoot surgery in the *American Journal of Orthopaedic Surgery* in 1904, reviewing his results of surgical treatment of hallux valgus deformities in 152 feet.[24] He had observed that the popular Keller operation, consisting of resection of the proximal part of the proximal phalanx of the great toe, left patients worse off than they were preoperatively. He performed exostectomies to remove the bony prominence of the bunion, then reduced any such displacement of the great toe on the shaft of the first metatarsal.

During the mid-20th century an operation devised by Earl D. McBride[25] of Oklahoma City captured the attention of most orthopaedists surgically treating bunion deformities. McBride based his operation on the concept that the adductor hallucis muscle and the lateral half of the flexor hallucis brevis produced "an abnormal mechanical force" on the lateral sesamoid and base of the great toe. Unfortunately, the procedure too often overcorrected the deformity and left patients with a hallux varus deformity, a problem worse than their original complaint. The once-popular McBride operation understandably has fallen from favor. Keller's operation, the resection of the base of the proximal phalange of the great toe, too often left patients with a short, stubby, unwieldy hallux, as did the Mayo procedure, which produced the same kind of deformity by resecting the head of the first metatarsal. Fusion of the joint, when successful, relieved pain but often made normal toe-off impossible. In the mid-20th century, C. Lesley Mitchell and his associates[26] at the Henry Ford Hospital in Detroit addressed these issues in the publication of their results in 400 osteotomies to the first metatarsal. Mitchell concluded that a congenital shortening and varus alignment of the first metatarsal caused the problem. The Mitchell osteotomy, however, led to complications postoperatively when large numbers of other orthopaedic surgeons adopted it. These complications included osteonecrosis of the distal fragment, loss of position of the osteotomy site with recurrence of deformity, and shortening of the first metatarsal with transfer of weight-bearing stresses to the adjacent metatarsal heads. Modification of the Mitchell osteotomy followed, with debates over the location of the osteotomy and how it should be stabilized. The Chevron osteotomy, devised by Jay Corless[27] and later reported by Austin and Leventen,[28] divides the bone in more or less the same location as the Mitchell procedure, but its V-shaped configuration produces a more stable construct. Osteotomy at the proximal metatarsal is the currently favored location, usually requiring screw fixation.[29] Some surgeons have devised osteotomies through the first cuneiform, and Akin[30] in 1925 described an osteotomy through the proximal part of the proximal phalanx of the great toe. Consensus among foot surgeons is that bony alignment trumps adjustment of soft tissues in the treatment of bunions and hallux valgus deformities.[31]

As orthopaedic surgery matured in the second half of the 20th century, an increasing number of its practitioners specialized in foot and ankle surgery. Many of them earned justified recognition and stature. An incomplete list of these individuals would include Henri Duvries, Verne Inman, and Roger Mann of the University of California in San Francisco; Melvin Jahss, Francesca Thompson, and William Hamilton of New York; Mark Morrison of Baltimore; James Drennan of Albuquerque; Michael Coughlin of Boise, Idaho; Nicholas Giannestras of Cincinnati; and Leonard Goldner of Durham, North Carolina. These notable orthopaedic surgeons interested in foot and ankle surgery formed the American Orthopaedic Foot Society in 1969. The name was changed to the American Orthopaedic Foot and Ankle Society (AOFAS) several years later. The society holds its own annual meetings, but as an official affiliate of the AAOS it also participates in the Academy's educational activities, such as Specialty Day at the AAOS Annual Meeting. Since 1980, the AOFAS has published a journal, *Foot and Ankle International*. As the journal name implies, the AOFAS has developed relationships with other similar organizations in other countries. Melvin Jahss took on the daunting task of editor-in-chief for the first eight years of the journal's existence, succeeded by Ken Johnson of the Mayo Clinic in Scottsdale in 1988. Volume 1 contained an editorial by Leonard Goldner[32] entitled "Why Another Journal?" in which he proclaimed that the members of the sponsoring organization, the AOFAS, had a responsibility "to collect and record information to provide benefit for those who need advice and treatment about foot and ankle problems." He acknowledged that improvements in the surgical treatment of foot disorders developed too slowly, announcing that the Foot and Ankle Society had assumed the obligation to correct this by means of "clinical and laboratory investigations into disorders of the foot."

The early issues of the journal had a clinical slant with few basic science articles. Topics such as ankle fusion with a Hoffman device, peg-and-dowell fusion of the proximal interphalangeal joint, and dislocation of the first toe confirmed the strong orientation of the first issues of *Foot and Ankle International* toward clinical subjects. With time, however, extensive analyses of the biomechanics and pathophysiology of the foot and ankle appeared in increasing numbers. Twenty-five years later, after continuous publication under four editors-in-chief (Jahss, Kenneth Johnson, Lowell Lutter, and the current editor, E. Greer Richardson), the journal's titles imply greater sophistication in diagnosis, surgical techniques, and basic science. The volume published in 2005 contained 181 articles compared to the 50 articles of volume 1, published in 1980–1981.

Understandably, the AOFAS and its journal have taken considerable interest in the subject of the diabetic foot. In a recent issue, Michael Pinzur[33] of Loyola University Medical Center in Chicago recounted statistics that underscore the magnitude of the problem. Sixteen million Americans have diabetes, and the most common reason for hospitalization is a foot ulcer or infection, complications that currently result in 50,000 lower extremity amputations a year. Pinzur emphasized the importance of proactive care, which should include patient education and protective footwear, because patients with diabetic neuropathy often do not have enough sensation in their feet to appreciate the fact that they are developing ulcers, infections, or fractures. The journal publishes papers on such topics as the measurement of dynamic shear and vertical pressures on the diabetic foot, how orthotics of varying materials can influence them, microvascular responses of the skin of diabetics, the use of walking braces versus total contact casts in an effort to prevent skin breakdown and infection, and how to treat an infection once it has occurred.

At this point, the AOFAS has not sought formal certification of orthopaedic surgeons as have the ASSH and the AOSSM. Nevertheless, membership in the AOFAS and related organizations gives useful credentials in the diagnosis and treatment of foot disorders to physicians with medical degrees and orthopaedic certification. This important level of recognition differentiates them from non-physician suppliers of foot care services. The American Association of Colleges of Podiatric Medicine now lists eight institutions in the United States that award degrees in podiatry. They are located in Glendale, Arizona; Miami, Florida; Oakland, California; Des Moines, Iowa; New York, New York; Chicago, Illinois; Cleveland, Ohio; and Philadelphia, Pennsylvania. The American College of

Foot and Ankle Surgeons (ACFAS), the professional organization for podiatrists, now has over 6,000 members.

The Musculoskeletal Tumor Society

In 1977, the small group of orthopaedic surgeons specializing in musculoskeletal pathology and tumors decided to form the Musculoskeletal Tumor Society (MSTS). At that time, the mortality caused by malignant musculoskeletal tumors was appalling. The founders of the MSTS hoped that by pooling their data they could formulate better treatment strategies to achieve higher survival rates. In the ensuing 30 years, they have realized these goals.

When the MSTS was founded, only 20 percent of patients with osteosarcomas survived for five years after diagnosis. Throughout most of the first half of the 20th century, amputation was the universal treatment. A Philadelphia surgeon, Samuel W. Gross,[34] (son of Samuel D. Gross) established amputation as the best and only way to treat osteosarcomas, stating: "General measures being worthless, no time should be lost in resorting to amputation." He advocated amputation even though "surgical interference has been followed by a mortality of 31.25 percent"; for the patients who did survive the operation, the specter of dying with a massive fungating tumor protruding from the leg was avoided. Those patients died from pulmonary metastases, but for some (up to 20 percent), the amputation appeared curative. The approach to osteosarcomas began to change in the early 1950s when Stanford Cade,[35] a British radiologist, published several papers on the possibilities of combining radiation therapy with amputation. He pointed out that at the Memorial Hospital in New York (later Memorial Sloan-Kettering), amputation alone attained a survival rate of 4 $\frac{1}{2}$ percent, whereas irradiation followed by amputation produced a 46 percent five-year survival rate. Cade suggested a course of radiation therapy with a total tumor dose of 3,000 rads as the first treatment of osteosarcoma patients, followed by four to six weeks of observation. Cade advised amputation for the patients who did not improve with this regimen. For patients who experienced marked improvement, Cade advised further observation, noting that if the tumor started to grow again, amputation could be performed at that time. If the patient already had pulmonary metastasis, Cade claimed that palliative radiation therapy would shrink the primary tumor of the limb and spare the patient from mutilation, with the expectation that death was imminent from pulmonary metastasis rather than the primary site.

In the mid-1970s, orthopaedists and oncologists reassessed chemotherapy as a critical adjunctive treatment of osteosarcoma. Until that time, they found that chemotherapy had little long-term benefit. In the later decades of the 19th century, Coley[36] observed that some patients with osteosarcomas experienced remission of malignancy following a severe streptococcal infection. This inspired Coley to use the toxins of the streptococci to inhibit growth of osteosarcomas. "Coley's toxins" were found to be ineffective, and the idea was abandoned. The development of chemotherapeutic agents persisted, however, and their use brought a marked decline in mortality rates and the advent of "limb salvage" surgery in osteosarcoma patients (Figure 47). Lucius Sinks and Eugene Mindell[37] at Roswell Park Memorial Institute in Buffalo, New York, administered adriamycin as adjunctive therapy for osteosarcoma, and Norman Jaffe and associates[38] of Boston Children's Hospital used a high-dose methotrexate with citrovorum rescue and vincristine upon amputation. During the 1970s, other investigators published several variations of these protocols. They found that chemotherapy produced a profound response in the primary tumor. With necrosis of up to 90 percent of the malignant cells in the lesion, the tumor stopped growing and developed distinct margins. The tumor shrank, becoming less swollen and more defined, although none claimed that the tumor had been definitively cured by these drugs. Coincident with the development of chemotherapy, CT and MRI began to supplant plain radiographs in the evaluation of patients with osteosarcoma. These imaging modalities allowed accuracy in staging tumors previously not thought possible. During the first two decades after World War II, surgeons such as Lemuel Bowden and Robert Booher[39] of Sloan-Kettering showed that patients could survive indefinitely after removal of sarcomas when they excised the entire tumor with the entire compartment of normal tissue about the lesion. Judging from their illustrations, surgery left their patients considerably deformed, but complete extirpation of tumors such as fibrosarcomas and rhabdomyosarcomas proved to be life-saving. William Enneking[40] of the University of Florida in Gainesville proposed a staging system that provided uniformity for surgeons interested in performing limb-salvage procedures in patients with sarcomas of the musculoskeletal system, including osteosarcomas. Enneking's surgical staging system is now widely accepted. The system cross-references the degrees of a tumor's malignancy with its location (intracompartmental or extracompartmental) or whether the tumor has metastasized.

The combination of adjunctive chemotherapy (a staging system based on new technologies such as MRI) and long experience with grading sarcomas cystologically has saved the limbs of many patients with malignant tumors such as osteosarcomas and has lowered alarmingly high mortality rates.

Enneking and his associates in the MSTS have applied the staging system to collaborative research beginning with a validation of interobserver reliability at the M. D. Anderson Hospital in Houston, Texas, Roswell Park Cancer Center in Buffalo, New York, University of California at Los Angeles, University of California in San Francisco, Case Western Reserve University, University of Chicago, University of Iowa, Massachusetts General Hospital, Mayo Clinic, Sloan-Kettering Memorial Hospital, University of Miami, University of Minnesota, and the Rizzoli Institute of Orthopaedics in Bologna, Italy. The physicians at these institutions have been vital in the fight against malignancy of the musculoskeletal system, which has helped preserve the lives and limbs of many patients who in the past would have died.

Orthopaedic tumor surgeons have displayed remarkable ingenuity in devising numerous kinds of limb-salvage operations, such as developing prostheses to replace not only joints but also large segments of bone. For the last few years, members of the MSTS have published selected papers presented at their annual meeting in *Clinical Orthopaedics and Related Research*, reporting the results of using these devices. For example, Michael Neel and his associates[41] published a paper on the use of a "noninvasive expandable prosthesis" in skeletally immature children. Their device consists of a polyester ketone prosthetic replacement of a distal femur. The device contains a cylinder, which in turn has a spring and titanium stem. Heating the device with electromagnetic energy melts a cuff of polyester to allow the spring to expand and push the metal rod out of the prosthesis, thereby lengthening the limb. Neel and his colleagues reported that the device permits multiple lengthenings at intervals to keep up with the expected growth of the child's limb.

Wear, loosening, and breakage of these increasingly complicated prosthetic devices led to a much more extensive use of bone allografts to replace large segments removed for treatment of tumors. Fox and associates[42] at Massachusetts General Hospital have reported on large numbers of patients in whom allografts were used as osteoarticular or intercalary grafts or as an allograft/endoprosthesis composite. The allografts carry the advantage over prostheses of allowing healing between host and donor bone, preserving bone stock for later reconstruction, and providing ligamentous and tendinous insertions to which the surgeon could secure the patient's own soft tissues. The risk of transmission of diseases has been recognized and is almost completely controlled by screening and processing. Overall, limb-salvage surgery for patients with osteosarcomas and other malignant musculoskeletal tumors has led to improvements in quality of life and less self-dissatisfaction than that experienced by amputees after surgery for similar lesions.

A discussion about the MSTS would not be complete without mentioning its role in alerting the broader fellowship of orthopaedic surgeons about the hazards of biopsy. In 1979, before the advent of modern chemotherapy, staging, and limb-salvage surgery, Broström and associates[43] reported that a biopsy of malignant bone lesion had no effect on survival. Since then, members of the MSTS have received patients referred from physicians who have performed biopsies that adversely affect the outcomes of treatment on a musculoskeletal malignancy. In 1982, Enneking[44] published an editorial about this matter in *JBJS*, commenting on a paper by Henry Mankin and associates.[45] The MSTS members studied patients they believed were harmed by a biopsy and made a list of recommendations that Mankin and his associates passed on to the readers of the journal. The study revealed an 18 percent major error in diagnosis, a 10 percent "nonrepresentative" or "technically poor" biopsy, and a 4 ½ percent unnecessary amputation rate resulting from the biopsy, along with other complications associated with the procedure. Enneking and Mankin and his associates urged their nonspecialist colleagues to refer the patients with sarcomas before the biopsy for four reasons: (1) staging should be done first; (2) indications for open versus percutaneous biopsies vary; (3) placement of the incisions had critical implications; and (4) proper diagnosis often required fresh tissue, among other necessary aspects of treatment.[44,45]

Regrettably, the recommendations were not followed. Fourteen years later, Mankin and associates[46] published a paper that echoed the findings of the 1982 article. The MSTS had performed a similar study looking for adverse biopsy outcomes. They found in a review of 597 patients diagnostic errors in 17.8 percent, similar percentages of unnecessary amputations resulting from the biopsy, and nearly 20 percent incidence of problems with the biopsy that forced the treating surgeon to perform a more complex operation in an attempt to save the limb. Dempsey Springfield and Andrew Rosenberg[47] of Boston commented editorially on the 1996 paper by Mankin and associates, finding it "especially frustrating" that their nontumor specialist colleagues continued to do biopsies on patients with sarcomas and ignored the admonition, "Do not biopsy what you are not going to treat." They also commented on problems with percutaneous procedures using needles, trochars, and cannulas popularized by Ottolenghi and Schajowicz of Buenos Aires and Frederick Craig of the New York Orthopaedic Hospital. The MSTS study showed that 40 percent of all needle biopsies led to diagnoses that were incorrect. To date, the MSTS has not revisited the issue of orthopaedic generalists performing biopsies. In the same issue, Michael Skrzynski and associates[48] reported that needle biopsy produced less accurate diagnoses than open biopsy of musculoskeletal tumors.

In discussing musculoskeletal tumor surgery and the MSTS, the influence of Dallas Phemister[49] of the University of Chicago should be considered. The University of Chicago was founded in 1890 by wealthy philanthropist John D. Rockefeller. Philanthropists also founded Johns Hopkins, Stanford University, and other institutions of higher learning during the late 19th and early 20th centuries. These successful institutions all had strong first presidents: Daniel Coit Gilman at Hopkins, Daniel Starr Jordan at Stanford, and David Harper at the University of Chicago. Harper established a year-round core curriculum and supervised the actual building of the university, which welcomed all qualified applicants—including women and minorities—at a time when such policy was not in fashion. Harper shaped the spirit and expectations of the university that eventually led to a plethora of Nobel Prize winners as well as other high achievers such as physicist Enrico Ferme, who led the research that resulted in the first controlled, self-sustaining nuclear chain reaction; economist and Nobel Laureate Milton Friedman, who revolutionized economic theory; and Howard Ricketts, who discovered that a class of microorganisms, now called *Rickettsiae*, were responsible for tick-borne diseases. The medical school at the University of Chicago (now the Pritzker School of Medicine because of a large endowment from that family) was founded in 1924, and Dallas Phemister was appointed to its faculty as the first chairman of the Department of Surgery.

Phemister was born in Carbondale, Illinois, in 1882. He learned to speak French and German fluently in grade school and was admitted to Valparaiso University in Indiana at the age of 16. After two years, he transferred to the

University of Chicago. By 1904, at 22 years of age, Phemister graduated from the Rush Medical School with a medical degree. Private practice and surgical training in Paris and Vienna qualified him to join the army as a major in 1917; he served in France during the last year and a half of World War I. Dean Lewis, a fellow officer with him in the Presbyterian Hospital unit, was earmarked for the position of Chairman of Surgery at the University of Chicago, but after Lewis accepted the position of Chairman of Surgery at Johns Hopkins he suggested to the administration at the University of Chicago that they appoint Phemister to that post. Phemister accepted the appointment and remained there until his death in 1952. He was a general surgeon but had a profound interest in orthopaedics, especially in diagnosis and treatment of musculoskeletal system tumors. Phemister used bone autografts extensively to reconstruct segmental bone defects. He published important papers on the biology of bone grafts for nonunion of fractures and treatment of tuberculosis infections in the musculoskeletal system. Although he was a general surgeon who also performed abdominal and thoracic surgery, he greatly influenced orthopaedics and developed a division of orthopaedics in the Department of Surgery at the University of Chicago that achieved great prominence. Howard Hatcher was the first resident in orthopaedics at the University of Chicago in 1930; he developed an intense interest in the pathology of bone tumors and studied them over a period of 30 years. During that time, Hatcher rose from resident to full professor and chief of the Division of Orthopaedics at the university. He, like Phemister, produced a legacy of intellectual heirs who have become the leaders of modern orthopaedic oncology, including James S. Miles (Denver), J. Crawford Campbell (Boston), William F. Enneking (Gainesville, Florida), Michael Bonfiglio (Iowa), Eugene Mindell (Buffalo), Thomas D. Brower (Kentucky), Henry Mankin (Boston), John Fahey (Chicago), Mary Sherman (New Orleans), and Eugene Bleck (Los Angeles). Due to these pioneering physicians, orthopaedic surgery has evolved into a specialty that has saved the lives and limbs of thousands of people with musculoskeletal tumors. Interestingly, the Phemister/Hatcher/Enneking tradition continues at the University of Chicago Pritzker School of Medicine, Division of Orthopaedics, headed by Michael Simon. Philanthropist John D. Rockefeller commented late in his life that founding the University of Chicago was his best investment.

Musculoskeletal Infection Society

Hematogenously spread *Staphylococci* and *Streptococci* produced most acute infections of the musculoskeletal system up until the last quarter of the 20th century. Physicians and surgeons trained in medical science before the late 20th century understood the principles of incision, drainage, sequestrectomy, and immobilization very well. Nevertheless, both physicians and patients justifiably feared these infections. Osteomyelitis and septic arthritis, for example, caused mortality rates between 20 percent and 60 percent in young children, and those who survived faced the probability of lifelong deformity as well as locally recurring abscesses (Figures 48 and 49). Virgil Gibney[50] described this in his 1884 book *The Hip and Its Diseases*:

> In no one of the inflammatory lesions in and about the hip is there a greater call for the employment of sound surgical principles. If abscess forms, the pus should be promptly evacuated . . . I made a diagnosis of periarthritis and advised an incision. The advice was not taken—two and a half months later the abscess extended through the whole of the gluteal region. It opened spontaneously, extensive sloughing followed . . . she died of exhaustion a year after the first appearance of the disease.

The arrival of antibiotics in the mid-20th century brightened the picture for patients with acute musculoskeletal infections. Patients with chronic draining sinuses and deformities caused by acute bacterial infections became unusual, if not rare. Later in the 20th century, however, total joints and the nearly universal use of internal fixation for fractures and spine surgery led to the creation of whole new patient groups with new kinds of musculoskeletal infections. The members of the Musculoskeletal Infection Society (MSIS) determined to address these issues in founding their organization in 1989. The group of founders included Carl Nelson of Little Rock, Arkansas; Jeannette Wilkins and Michael Patzakis of Los Angeles; Richard Evans of Denver; David Seligson and Steven Henry of Louisville; Bruce Heppenstall and John Esterhai of Philadelphia; George Cierny and John T. Mader of Galveston; and Kevin Garvin and Arlen Hanssen of Rochester, Minnesota. The society met annually and published some of the papers presented at its meetings in *Clinical Orthopaedics and Related Research* (*CORR*). *CORR* recently became its official journal, publishing these papers once a year in a symposium format.

The MSIS fills an important niche in orthopaedics, bringing together orthopaedists, microbiologists, epidemiologists, and other basic scientists. At its meetings and in its publications, members of the society developed a system for staging musculoskeletal infections, an essential guide to treatment.

Soon after Fleming, Chain, and Florey discovered penicillin in the late 1930s, bacteria began to develop enzymes that would prevent penicillin from breaking down the cell walls of the bacterial organisms. By the late 1950s, half of the identified *Staphylococci* strains could produce penicillinase, thus were resistant to the drug. Science countered with methacillin and methacillin-like antibiotics, but within a year after the formulation of methacillin, *Staphylococci* began to develop resistance to these drugs as well. Since then, infecting organisms have manifested a nearly infinite capacity to mutate and develop resistance to antibiotics. Furthermore, as the numbers of infected total joint revisions increased, orthopaedists began to recognize the adhesive properties of bacteria and their ability to elaborate a protective biofilm around the prosthetic components. The MSIS has been in the forefront of investigating these issues.[51] Recent papers by members at its annual meetings published in *CORR* also report studies of the rapid and precise identification of bacteria using polymerase chain reaction technology and the development of antibiofilm strategies to disrupt adherent bacteria.

Limb Lengthening and Reconstruction Society

The Limb Lengthening and Reconstruction Society was organized after orthopaedic surgeons realized the potential of Ilizarov's distraction osteogenesis in treating musculoskeletal deformities. In the early decades of the 20th century, little attention was paid to the subject of limb-length equalization. Patients with severe discrepancies had to make do with a high platform attached to the sole of the shoe on the short side or accept an amputation and wear a prosthesis. For patients who could not accept either approach, they had the option of shortening the long leg or lengthening the short one. For tall adults, shortening the limb on the long side occasionally seemed like the better alternative; orthopaedic literature of the mid-20th century described several surgical techniques to accomplish this. In children, a surgeon could slow down or stop the growth of the longer leg to allow the short leg to catch up, providing legs of equal length at maturity. William T. Green and M. Anderson[52] studied this issue extensively, publishing growth charts in the 1940s and 1950s that surgeons subsequently have used to estimate the remaining contribution to growth that a distal femoral or proximal tibia epiphyseal plate could make. When the time was right, the surgeon could select one of several techniques to operate on the growth plate to prevent it from making the bone elongate further. Phemister,[53] for example, published a technique in which he placed a bone graft across the growth plate on the medial and lateral sides of the bone. Walter Blount[54] stapled the plate, assuming that the metal bridge across it would prevent it from growing. Epiphyseal arrest is still an important technique of limb-length equalization.

Lengthening the short leg, however, obviously has greater appeal than shortening or stopping the growth of the longer limb. Two European surgeons, Codovilla[55] (in 1905) and Putti[56] (in 1934), described limb-lengthening methods, but American orthopaedic surgeons had too many complications with these procedures and advised against them. H. A. Sofield[57] and E. L. Compere[58] published articles in the 1930s that essentially ended attempts at limb lengthening until H. Wagner[59] developed a technique in the late 1970s using an external fixator. The Wagner operation consists of inserting two heavy pins in the upper and lower femur or tibia and securing them to a turn buckle. At the same sitting, the surgeon performs a "corticotomy," that is, cutting through the bone to permit an immediate lengthening of about 1 cm. Thereafter, the surgeon usually turns the knob on the turn buckle daily to lengthen the leg gradually by 1 or 2 mm, up to a total of 6 to 7 cm. During the process, new membranous bone fills in the gap (distraction osteogenesis); upon completion, the surgeon applies a plate and bone graft along the lengthened femur and removes the external fixator. The simplicity of the description belies the difficulties and numerous complications that can occur, ranging from infection, impairment of nerve conduction, fractures and angulation of the lengthened bone, and dislocations of joints above or below the corticotomy. These techniques can also be applied bilaterally to the lower extremities to gain height in patients with dwarfism or very short stature—often to both the femur and tibia bilaterally, which presents a very high risk for complications. Nevertheless, members of the Limb Lengthening and Reconstruction Society describe undertaking these procedures with impressive success. In an effort to minimize complications associated with lengthening a bone through its shaft, several investigators studied the possibilities of distraction through the growth plate. These efforts showed that there were practical and theoretical reasons why "chondrodiatasis" or "distraction epiphysiolysis"[60-63] had little applicability to clinical practice. The preferred method of "callotasis" (distraction through a corticotomy in the shaft of the bone)[64] is safer; when done carefully callotasis can achieve quite useful lengthening of the limb.[65-67] Inevitably, orthopaedists have looked for other and possibly better ways to do this, including inserting a long intramedullary rod into a femur and distracting the corticotomy over the rod. After achieving the desired lengthening, the surgeon can interlock the rod with transverse screws.

The American Society for Reconstructive Microsurgery

The fifth edition of *Campbell's Operative Orthopaedics* published in 1971 did not include the word "microsurgery." Nine years later, in 1980, the sixth edition of *Campbell's* devoted nine pages of text to it, beginning with the sentence: "Microsurgery includes surgical procedures for structures so small that magnification by an operating microscope is required for their performance." Lee Milford, the author of the chapter on hand surgery in the sixth edition of *Campbell's*, briefly reviewed the usefulness of microsurgery in the repair of nerve injuries in hands, replantation, and the transposition of free flaps. The seventh edition of *Campbell's*, published in 1987, devoted an 85-page chapter to the general topic of microsurgery, with particular focus on hand injuries. Microsurgery—and the replantation, repairs, and tissue transfers it makes possible—is a fairly recent innovation in extremity surgery. One of the first reports of successfully using small-vessel and nerve repair, although not necessarily with a microscope, appeared in the 1963 *Journal of Bone and Joint Surgery*. Harold Kleinert, Morton Kasdan, and Jose Romero[68] of Louisville described their reattachment of four dysvascularized upper extremities in which they repaired transected bones, tendons, blood vessels, and nerves. In 1964, R. A. Malt and C. F. McKhann[69] reported on the successful replantations of the arm of a 12-year-old boy and the arm of a 44-year-old man, both of whom experienced transection of their upper arm when struck by a train. Since then, there have been numerous reports of replantation of parts or complete upper extremities as well as microvascular repair of small vessels and nerves and transplantation of revascularized tissue.

The replantation of a whole limb transected in the upper arm presented enormous difficulties, but in these patients the vessels were large enough that they could be repaired without the use of a microscope.[70] In 1960, Jules Jacobson and E. L. Suarez found that a microscope used by otolaryngologists for middle ear surgery gave sufficient magnification to repair blood vessels as small as 1.4 mm. Jacobson coined the term "microvascular surgery."[71] Kleinert and Kasdan,[68] however, were the first to report the successful revascularization of a severed digit, in 1963. The American Society for Reconstructive Microsurgery was founded in 1985 by James B. Steichen, Barish Strauch, Julia K. Tezis, James R. Urbaniak, and Allen Van Beek. The society now has approximately 475 members. The society's mission statement reads: "To encourage, foster, advance the art and science of reconstructive microsurgery, and to establish a forum for teaching, research, and free discussion of reconstructive microsurgical methods and principles among its members." Slightly less than half of the members of the society are orthopaedic surgeons.

The Rehabilitation Societies

Orthopaedics in its earliest manifestation centered exclusively on nonsurgical rehabilitation. During the late 19th century, American orthopaedists began to relinquish this aspect of the specialty as they turned more toward surgical solutions for problems associated with musculoskeletal deformities, injuries, and diseases. The gradual changeover to surgery in orthopaedics did not happen without resistance from several prominent early orthopaedists, including James Knight of the Hospital for the Ruptured and Crippled in New York and Charles Fayette Taylor of the New York Orthopaedic Hospital. Despite this resistance, modern orthopaedics has become largely a surgical specialty. Rehabilitation remains a critical component of orthopaedics; the rehabilitation societies discussed below keep the specialty of orthopaedics true to its origin.

The Orthopaedic Rehabilitation Association, founded in 1990, attempts to bridge the surgical and rehabilitative aspects of orthopaedics in its meetings and presentations. The program for the association at the 2006 AAOS Specialty Day program, for example, consisted of two sections. One was devoted to papers on the surgical treatment of deformities caused by neurologic injury, such as cerebral palsy and cerebral spastic deformities; the second half of the program consisted of papers on prosthetics for patients with amputations, especially those considered difficult to fit with usable devices (e.g., upper arm amputations and hip disarticulations). This and other programs suggest that surgery of the musculoskeletal system remains at the center of orthopaedics, and that even orthopaedists with an interest in the rehabilitative aspects of the specialty still emphasize the surgical side.

The Association of Children's Prosthetic-Orthotic Clinics (ACPOC) originated 50 years ago in a subcommittee formed by the National Academy of Sciences and the Prosthetic Research and Development Committee. Selected clinics host annual conferences sponsored by ACPOC for evaluating experimental designs and establishing standards and criteria. ACPOC assumed its own identity as an independent group and not a subset of the National Science Foundation in 1970. Its main office and administrative staff now reside in Rosemont, Illinois, in the AAOS headquarters building. ACPOC published a journal for several years, but it was discontinued in 1994. Topics covered by the journal reflected the organization's mission.

The American Spinal Injury Association was founded in 1973 for the purpose of promoting and establishing standards of excellence for all aspects of healthcare of individuals with spinal cord injury from onset throughout life.[72] Edwin Carter of Houston was the first president of the American Spinal Injury Association (ASIA), and was succeeded by Paul Meyer (Chicago). The society sponsors research into the prevention of spinal cord injury (SCI), emergency management of SCI, neurologic recovery, rehabilitation, medical complications of autonomic dysreflexia (bladder and bowel, cardiovascular), pulmonary complications, limb contracture, skin problems, spasticity, sexuality, psychology, mortality, causes of death, and economic impact.

SCI is an enormous problem in the United States. As many as 230,000 people may be disabled by SCI; most require continuing care until death.[72] To evaluate and treat these individuals, 25 states and the District of Columbia now have SCI centers. Physicians, researchers, therapists, and others throughout the system have largely adopted the ASIA scales and classifications to provide uniformity in assessment and treatment. Analysis of large numbers of SCI patients has made it possible to use this scale to predict fairly accurately the chances the patient has of regaining strength and sensation below the level of injury.

Research and papers presented by members at ASIA meetings available online and in the *Journal of Spinal Cord Medicine* also address the issues of chronic care of these patients.

References

1. Sterling Bunnell, 1882-1957. *J Hand Surg Am* 1982;7:217-220.

2. Newmeyer WL 3rd: Sterling Bunnell, MD: The founding father. *J Hand Surg Am* 2003;28:161-164.

3. Bunnell S: Presidential address (presented at the Annual Meeting of the American Society for Surgery of the Hand, Chicago, January 25, 1947). *J Bone Joint Surg Am* 1947;29:824-825.

4. Cutler CW: Plastic and hand surgery: First service command. Military department. United States Army. Surgery in World War II. Activities of surgical consultants, volume 1, in Heaton LD, Coates JB, Carter BN, McFetridge EM (eds): *Surgery in World War II*. Washington, DC, Office of the Surgeon General, Department of the Army, 1962, p 187.

5.   Bunnell S: *Surgery of the Hand*, ed 3. Philadelphia, PA, JB Lippincott, 1956.

6.   Boyer MI: Flexor tendon injury: Acute injury, in Green DP, Pederson WC, Hotchkiss RN, Wolfe SW (eds): *Green's Operative Hand Surgery*, ed 5. Philadelphia, PA, Elsevier, 2005, p 219.

7.   Verdan CE: Primary repair of flexor tendons. *J Bone Joint Surg Am* 1960;42:647-657.

8.   Kessler I, Nissim F: Primary repairs without immobilization of flexor tendon division within the digital sheath: An experimental and clinical study. *Acta Orthop Scand* 1969;40:587-601.

9.   Strickland JW: Development of flexor tendon surgery: Twenty-five years of progress. *J Hand Surg Am* 2000;25:214-235.

10.   Hunter JM, Schneider LN, Mackin EJ (eds): *Tendon Surgery in the Hand*. St. Louis, MO, CV Mosby, 1987.

11.   Flatt AE: *The Care of the Arthritic Hand*. St. Louis, MO, Quality Medical, 1995.

12.   Flatt AE: Restoration of rheumatoid arthritis finger-joint function: Interim report on role of prosthetic replacement. *J Bone Joint Surg Am* 1961;43:753-774.

13.   Swanson AB: Flexible implant arthroplasty for arthritic finger joints: Rationale, technique, and results of treatment. *J Bone Joint Surg Am* 1972;54:435-455.

14.   Feldon P, Terrano AL, Nalebuff EA, et al: Rheumatoid arthritis and other connective tissue diseases, in Green DP, Pederson WC, Hotchkiss RN, Wolfe SW (eds): *Green's Operative Hand Surgery*, ed 5. Philadelphia, PA, Elsevier, 2005, p 2049.

15.   Vedder NB, Hanel DP: The mangled upper extremity, in Green DP, Pederson WC, Hotchkiss RN, Wolfe SW (eds): Green's Operative Hand Surgery, ed 5. Philadelphia, PA, Elsevier, 2005, p 1587.

16.   Goldner RD, Urbaniak JR: Replantation, in Green DP, Hotchkiss RN, Pederson WC, Wolfe SW (eds): *Green's Operative Hand Surgery*, ed 5. Philadelphia, PA, Elsevier, 2005, pp 1569-1586.

17.   Omer GE: The Joint Committee for Surgery of the Hand: Guest editorial. *J Hand Surg Am* 1982;7:221-223.

18.   Omer GE Jr, Graham WP III: Development of certification in hand surgery. *J Hand Surg Am* 1989;14:589-593.

19.   Lovett RW: The occurrence of painful infections of the feet among trained nurses: A series of observations upon normal and disabled feet. *Am J Orthop Surg* 1903;1:41.

20.   Freiberg AH, Schroeder JH: A note on the foot of the American negro. *Am J Orthop Surg* 1903;1:164-167.

21.   Townsend W: The abuse of flat-foot supports. *Am J Orthop Surg* 1903;1:71-76.

22.   Whitman R: The importance of supplementing tendon transplantation in the treatment of paralytic talipes by other procedures designed to assure stability. *Am J Orthop Surg* 1903;1:77-82.

23.   Whitman A: Astrogolectomy and backward displacement of the foot. An investigation of its practical results. *J Bone Joint Surg Am* 1922;4:266-278.

24.   Wilson HA: An analysis of 152 cases of hallux valgus in 77 patients with a report of an operation for its relief. *Am J Orthop Surg* 1905-1906;3:214-230.

25.   McBride ED: Hallux valgus bunion deformity: Its treatment in mild, moderate and severe stages. *J Int Coll Surg* 1954;21:99-105.

26. Mitchell CL, Fleming JL, Allen R, Glenney C, Sanford GA: Osteotomy-bunionectomy for hallux valgus. *J Bone Joint Surg Am* 1958;40:41-60.

27. Corless J: A modification of the Mitchell procedure. Canadian Orthopaedic Association Proceedings. *J Bone Joint Surg Br* 1976;58:138.

28. Austin DW, Leventen EO: A new osteotomy for hallux valgus: A horizontally directed "V" displacement osteotomy of the metatarsal head for hallux valgus and primus varus. *Clin Orthop Relat Res* 1981;157:25-30.

29. McCluskey LC, Johnson JE, Wynarsky GT, Harris GF: Comparison of stability of proximal crescentric metatarsal osteotomy and proximal horizontal "V" osteotomy. *Foot Ankle Int* 1994;15:263-270.

30. Akin O: The treatment of hallux valgus: A new operative procedure and its results. *Med Sentinel* 1925;33:678.

31. Mitchell LA, Baxter DE: A Chevron-Akin double osteotomy for correction of hallux valgus. *Foot Ankle* 1991;12:7-14.

32. Goldner JL: Why another journal? *Foot Ankle* 1980;1:2.

33. Pinzur M: Surgical versus accommodative treatment for Charcot arthropathy of the midfoot. *Foot Ankle Int* 2004;25:545-549.

34. Gross SW: Sarcoma of the long bones: Based upon a study of 165 cases. *Am Med Sci NS* 1897;78:17.

35. Cade S: Primary malignant tumors of bone. *Br J Radiol* 1947;20:10.Y

36. Coley WB: The treatment of malignant tumors by repeated inoculations of erysipelas: With a report of ten cases. *Am J Med Sci* 1893;105:487.

37. Sinks LF, Mindell ER: Chemotherapy of osteosarcoma. *Clin Orthop Relat Res* 1975;111:101-104.

38. Jaffe N, Frei E, Traggis D, Bishop Y: Adjuvant methotrexate and citrovorum-factor treatment of osteosarcoma. *N Engl J Med* 1974;291:994-997.

39. Bowden L, Booher RJ: The principles and technique of resection of soft parts for sarcoma. *Surgery* 1958;44:963-977.

40. Enneking WF, Spanier SS, Goodman MA: A system for the surgical staging of musculoskeletal sarcoma. *Clin Orthop Relat Res* 1980;153:106-120.

41. Neel MD, Heck R, Britton L, Daw N, Rao BN: Use of a smooth press-fit stem preserves physeal growth after tumor resection. *Clin Orthop Relat Res* 2004;426:125-128.

42. Fox EJ, Hau MA, Gebhardt MC, Hornicek FJ, Tomford WW, Mankin HJ: Long-term followup of proximal femoral allografts. *Clin Orthop Relat Res* 2002;397:106-113.

43. Broström LA, Harris MA, Simon MA, Cooperman DR, Nilsonne U: The effect of biopsy on survival of patients with osteosarcoma. *J Bone Joint Surg Br* 1979;61:209-212.

44. Enneking WF: Editorial: The issue of the biopsy. *J Bone Joint Surg Am* 1982;64:1119-1120.

45. Mankin HJ, Lange TA, Spanier SS: The hazards of biopsy in patients with malignant primary bone and soft-tissue tumors. *J Bone Joint Surg Am* 1982;64:1121-1127.

46. Mankin HJ, Mankin CJ, Simon MA: The hazards of the biopsy, revisited: Members of the Musculoskeletal Tumor Society. *J Bone Joint Surg Am* 1996;78:656-663.

47.   Springfield DS, Rosenberg A: Biopsy: Complicated and risky. *J Bone Joint Surg Am* 1996;78:639-643.

48.   Skrzynski MC, Biermann S, Montag A, Simon MA: Diagnostic accuracy and charge-savings of outpatient core needle biopsy compared with open biopsy of musculoskeletal tumors. *J Bone Joint Surg Am* 1996;78:644-649.

49.   Dallas Burton Phemister 1882-1951. *J Bone Joint Surg Am* 1952;34:746-747.

50.   Gibney V: *The Hip and its Diseases*. London, England, Bermingham Company, 1884, pp 107-108.

51.   Patzakis MJ, Holtom PD: Editorial comment: Orthopedic infections: Symposium presented by the Musculoskeletal Infection Society. *Clin Orthop Relat Res* 2002;403:2.

52.   Green WT, Anderson M: Epiphyseal arrest for correction of discrepancies in length of the lower extremities. *J Bone Joint Surg Am* 1957;39:853-872.

53.   Phemister DB: Operative arrestment of longitudinal growth of bones in the treatment of deformities. *J Bone Joint Surg Am* 1933;15:1-15.

54.   Blount WP, Clarke GR: Control of bone growth by epiphyseal stapling: A preliminary report. *J Bone Joint Surg Am* 1949;31:464-478.

55.   Codovilla A: On the means of lengthening in the lower limb, the muscles and tissues which are shortened by deformity. *Am J Orthop Surg* 1905;2:353.

56.   Putti V: Operative lengthening of the femur. *Surg Gynecol Obstet* 1934;58:318.

57.   Sofield HA: Limb lengthening. *Surg Clin North Am* 1939;19:69.

58.   Compere EL: Indications for and against the leg-lengthening operation: Use of the tibial bone graft as a factor in preventing delayed union, non-union or late fracture. *J Bone Joint Surg Am* 1936;18:692-705.

59.   Wagner H: Operative lengthening of the femur. *Clin Orthop Relat Res* 1978;136:125-142.

60.   Letts RM, Meadows L: Epiphysiolysis as a method of limb lengthening. *Clin Orthop Relat Res* 1978;133:230-237.

61.   Bjerkreim I: Limb lengthening by physeal distraction. *Acta Orthop Scand* 1989;60:140-142.

62.   Ring PA: Experimental bone lengthening by epiphysial distraction. *Br J Surg* 1958;46:169-173.

63.   Gelbke H: Influence of pressure and tension on growing bone in experiments with animals. *J Bone Joint Surg Am* 1951;33:947-954.

64.   Frierson M, Ibrahim K, Boles M, Bote H, Ganey T: Distraction osteogenesis: A comparison of corticotomy techniques. *Clin Orthop Relat Res* 1994;301:19-24.

65.   Paley D, Maar DC: Ilizarov bone transport treatment for tibial defects. *J Orthop Trauma* 2000;14:76-85.

66.   Paley D: Problems, obstacles, and complications of limb lengthening by the Ilizarov technique. *Clin Orthop Relat Res* 1990;250:81-104.

67.   Faber FW, Keessen W, van Roermund PM: Complications of leg lengthening: 46 procedures in 28 patients. *Acta Orthop Scand* 1991;62:327-332.

68.   Kleinert HE, Kasdan ML, Romero JL: Small blood-vessel anastomosis for salvage of severely injured upper extremity. *J Bone Joint Surg Am* 1963;45:788-796.

69. Malt RA, McKlann CF: Replantation of several arms. *JAMA* 1964;189:716-722.

70. Hall RH: Whole upper extremity transplant for human beings: General plans of procedure and operative technique. *Ann Surg* 1944;120:12.

71. Jacobson JH II, Suarez EL: Microsurgery in anastomosis of small vessels. *Surg Forum* 1960;11:243.

72. Dawodu ST: Spinal cord injury: Definition, epidemiology, pathophysiology. American Spinal Injury Association Standards for Neurological Classification of Spinal Injury Patients, Chicago, IL, American Spinal Injury Association, 1982. Available at: www.emedicine.com/pmr/topic 182.htm.

CHAPTER 9
ORTHOPAEDIC DEVICE MANUFACTURERS

HISTORY

DePuy

The DePuy Manufacturing Company claims the title of "the first commercial orthopaedic manufacturer in the world."[1] Revra DePuy of Warsaw, Indiana, established his company in 1895 to supply physicians with fiber splints for the treatment of fractures. The enterprise prospered, and when DePuy died in 1921, his wife Winifred assumed control.

Although DePuy Manufacturing was successful, she made two important errors while running the company. When J. O. Zimmer, DePuy's first sales representative, hired by Revra in 1905, suggested that the company should expand its line of fracture splints by making new ones out of aluminum, she vetoed the idea. Zimmer then left the company and opened his own orthopaedic supply business, also in Warsaw, in direct competition with his former employer. In 1934, another sales representative at odds with DePuy left the company, again to establish his own business. That representative, J. Dan Richards, set up the Richards Manufacturing Company in Memphis, Tennessee. Although physically removed from Warsaw, it too was in direct competition with DePuy.

After going through a series of owners, DePuy Manufacturing was sold to another Indiana-based company, Biodynamics, in 1968, which sold DePuy to the German firm Boehringer Mannheim in 1974. DePuy remained in Warsaw, although it did relocate its headquarters. In 1968, the new owners of DePuy acquired the marketing rights to the Müller total hip developed by the Swiss surgeon Maurice Müller. The Müller hip had an extremely successful run in the United States in competition with the Charnley prosthesis, but after ten years the focus switched to implant fixation with cementless techniques. DePuy brought its anatomic modular locking (AML) total hip system into the hip prosthesis marketplace in 1979, featuring metal sintered porous-coating technology. Five years later, it introduced the first mobile-bearing total knee prosthesis.

Since the late 1960s, Revra DePuy's company has gone through multiple transformations. In 1968, DePuy purchased Kellogg Industries of Jackson, Michigan. Kellogg, like DePuy, manufactured soft goods, braces, foundations, and splints. DePuy eventually moved this part of its operation to Tracy, California, where it continues its operation under the name DePuy Orthotec.

In 1987, under the ownership of the Boehringer Mannheim Group, DePuy formed the DePuy-DuPont Corporation in a joint venture with

DuPont to manufacture new kinds of polyethylene for prosthetic joint implants. In 1990, it acquired the British firm, Charles F. Thackray Ltd., which had manufactured the Charnley total hip system since 1963; this company was renamed DePuy International. In 1992, still under Boehringer Mannheim, DePuy developed an alliance with Genentech for research into and marketing of biologic products. In the same year, DePuy entered the arthroscopy arena in a complicated arrangement with Extended Optics of Westminster, California. In 1993, still under Boehringer Mannheim, DePuy formed a new company with Biedermann Motech, a German producer of spine products. From 1994 to 1998, DePuy acquired or co-ventured with ACE Medical (trauma products), Orthopaedic Technology Inc. (sports medicine equipment, including arthroscopy), and Landanger-Camus (the largest French manufacturer of hip implants). In 1997, Boehringer Mannheim, which had actually owned DePuy through its Bermuda-based company Corange, Inc. sold Corange to the French firm Roche Inc. for $11 billion. A year later, in 1998, DePuy, now part of Roche, purchased AcroMed, of Cleveland, Ohio, making DePuy the second largest manufacturer of spinal surgery implants and equipment. Later in 1998, Roche sold DePuy to Johnson & Johnson. In 1999, Johnson & Johnson, which owned the Ethicon Corporation, manufacturers of suture material and other surgical equipment, decided to transfer the DePuy Orthotech product line to another Johnson & Johnson subsidiary called Mitek, which was a division of Ethicon. Mitek is a leading manufacturer of arthroscopy equipment and suturing material used in arthroscopic surgery. In 2001, Johnson & Johnson spun off what was left of DePuy Orthotech to DJO Inc. of San Diego, allowing that company to enhance its position as a supplier of braces, splints, and other soft goods that ironically had been Revra DePuy's original product in 1895. In 2003, management decided to drop the name AcroMed from its company name, DePuy AcroMed; it is now known only as DePuy Spine.

Johnson & Johnson

Johnson & Johnson, now the owner of a major supplier of orthopaedic products, has its own interesting history.[2] In 1876, Robert Wood Johnson heard Sir Joseph Lister speak about antiseptic surgery. Lister's methods had gained slow recognition, but by the time Johnson heard Lister's lecture, surgeons in the United States had come to accept his principles. Lister's methods were time-consuming and expensive during surgery, requiring washing the incision with carbolic acid and spraying the air with a continuous carbolic acid mist. Listerism also mandated carbolic-acid–soaked dressings and special tin foil coverings for care of the incision. Johnson had the idea of prepackaging sterile dressings for surgical use, and in partnership with his two brothers he opened a business specializing in surgical dressings. It began with 14 employees on the fourth floor of a former wallpaper factory in New Brunswick, New Jersey, in 1885. Within a few years, Johnson & Johnson was the major supplier of sterile dressings in the United States. The company soon branched out into manufacturing scented talcum powder to soothe the rashes caused by carbolic acid in the sterile dressings. This product morphed into Johnson's Toilet and Baby Powder, hugely successful in the late 1890s and early 1900s. Johnson & Johnson also developed processes to mass-produce sterile dressings with new steam and pressure methods; developed and manufactured adhesive tape; and devised methods for producing, sterilizing, and marketing sterile cat-gut sutures. By the 1920s, Johnson & Johnson developed the Band-Aid, another enormously profitable consumer-oriented product. By then, Johnson & Johnson was an international company well on its way to becoming the behemoth it is today. Upon going public in 1944, Johnson & Johnson developed several consumer products, as well as medical and surgical equipment and well-known medications. In 1977, Johnson & Johnson bought McNeil Pharmaceuticals, manufacturers of Tylenol, another product with very high public recognition. Since then, the company has made several strategic acquisitions, including DePuy in 1998. Johnson & Johnson has also branched out into the managed care market, supplying managerial expertise for hospitals, health maintenance organizations, physician practices, government, and government employees. It is, in fact, involved in every niche of medical care, not only in the United States but internationally; it is a vast, highly successful health care conglomerate.

Zimmer

J. O. Zimmer[3] started his own business with his own money and that supplied by a few friends. He set up shop in the basement of his house, where he developed and manufactured a variety of aluminum splints and other orthopaedic products throughout the 1930s. Surprisingly, his business did not fail during the Depression years, although Zimmer did have to shorten the workweek a few times to avoid layoffs. Zimmer's products during the 1930s and 1940s were mostly splints and braces, as Zimmer had not yet sought a place in the competitive surgical instruments market. Zimmer prospered during the war years, and in 1950 the company decided to manufacture and market the Eicher hip prosthesis. This device consisted of a large femoral head mounted on a fluted intramedullary bar. To achieve any chance of fixation of the implant, surgeons had to select the bar that matched the dimensions of the femoral canal. Reaming techniques in 1950 had not progressed to the point that this could be successfully accomplished on a consistent basis; as a result, the prosthesis too often split the femoral shaft and the design was not successful. In the early 1970s, Zimmer introduced Paul Harrington's spinal instrumentation for the treatment of scoliosis. By 1970, the company reached $27.2 million in annual sales. A year later, Zimmer developed and marketed its own Charnley type of total hip prosthesis, and in 1972 the company sold out to Bristol-Myers, the New York–based pharmaceutical giant. The next year, Zimmer began marketing its own total knee device. Over the ensuing 10 to 12 years, it continued to develop and refine its products in the total joint market. By the mid-1980s, the company had annual sales of $500 million, manufacturing and selling more than 7,000 products. Zimmer and its parent company Bristol-Myers became heavy contributors to research in orthopaedics, donating millions of dollars to the Orthopaedic Research and Education Foundation and making generous grants to other research done under the auspices of subspecialty societies. In 2000, Bristol-Myers divested itself of Zimmer. In 2006, the company's financial statements reported that Zimmer Holdings, Inc, had a market cap of nearly $17 billion.

Richards, Wright, and Smith & Nephew

In 1934, Winifred DePuy, by then running her late husband's company, parted ways with J. Dan Richards, who enjoyed moderate success manufacturing and selling braces and splints in his home city of Memphis, eventually expanded his product line to otology and orthopaedic surgical equipment. His company went through several buyouts, and in 1986 was absorbed into the Smith & Nephew Corporation.

Smith & Nephew has had a long history in medical supplies as well.[4] Thomas James Smith opened a pharmaceutical shop in Hull, England, in 1856. In 1896, Smith's nephew became his partner, naming their business T. J. Smith & Nephew. They expanded their pharmaceutical enterprise into the manufacture and sale of medical dressings, as Joseph Lister's principles of antisepsis and then asepsis were finally adopted almost universally. During World War I, the company greatly expanded its scope, and after the war extended its operations into Canada, South Africa, Australia, and New Zealand. It also began manufacturing elastic adhesive tape (Elastoplast), and developed a line of plaster of Paris bandages (Gypsona). Smith & Nephew then entered the orthopaedic market in many other countries, including Italy, Germany, Spain, and, in 1986, the United States. It entered the American market by purchasing the Richards Manufacturing Company and at the same time Dionics, a manufacturer of arthroscopic surgical equipment. A year after absorbing Richards and Dionics, Smith & Nephew purchased DonJoy, Inc. as well as two French companies that manufactured an array of orthopaedic devices. By 1987, Smith & Nephew (including its new companies) showed a profit of £109.6 million. Additional acquisitions during the 1990s included the Acufex Company. Acufex manufactured arthroscopy-related equipment. In 1999, Smith & Nephew purchased the hip and shoulder implant business of the 3M Corporation and started the development of hyaluronate for joint lubrication. Since the year 2000, Smith & Nephew has entered almost every part of the orthopaedic market through acquisitions and partnering arrangements.

Smith & Nephew is a British company, with headquarters in London. Its American base is Memphis, the home city of J. Dan Richards of the Richards Manufacturing Company.

Stryker

In 1941, Homer Stryker, an orthopaedic surgeon from Kalamazoo, Michigan, and a 1925 graduate of the University of Michigan Medical School, started a company to produce some of his innovations, such as, a rubber heel to incorporate into a leg cast so that a patient could walk on the cast without breaking it apart.[5] Stryker (Figure 50) also developed the Stryker frame to turn patients face up or face down without difficulty. Although these two straightforward inventions were not high-tech, they were very useful and could be found in almost every orthopaedic practice. In 1947, Stryker patented the Stryker saw. Its blade oscillated instead of rotating, making it possible for orthopaedic surgeons to remove a cast without cutting the patient's skin. Before this invention, removing a cast required using long-handled cast-cutters that often did cut the patient's skin. The company sold thousands of Stryker saws, and they became a standard fixture in virtually every orthopaedic surgeon's office and hospital in the country.

In 1979, Stryker acquired the Osteonics Corporation, entering into the manufacture and sale of hip and knee replacements and other orthopaedic implants. The company has made multiple other strategic acquisitions: Syn-Optics (arthroscopy equipment) in 1976; Dinsao SA (spinal fixation products) in 1992; Osteo AG (trauma) in 1996; and in 1998, Howmedica, a large manufacturer of orthopaedic equipment products. The next year, Stryker sales reached $2.1 billion. In 2002, Stryker acquired Surgical Dynamics and in 2004 it bought Spine Care, a manufacturer of artificial disks. In 2004, sales reached $4.3 billion. Although the company headquarters are still in Kalamazoo, Stryker has divisional centers in various locations in the United States and around the world. Stryker Orthopaedics is located in Mahwah, New Jersey, not far from Rutherford, New Jersey, the former corporate headquarters of Howmedica.

Howmedica's corporate lineage originated in the Austenal Corporation, which Reiner Erdle and Charles Prange founded in 1983. Erdle and Prange attempted to make corrosion-resistant dentures with austenitic stainless steels. In their work with various alloys, they came upon one that combined cobalt, chromium, and molybdenum. It showed virtually no deterioration in dental use. They named the new alloy Vitallium. The Austenal Corporation sold out to the Howe Sound Company in 1958, and the name was changed to HowMet in 1964. In 1969, it was changed to Howmedica. In 1972, Howmedica was acquired by Pfizer and was sold to Stryker in 1998.[5]

Biomet

DePuy and Smith & Nephew date back to the 19th century. Biomet, founded in 1977, is at this writing the newest arrival in the competitive orthopaedic marketplace. Four entrepreneurial bioengineers—Dane Miller, Niles Noblitt, Jerry Ferguson, and Ray Harroff—left Zimmer to found Biomet.[6] They perceived that joint arthroplasties, dramatic changes in fracture management, arthroscopy, and other unforeseen changes in orthopaedics might create vast new opportunities. Biomet absorbed another older company, Orthopaedic Equipment Company (OEC) in 1984, and then Electro-Biology, Inc (EBI), a supplier of electrical stimulating equipment. In 1990, Biomet acquired Arrow Surgical Technologies and merged it into its Arthrotek division to enhance their capabilities in the arthroscopy arena. With several other strategic acquisitions, it is now a strong player in the orthopaedic market, with annual sales exceeding $1.6 billion. The original founders are still involved in the Warsaw, Indiana-based company 30 years later. Biomet is one of the few companies created specifically for the orthopaedic market in the late 20th century.[6]

Medtronic

Medtronic, on the other hand, started out very modestly as a part-time, two-person business that fixed broken electrical equipment in Minneapolis hospitals. The founders were Earl E. Bakken and Palmer J. Hermundslie.[7] Earl was a graduate student in electrical engineering at the University of Minnesota in 1949. His wife, who worked as a medical technologist in a local hospital, occasionally asked him to repair electronic hospital equipment. Earl was good at it, and soon it became a nearly full-time job. Earl's brother-in-law, Palmer, saw an opportunity in Earl's engineering skills, forming a medical equipment repair company with him that they called Medtronic. They started out using secondhand benches and equipment in a garage heated in the winter with pot-bellied stoves. After a slow start, they began to prosper, and began to manufacture custom-made electronic devices to clients' specifications. In the mid-1950s, Walton Lillehei began his groundbreaking work on cardiac pacemakers. He asked Bakken and Hermundslie to help him in the design and manufacture of these devices. By then they had enlarged their working facilities and hired engineers and technicians so that they were well positioned to participate in the explosion of the pacemaker market. They progressed through the evolution of external pacemakers to implantable pacemakers, obtaining exclusive rights to manufacture and distribute them as well as other heart-monitoring equipment. Throughout the 1980s, Medtronic expanded its business and core product line with multiple purchases, including the Johnson & Johnson cardiovascular division, and aggressively pursued foreign markets. By the 1990s, their scientists and engineers developed implantable stimulation devices for control of chronic pain and motion disorders such as Parkinson's disease. Through the acquisition of "market-leading companies" they expanded into ear, nose, and throat surgery, peripheral vascular surgery, and spinal and orthopaedic surgery.[7] The orthopaedic and spine venture required the takeover of the Sofamor-Danek Company, created quite recently through the merger of two French companies, Sofamor and Danek. Medtronic Sofamor-Danek has become an aggressive participant in the spine surgery market in a short period of time. The company intends to maintain the small-business image of its entrepreneurial founders: Earl with screwdriver in hand, tending to electrical problems in local operating rooms, and Palmer flying his small-engine airplane to make emergency deliveries of the company's pacemakers. In reality, Medtronic now operates in 120 countries and employs 33,000 people worldwide.

The Wright Medical Group

In 1895, when the DePuys started their orthopaedic business in Warsaw, Indiana, they could not have imagined the generation of so many competing enterprises out of their company. Zimmer, Richards, and Smith & Nephew all began because of the DePuys, and indirectly so did the Wright Medical Group. In 1944, ten years after Dan Richards set up shop for himself in Memphis, he hired Frank Wright as his Memphis-area sales representative. Six years later, Wright pulled out of the Richards Manufacturing Company and started the Wright Manufacturing Company, also in the Memphis area, specializing in orthopaedic products. Twenty-seven years later, Wright Manufacturing was sold to Dow Corning, which then became Dow Corning Wright. Since then, the company has gone through several other buyouts by private investors, most recently the Warburg Pincus Equity Partners (a New York investment firm). In the past several years, Wright has invested in the development of ceramic-on-ceramic total joints, small-joint silicone implants, and synthetic and human tissue–based materials. The ceramic-on-ceramic hip system recently went through an investigational device exemption study to determine the safety and effectiveness of this technology in total hip replacement.[8]

Manufacturing Orthopaedic Implants

The manufacturers of orthopaedic implants employ the time-honored processes of casting, forging, machining, and finishing. The basic technique for production of femoral head prostheses, for example, includes the lost-wax method of casting, in which workers fill a mold of the femoral head with hot wax. After the wax hardens, workers remove the mold and encase the wax model of the prosthetic femoral head in plaster. Running trays of the plaster casts through a kiln melts the wax, which runs out of the cast, while in an adjacent area other workers prepare ingots of cobalt-chromium alloy. They melt the alloy in an electric furnace and pour it into the casts. After the alloy cools and hardens, they break off the casting material, leaving the rough, unfinished component. The unfinished prosthesis is then taken through the finishing and polishing processes, performed by hand or robotically. Company inspectors then examine the components and x-ray the product before it proceeds through packaging and sterilization.

Manufacturers also use forges to create some prosthetic implants and most surgical instruments and fracture plates. In the forging process, metal is heated, pounded, hammered, or stamped into the desired configuration. Many implants also require milling, turning, and drilling to make them usable. Once the implants pass the final inspection, packaging and sterilization follow.

Descriptions of the processes do not convey the visual image of a vast 11,000-square-foot factory floor populated by hundreds of employees engaged in the production of thousands of beautiful, gleaming implants and instruments. The organization of large numbers of employees with varying skills and backgrounds requires tremendous engineering and administrative expertise.

Companies must continuously adapt to changing circumstances, new ideas, and the demand for new products. As a result, all of the successful companies have large research and development departments in which engineers, chemists, and orthopaedic surgeons work on improving existing products and search for new ones. Although the profession and its suppliers can claim many innovative solutions, they have also encountered several dead ends. For example, the search for a better polyethylene resulted in the development of a carbon fiber–polyethylene composite. This product had poor wear characteristics, however, and was discontinued.

Manufacturers continue to seek new alloys as they relate to component strength and bearing characteristics, new porous ingrowth technologies, new coatings for the implants to increase the strength of fixation, and navigation systems to facilitate minimally invasive surgical procedures. Manufacturers must anticipate their customers' changing needs to remain competitive, yet remain in compliance with federal requirements.

The U.S. Food and Drug Administration

The Federal Food and Drug Bureau originated in a small office within the Department of Agriculture in 1862.[9] It began with a single chemist who investigated the adulteration and mislabeling of foods and drugs. The department hired additional personnel over the next several years and created first the Division of Chemistry and then, as that grew larger, the Bureau of Chemistry. In 1883, Harvey W. Wiley assumed the position of Chief Chemist in the bureau, which grew rapidly in size and importance under his watch. Unscrupulous purveyors of adulterated foods and drugs kept the bureau very busy. It had no real regulatory or enforcement powers, however, and abuses continued despite the efforts of Wiley and his staff. Gradually, public outrage, fanned by such authors as Upton Sinclair in his book *The Jungle* (an exposé of the meat-packing industry in Chicago), caught the attention of Congress, which considered new laws to better protect the public at the end of the 19th century. Photographs of Wiley during those years reveal him to be a tall, solemn, and impressive gentleman, and he apparently was a formidable opponent to those intent on misleading the public. Wiley enjoyed considerable support in his crusade from important allies such as the American Medical Association, the National Organization of Women's Clubs, pharmacists' organizations, and others. In 1906, at the height of the Progressive movement, Congress passed the Food and Drugs Act, also known as the "Wiley Act." It empowered the Bureau of Chemistry to identify and seize questionable food and drug products and to prosecute the parties responsible. The 1906 law did not require pre-market approval of drugs and only gave the bureau the power to enforce honest labeling; absence of adulterants; and requirements related to purity, cleanliness, and full measure. It also mandated that the label of a food or drug product should disclose the presence and amounts of any dangerous substances such as alcohol, cocaine, or heroin.

Enforcement of the Wiley Act created confusion and multiple lawsuits, which resulted in new laws that tried to establish less vague standards for foods and drugs. Congress created new agencies that lessened Wiley's authority, and when the Supreme Court ruled that his bureau did not have authority over false therapeutic claims for drugs, he resigned.

This weakness in the law caused several well-publicized disasters. After the Curies discovered radium, several companies included it in their elixirs and tonics, claiming that radium was curative for several illnesses. Deaths from radiation ensued in people who believed the claims and bought the products. In addition, women using cosmetics containing corrosive substances lost their eyesight, and in the 1930s a company manufacturing and selling sulfanilamide contaminated their product with antifreeze. One hundred people, mostly children, died. As a result of these and other events, in 1938 Congress passed a new Food, Drug, and Cosmetic Act. The new law gave the bureau, now named the Food and Drug Administration (FDA), control over new drug products and medical devices. It mandated that the FDA subject them to pre-market approval and thus declared that false drug claims would henceforth be illegal.

Nevertheless, the new laws did not prevent additional drug-related tragedies such as the thalidomide event, in which women taking the drug for morning sickness in the first trimester of pregnancy had babies with phocomelia. This episode led to more stringent laws and eventually the establishment of a new agency, the Drug Enforcement Administration (DEA), in 1968.

The passage of these laws did not affect orthopaedic surgeons at first, as they did not prescribe drugs to the extent that internists and other physicians did. More important, the explosion in orthopaedic technology had not yet materialized. The FDA did have authority over medical devices, but orthopaedic surgeons in 1968 had not yet begun to use them extensively. In 1976, the Dalkon Shield episode caused Congress to revisit the FDA laws. The Dalkon Shield, an intrauterine contraceptive device, had a design flaw that caused severe, and in some cases fatal, pelvic infections. These cases received a great deal of publicity in the media and caused legislators to tighten their control over all medical devices, including those used by orthopaedic surgeons. The legislation created three classes of devices. Class I devices are subject to general control, such as registration and listing with the FDA and labeling in accordance with regulations. Class II devices are subject to these requirements plus special labeling and surveillance of performance. Class III devices receive the most scrutiny. The marketing of a class II device requires a 510(k) application, which means that the FDA would consider it to be essentially equivalent to one sold before the 1976 legislation. A class III device requires an investigational device exemption, which means that it undergoes evaluation of its efficacy and safety, usually under the auspices of an investigational review board (IRB) established locally as a "committee for the protection of human subjects." The FDA maintains very tight control over the testing of medical devices, and Congress empowered it to prosecute individuals and corporations that knowingly or inadvertently do not comply with its regulations. They risk severe civil penalties and fines that may exceed $1 million.

The FDA has had a demonstrable impact on orthopaedic surgeons and their partners in industry. An earlier chapter, for example, described the FDA's action in delaying approval of methylmethacrylate for fixation of total hip implants in the early 1970s. Orthopaedic surgeons who used PMMA for that purpose before 1971 could continue to do so, but other orthopaedic surgeons were not permitted to use it for several years. The FDA's action in this episode resulted in imbalances in providing care for patients with advanced arthritis of the hip.

The pedicle screw situation was also mentioned in an earlier chapter. Orthopaedic surgeons had used screws to secure plates to bone for many decades, and in fact used screws in spine surgery well before the 1976 device-class legislation became law. The FDA's decision to prohibit pedicle screws for use in spinal fusions resulted in the filing of several thousand lawsuits and the expenditure of millions of dollars in costs for the defendants in these actions, the overwhelming majority of which were subsequently dropped.

Orthopaedics, Industry, and the Anti-Kickback Laws

During the Great Depression of the 1930s, Congress passed laws prohibiting kickbacks. Workers in the steel and construction industries had won major concessions from employers with the passage of much of President Roosevelt's New Deal legislation. The prevailing wage laws, for example, required employers to pay a wage dictated by a federal commission. Employers, often cash-strapped themselves, tried to find ways around this mandate. By the mid-1930s, some employers hit upon the idea of forcing workers to pay for their jobs by taking deductions from the worker's salary. The workers therefore had to "kick back" a stated sum to remain employed. To counter this practice, Congress passed the "Anti-Kickback Law," with penalties up to $5,000 and imprisonment for up to 5 years if convicted of engaging in this practice. The government enforced this law aggressively, and in May 1935 convicted 12 contractors for violating it. In the 1950s, Congress reinforced this law with new legislation under the Davis-Bacon and Copeland anti-kickback laws.[10]

More recently, anti-kickback laws have been applied to physicians. These laws state that it is illegal to offer "something of value" for referral of a patient. These rules differ from the "Stark Amendments," named after Congressman Fortney "Pete" Stark (D-CA). Those amendments to the Medicare laws were designed to prevent referrals by physicians to entities in which the physician had a financial interest. Anti-kickback statutes also differ from "false claims," which were meant to deal with issues such as unbundling, upcoding, and billing for medical services provided by another individual such as an intern, resident, fellow, nurse, or professional assistant. The false claims acts were intended to prevent fraudulent billing.[11]

Anti-kickback laws codify what physicians in the past have referred to as "fee splitting." Doctors have always regarded this activity as unethical, and the early American Medical Association Code of Medical Ethics condemned it. Kickbacks have become more difficult to define, as relationships between fellow physicians as well as between physicians and corporate entities are now considerably more complex.[12] A salesman's gift of a pen or reflex hammer may be regarded as such. The value of the salesperson's gifts, however, can escalate quickly to lunch, then dinner, then a weekend at a resort, ostensibly to learn about the salesman's products.[13] If the orthopaedic surgeon accepts any of these gifts in return for using the salesman's products, one might have to conclude that such activity violates the anti-kickback violations.

On the other hand, the sales representative has an important place in an orthopaedic surgeon's practice. The sales representative makes it possible for the surgeon to handle instruments, prostheses, and other devices, and provides education and training in their use. This might include a session over a meal or even a weekend retreat to discuss surgical procedures and equipment, perhaps featuring the inventor of the operation or prosthesis.

The relationship between an orthopaedist and industry becomes more complex when the orthopaedist goes beyond merely using the company's equipment and starts improving upon it. This may progress to complete revision of a company's product line or even to the invention of a whole new concept for treatment of a musculoskeletal disorder. Orthopaedics has progressed remarkably during the past 50 years because of the inventions and innovations of its practitioners, and industry has been an essential partner in this revolution in orthopaedic care. Inventive surgeons require the support of industry, which provides technicians, engineers, joiners, turners, a sales force, managers, and others to develop their ideas into reality.[14,15]

Many concerns arise over the relationship between orthopaedic inventors and their industrial partners. These include such issues as patents and royalties, how the new product will be brought to the marketplace, and how it will be demonstrated to potential users. Because most new techniques and devices first reach the market through presentations at scientific meetings, inventors must guard against bias or an inclination to present the invention in the best possible light. Once the product reaches the market, inventors must also guard against a conflict of interest, that is, they should not use their inventions (from which they receive royalties) when another device or technique might better serve the patient's interests. The innovator/inventor therefore must make full disclosure of a possible bias or conflict of interest in presentations, product discussions, and to patients scheduled for treatment with that product.

References

1.   http://www.depuy.com/home.jhtml. (Accessed April 9, 2007)

2.   http://www.jnj.com/home.htm. (Accessed April 9, 2007)

3.   http://www.zimmer.com. (Accessed April 9, 2007)

4.   http://www.smith-nephew.com. (Accessed April 9, 2007)

5. http://www.stryker.com. (Accessed April 9, 2007)

6. http://www.biomet.com. (Accessed April 9, 2007)

7. http://www.medtronic.com. (Accessed April 9, 2007)

8. http://www.wmt.com. (Accessed April 9, 2007)

9. http://www.fda.gov. (Accessed April 9, 2007)

10. http://oig.hhs.gov/fraud/docs/safeharborregulations/safefs.htm. (Accessed April 9, 2007)

11. Spivack P: Understanding the anti-kickback statute. *Orthop Today* 1999;19:50-54.

12. Orlowski JP, Wateska L: The effects of pharmaceutical firms enticements on physician prescribing patterns: There's no such thing as a free lunch. *Chest* 1992;102:270-273.

13. Stryer D, Bero LA: Characteristics of materials distributed by drug companies: An evaluation of appropriateness. *J Gen Intern Med* 1996;11:575-583.

14. Wilkes MS, Doblin BH, Shapiro MF: Pharmaceutical advertisements in leading medical journals: Experts' assessments. *Ann Intern Med* 1992;116:912-919.

15. Wenger NS, Lieberman JR: The orthopaedic surgeon and industry: Ethics and industry incentives. *Clin Orthop Relat Res* 2000;378:39-43.

CHAPTER 10

EDUCATION AND RESEARCH IN ORTHOPAEDICS

Education

Orthopaedic training during the late 19th century was obtained mostly in a preceptorship. The few individuals interested in orthopaedics at that time usually signed on as assistants to established orthopaedists, who mentored them with no specific curriculum or plan. The pool of candidates for such positions varied considerably because standards for enrollment at medical schools were haphazard at that time and curricula were essentially unregulated. Furthermore, the public during most of the 19th century had not worried much about the state of medical education because it expected relatively little from physicians. But eventually, as science became more a part of medicine, physicians educated themselves and their patients regarding the advancements of Pasteur, Koch, Virchow, Bernard, Lister, and others. This changed the expectations of the lay public. In the late 1890s, several states passed laws establishing state boards of medical examiners (New York was the first in 1890), and influential people began to consider rectifying the perilous state of the educational system for physicians. At that time, there were too many doctors, most of whom had no real education in medicine, and far too many medical schools, most of which were merely diploma mills.

Toward the end of the 19th century, a wealthy benefactor named Johns Hopkins donated money to establish a university in Baltimore for the purpose of supporting a model medical college. Daniel Coit Gilman, the first president of the college, recruited the most outstanding physicians available to staff the new medical school. He set up William Welch[1,2] (the pathologist) as dean (Figure 51), William Osler as chairman of medicine, William Halsted as head of surgery, and Howard Kelly as head of obstetrics and gynecology. They were not only physicians, but also men of science, and subsequently they had a profound effect on medical education in the United States.

To improve the level of medical education, Hopkins, Welch, Gilman, and the others would have to effect the shutdown of the diploma mills. They had powerful allies to accomplish this objective, such as Andrew Carnegie and the American Medical Association (AMA) Council on Medical Education, among many others. However, they needed someone to observe medical schools nationwide and report on how poor the medical instruction was. They found their man in Abraham Flexner (Figure 52).[3,4]

Flexner began his famous tour of American medical schools in January 1909. The Carnegie Foundation for the Advancement of Teaching retained him to survey all of the medical schools' facilities, faculties, students, and administrations. Andrew Carnegie generously funded the foundation in response to a scathing report on medical education prepared by the AMA Council on Medical Education. Henry Pritchett, president of the Massachusetts Institute of Technology, read the report and discussed it with members of the AMA council. Pritchett's friendship with Carnegie enabled him to enlist Carnegie's help in funding the survey. Pritchett was also responsible for selecting the surveyor, and chose Flexner.

Flexner was a young professional educator known for enforcing high standards in the classroom. Once he flunked an entire class. As a non-physician, he could be objective and disinterested. Flexner probably became known to Pritchett through William Welch, the dean of the new Johns Hopkins Medical School. One of Welch's protégés there was Abraham Flexner's brother, Simon Flexner, a physician who had so impressed Welch that he had Simon appointed head of the newly organized Rockefeller Institute in New York. Abraham Flexner had in fact attended Johns Hopkins University as an undergraduate. He knew about the pathologist William Welch, who was probably the most influential physician in America. Welch agreed to spend time with Abraham Flexner before the survey and to explain what he should be looking for. Welch apparently dazzled Flexner. Flexner recalled in one of his two autobiographies: "The one bright spot was the Johns Hopkins at Baltimore. It possessed ideals and men who embodied them."[4]

Flexner went on a whirlwind tour, spending an average of an hour and a half at each school. His itinerary[4] reveals that he visited schools from November 4 to November 20, 1909, in Des Moines, Sioux City, Omaha, Kansas City, Lawrence (Kansas), St. Louis, northern Oklahoma, Oklahoma City, Dallas, Little Rock, Memphis, Vicksburg, Nashville, and Louisville. It took him 18 months by train to visit 155 medical schools around the country, but he spent most of his time in the Berkshires of western Massachusetts writing his lengthy Bulletin Number Four to the Carnegie Foundation.[5] This report was then made public in 1910, and according to Flexner: "Schools collapsed to the right and left, usually without a murmur. A number of them pooled their resources. The 15 schools in Chicago, which I had called 'the plague spot of the country' in respect to medical education, were shortly consolidated into three." Flexner's report was acerbic and sarcastic, which makes for very entertaining reading to this day. It was sensational and widely distributed and brought about the change in medical education that Welch, Andrew Carnegie, Pritchett, and the AMA Council on Medical Education desired. Flexner's report also made him famous. Later in life, he became the first head of the Institute for Advanced Research at Princeton. In that position, he successfully recruited Albert Einstein to join the institute and work there for the rest of his life.

As a result of Flexner's report, the AMA Council on Medical Education assumed considerable responsibility in guiding the accreditation process for existing and new medical schools. All modern American medical colleges now obtain their accreditation from the Liaison Committee on Medical Education (LCME), which is jointly sponsored by the American Association of Medical Colleges (AAMC) and the Council on Medical Education of the AMA. The U.S. Department of Education under the Higher Education Act of 1965 uses the accreditation of the LCME as the national standard for funding of medical student education, research, and patient care. The AAMC was founded in 1876 to work for reform in medical education. Apparently its early meetings were fractious, and some predicted it would not only fail in this mission but would cease to exist. The AAMC subsequently joined the AMA Council on Medical Education in forming the LCME, a relationship finalized in 1942. The AAMC currently operates the American Medical College application services, the National Resident Matching Service, and the Medical College Aptitude Tests (MCATs).

Upon graduation from an LCME-accredited medical college, a prospective orthopaedist must apply for an orthopaedic residency in a program accredited by the Accreditation Council of Graduate Medical Education (ACGME). In 1981, the ACGME replaced the LCGME (Liaison Committee for Graduate Medical Education), which was founded in 1972, to operate independently of the LCME. The ACGME's member organizations are the American Board of Medical Specialties (ABMS), the American Hospital Association, the AMA, the AAMC, and the Council of Medical Specialty Societies. Its purpose is to evaluate postgraduate programs such as residencies in orthopaedics and to accredit programs that meet predetermined standards. The ACGME appoints residency review committees responsible for establishing the standards and conducting the site visits that determine the status of a program.

An individual who successfully completes an accredited orthopaedic educational program becomes eligible to take the examination offered by the ABMS. The American Board of Orthopaedic Surgery (ABOS) is one of 24 medical specialty boards that compose the ABMS. The ABOS is the organization designated to administer the examination for certification, allowing orthopaedists to become board-certified in orthopaedics and diplomates of the ABOS. The ABOS comprises members nominated by the American Academy of Orthopaedic Surgeons (AAOS), the American Orthopaedic Association (AOA), and the AMA, and was established in the early 1930s at about the same time that the AAOS was established.

Melvin Henderson was the first president of the ABOS (Figure 53). In 1935, at his request, *The Journal of Bone and Joint Surgery* published a two-and-a-half-page statement about the ABOS.[6] Under general information, the statement notes: "The growth of specialism . . . has been accompanied by an insidious trend toward lower standards of qualification . . . Men with inadequate training and experience assume the title of specialist and by so doing degrade others who may be unusually well equipped to practice in a restricted field of medicine." This statement also pointed out that specialties in medicine should establish boards before the state licensing boards do, noting that ophthalmology, otolaryngology, obstetrics, gynecology, dermatology, pediatrics, radiology, and other specialties had already organized boards in their individual disciplines. To unify this effort, the AMA Council on Medical Education helped form the Association of

Examining Boards. Because three organizations—the AAOS, the AMA, and the AOA—had participated in the development of the ABOS, each group would appoint three members to the orthopaedic board. The ABOS was incorporated under the laws of Delaware in 1935. Henderson's 1935 statement declared that the existence of the boards was "to serve the public, physicians, hospitals, and medical schools by publishing lists of those who received a certificate of the board and thus assist in protecting the public against irresponsible and unqualified practitioners who profess to specialize in orthopaedic surgery."

Candidates for the board examination in 1935 needed recommendations from two orthopaedic surgeons "acceptable to the board." Applicants also had to document membership in the AMA and prove that training requirements were completed. An applicant's training included a one-year internship, two years of concentrated instruction in orthopaedic surgery "acceptable to the board," and two years of practice limited to orthopaedics. Because the board had just been established, however, the statement also contained notification that the board could waive any of these qualifications. An applicant had to pay a fee of $25 to cover the expenses of the board members (who served without compensation), but if "unable to meet the requirements of the board after three appearances before it, he would get half of the money back."

Besides Henderson, the other original members of the ABOS were Edwin Ryerson (Chicago), Henry Meyerding (Rochester, Minnesota), Fremont Chandler (New York), Samuel Kleinberg (New York), Philip Lewin (Chicago), W. Barnett Owen (Louisville), John C. Wilson (Los Angeles), and Hulett Wyckoff (Seattle). In 1935, the members of the ABOS did not specify how they would evaluate candidates for orthopaedic certification. In 1936, the board certified 84 candidates but reported that 10 percent had failed to meet the requirements. There was no mention in the announcement that an examination was offered. In contrast, the 2006 statement notes that board certification means qualifying to take the examination by satisfactory completion of 60 months of training in an approved orthopaedic residency, passing a 7-hour examination of 300 questions, practicing for up to 5 years, and then passing an oral examination based on the candidate's practice. Having run that gauntlet successfully, individuals can then consider themselves board-certified for ten years.

For many years, the ABOS certification was considered lifelong, but in 1985 the board determined that it should be time-limited, and effective immediately diplomates would be required to take a second examination to maintain ABOS certification. This decision was hotly contested by many orthopaedists, although those who were board-certified before that time were grandfathered and did not have to take another examination. Furthermore, candidates for recertification were given options to take a specialized examination, considering the fact that orthopaedics had evolved into many subspecialties.

The education of an orthopaedic surgeon in the United States now consumes more than 22 years of that individual's life. From grade school through high school takes 12 years, at which point the would-be orthopaedist spends 4 years of college earning a bachelor's degree, a year of internship, 4 years of residency, and for most practitioners at least 1 year of additional fellowship training. Entering medicine as a profession in the first place is highly competitive and securing a position as an orthopaedic resident is at this time even more so. The whole process is standardized and highly regulated, in sharp contrast to the chaos that characterized medical and orthopaedic education in 1910 when Flexner made his final report in Bulletin Number Four.

At this time, there are 149 orthopaedic residencies and the majority of these residencies have departmental status in medical schools and hospitals, but some are still divisions of surgery, an issue that remains a concern to department chairmen and program directors who seek greater independence and self-sufficiency within the academic framework of orthopaedic education. The orthopaedic residency program at the University of Pennsylvania lays claim to being the first and its academic orthopaedic department the longest in continuous operation.[7] Lewis A. Sayre organized the first orthopaedic department in America at the Bellevue Medical College in 1861, but that school has long since been absorbed into the New York University College of Medicine, and Sayre's program per se no longer exists.

Today, orthopaedic surgeons fully certified by the ABOS must document the fact that they continuously fulfill the requirements of continuing medical education as defined by the Accreditation Council on Continuing Medical Education (ACCME). This organization has seven members, one representative from each of the following organizations: the ABMS, the American Hospital Association, the AMA, the Association for Hospital Medical Education, the AAMC, the Council of Medical Specialty Societies, and the Federation of State Medical Boards. The federal government is also involved in the ACCME; the Secretary of the Department of Health and Human Services appoints a member of the board of directors. The ACCME is the agency that accredits institutions and organizations as official providers of continuing education, including state medical societies and the AAOS. Accredited entities must keep standards set by the ACCME, and because many state licensing boards and hospital membership committees require documentation of at least 50 hours of continuing medical education annually, physicians trying to comply with these requirements prefer to take courses offered by accredited providers. There is no shortage of accredited courses, and orthopaedic surgeons can obtain the necessary hours at accredited events presented by almost any accredited entity. Continuing medical education, however, does take time and is expensive, not only in terms of course fees, but in terms of lost income during the time away from practice.

Journals and Books

Journals
The Journal of Bone and Joint Surgery, American volume has been an integral part of the history of orthopaedics, and its early history sheds light on the origins of orthopaedics in America. The publication began as the

Transactions of the American Orthopaedic Association in 1887; in 1903, the association decided to turn the *Transactions* into *The American Journal of Orthopaedic Surgery*. The name was changed in 1918 to the *Journal of Orthopaedic Surgery* at the founding of the British Orthopaedic Association just after World War I; the members of the AOA believed it was appropriate to drop the designation "American" out of courtesy to their British colleagues. In 1922, the publication took its current name, *The Journal of Bone and Joint Surgery*.

Initially, the journal was run by an editorial committee, but in 1916 the AOA turned the responsibility over to a single individual, Mark Rogers of Boston. Rogers held the position of editor until 1919. H. Winnett Orr of Lincoln, Nebraska, succeeded Rogers in 1919, moving the journal from Boston to Lincoln. Jonathan Cohen, deputy editor emeritus, and James Heckman, the current editor-in-chief, wrote an essay on the history of *The Journal of Bone and Joint Surgery* in 2003 to mark the centennial of the *JBJS*. Regarding Orr's term in office, they stated this: "During Orr's tenure he wrote and published one article about his famous regimen for the treatment of infected bone resulting from war injuries. He did not introduce much to the journal in the way of innovative content, format, or processing."

After Orr stepped down in 1921, *JBJS* was promptly brought back to Boston and turned over to Elliott Brackett, "the first true editor in the modern sense." Brackett's editorship coincided with the increase in the number of orthopaedic surgeons in the United States after World War I. Readership expanded exponentially from 797 subscribers in 1921 to 3,300 in 1942 when Brackett retired. The AAOS was founded in 1933, and by 1945 the Academy became the cosponsor of the journal with the AOA. *JBJS* was still owned by the AOA, however, and the Academy's contribution of funds varied considerably from year to year. As a result, the journal's finances were precarious; its survival appears to have depended on the selfless dedication of Brackett during those years. The Academy attempted to fund the publication in several ways, such as establishing a requirement that all members had to subscribe or forfeit membership in the Academy, and it offered to pay for the journal pages devoted to AAOS transactions or announcements. Despite these and other measures, the journal continued to lose money. Brackett, who also maintained an active orthopaedic practice during his editorial tenure, found the combination too taxing. He resigned in 1942, after 21 years at the post. Murray Danforth was appointed editor in 1942 but died a few months later, and was replaced by Charles Painter, who served as acting editor until William A. Rogers took over in 1944. Dr. Rogers had an engineering background, and brought an appreciation of the hard sciences to the editorship. The finances of *JBJS* remained problematic, however. The AOA membership continued to express concern regarding the drain on its treasury because the organization still wholly owned the journal, although it shared some of the control with the AAOS. Finally, in 1953, the AOA relinquished ownership to an independent, nonprofit corporation in "joint direction" with the Academy. The new corporation would have a six-member board of trustees, three appointed by the AOA and three by the AAOS. The six trustees would elect the editor, who would be the seventh member ex officio. Rogers remained editor of the journal until 1958, succeeded by Thornton Brown. Brown remained editor until 1978. During Brown's tenure, orthopaedic surgery in the United States changed completely; as the editor of the journal of record for orthopaedics, he guided the changes to a large extent. As he relinquished his position in 1978, he said: "In recent years the orthopaedic literature has entered a period of rapid growth. There has been tremendous growth of the specialty of orthopaedic surgery, the development of the subspecialties, the accelerating rate of the advancement of knowledge, the broadening scope of orthopaedic research . . . the global extent of information exchange." In Cohen's and Heckman's centennial history of the journal, they commended Brown's performance: "The previous editor contributed so much to the establishment of the *JBJS* as the outstanding, internationally recognized organ of orthopaedic surgery."

Cohen and Heckman regarded the period following Brown's tenure as "the modern era" for *JBJS*, including the editorial leadership of Paul Curtiss, Jr, Henry Cowell, and James Heckman. During the nearly 30 years since Thornton Brown stepped down, Curtiss, Cowell, and Heckman have presided over all of the literature reporting new developments. The editors have attempted to control the editorial process by relying on peer review of submissions. The submitted papers are read by the editorial board or consultant reviewers, and the papers are graded. Those with the highest grades are published. Since the reviewers of the papers are not given the names of the authors, the process is as fair as it can be.

JBJS has become extremely successful because of the orthopaedic revolution; it is a benefit of membership for all active Fellows of the American Academy of Orthopaedic Surgeons, and attracts paying subscribers and large numbers of advertisers. Nevertheless, *The Journal of Bone and Joint Surgery* is only one journal and cannot publish all of the papers it receives. Furthermore, it is a general publication that accepts and publishes papers on a variety of subjects. These limitations have led to the growth of numerous other journals in orthopaedics, of both general and specialized interest.

In 1947, some orthopaedic surgeons wanted to increase the opportunities for getting their papers published.[8] They believed that *JBJS*, the only orthopaedic publication at that time, received too many worthy submissions to publish all of them, and "found it frustrating" that it was the only American orthopaedic journal available for publishing their papers. Many of these individuals also noted that there were only three "organized orthopaedic organizations." Thus, Earl McBride of Oklahoma City and others believed that another organization was needed "to hold small, intimate meetings to exchange professional ideas." McBride, with Garrett Pipkin, Duncan McKeever, Judson Wilson, Fritz Teal, Louis Breck, Henry L. Green, Howard Shorbe, Theodore Vinke, Paul Williams, Eugene Secord, and Frank Hand, met in 1949 at the annual AAOS convention to form the Association of Bone and Joint Surgeons (ABJS).[8]

A group photograph from the first meeting of the ABJS shows the 12 founders. The photo's caption states that the first meeting was in Oklahoma City (notably distant from Boston or New York), and McBride is wearing scrubs and rubber gloves, apparently having just left the operating room. "The idea for a journal was conceived at the inception of the organization,"[8] and at the association's second meeting in Lincoln, Nebraska, the group voted to create one. McBride was sent to Boston to confer with William Rogers, the editor of the well-established *JBJS*, and according to the history of the ABJS written by Robert Derkash,[8] McBride "sat in the office of Dr. Rogers until Dr. Rogers gave his approval to establish another English-language journal of orthopaedic surgery." Two years later, McBride and Anthony DePalma of Philadelphia negotiated a contract with the medical publisher J. B. Lippincott; the ABJS would own the title of the journal, which the association named *Clinical Orthopaedics*, while Lippincott would own the copyright. Dr. DePalma was named the first editor-in-chief and the first issue of *Clinical Orthopaedics* was published the next year, in 1953. Lippincott and the ABJS planned at first to offer one issue annually, but so many papers were submitted that this number was promptly increased. The journal had a symposium format, concentrating on a single subject in each issue. Publishing clusters of papers on topics such as children's orthopaedics in the first volume turned out to be popular for both readers and authors, propelling *Clinical Orthopaedics* to financial self-sufficiency and profitability early on. In 1962, less than ten years after the first issue was published, the association decided that the journal's title did not reflect the large numbers of research papers published and thus renamed it *Clinical Orthopaedics and Related Research (CORR)*.

DePalma stayed on as editor-in-chief for 16 years. Marshall Urist succeeded DePalma in 1966 as editor-in-chief, holding the position for 27 years. Carl Brighton of Philadelphia (the former long-time Chairman of the Department of Orthopaedic Surgery at the University of Pennsylvania) succeeded Urist. Upon Brighton's retirement, Richard Brand assumed the editorship.

Clinical Orthopaedics and Related Research began publishing at about the same time that orthopaedic surgery became established as a medical specialty. The serious young founders of the ABJS and their journal had just returned from World War II. Most of them had gained experience and confidence in trauma and fracture care and were ready to accept the new developments in orthopaedics, including total joints, new concepts in spinal surgery, and arthroscopy. The symposium format enabled them to offer concentrations of information and opinion in new developments as they occurred. *CORR* singularly contributed to making orthopaedics a vital grassroots national effort.

The success of *The Journal of Bone and Joint Surgery* and *Clinical Orthopaedics and Related Research* contributed to the creation of several other publications. The specialty societies, for example, often had so many papers presented at their meetings that neither *JBJS* nor *CORR* could accommodate them. As a result, the societies founded specialty journals on their own (most of which have been discussed in previous chapters). In addition, several general interest periodicals have also been published in the past 30 years. In 1970, W. B. Saunders started its own orthopaedic journal, the *Orthopaedic Clinics of North America*. J. Paul Harvey was the guest editor of volume 1, number 1, in July 1970. The subject of his symposium was "The Multiply-Injured Patient." *Orthopaedic Clinics of North America* competed with *Clinical Orthopaedics and Related Research* for decades as orthopaedics increased in importance and medical publishing flourished. Saunders has since been absorbed into the Dutch publishing conglomerate Elsevier, and Lippincott (J. B. Lippincott, subsequently merged with Williams & Wilkins) has been absorbed into the Wolters Kluwer publishing giant from The Netherlands.

In 1970, McNamara Publishing started its journal, *Orthopedic Review*, with an editorial board of prominent orthopaedists—Burr Curtis, M.A.R. Freeman, Alexander Garcia, Nicholas Giannestras, Ted Hartman, Carol Lauren, Robert Ray, and Robert Siffert. The price of a subscription was a modest $25 per year, but it carried a large number of advertisements for orthopaedic products. The *Orthopedic Review* became the *American Journal of Orthopedics* in 1995, and is currently published by Quadrant HealthCom of Chatham, New Jersey. Sixty-eight orthopaedic surgeons are on the editorial staff.

SLACK Inc. began publishing its journal, *Orthopedics*, in 1977. It also featured a long list of prominent editorial associate editors, a North American board of editors, an international board, and a consultant board. Andrew Wissinger of Pittsburgh was the first editor-in-chief. He was replaced later by Robert D'Ambrosia of New Orleans. Another journal named *Orthopedics* predates the SLACK publication. Founded in 1958, it was copyrighted by Bruce Cameron, of Houston. Its mission was to provide information about orthopaedic surgery to nonorthopaedists. It discontinued publication after only a few years of existence. The editorial advisory board for this first *Orthopedics* included well-known orthopaedists Ralph Gorman, G. W. N. Eggers, Hiram Kite, Daniel Riordan, Edward Henderson, G. E. N. Thomson, Robert Murray, Edward Singleton, and Maria Stone. The first *Orthopedics* journal sponsored the "Orthopedics Mercy Ship," a 110-foot shallow draft, former hospital station-keeping vessel. Cameron announced in the journal in 1959 that the ship would be supplied by air anywhere in the world where it might be needed. The name of the ship was the SS Dorin.[9]

There are now too many journals related to orthopaedic surgery to describe them in detail. The AAOS in 1993 began publication of its own journal, the *Journal of the American Academy of Orthopaedic Surgeons* (see Chapter 11). *JAAOS* is devoted to clinical reviews and is provided as a member-benefit to all of its members, including residents. The market for medical journals is complex, competitive, fickle, and increasingly subject to inroads by non-print media. Almost certainly, orthopaedic surgeons will depend more on the Internet and other electronic delivery mechanisms for their information as they become more comfortable with these media, challenging the dominance of print publications. (See the discussion in Chapter 11 about AAOS developments in electronic education.)

For modern orthopaedic surgeons, the problem is not lack of information, but perhaps too much material and so little time. Large professional societies such as the AAOS, smaller orthopaedic societies, the major publishers, and smaller start-ups all have crowded into the orthopaedic information market, giving orthopaedic surgeons access to hundreds of sources of new and review information.

Textbooks

Up until the last quarter of the 20th century, books had the predominant role in transmitting medical knowledge. For orthopaedic surgeons, serious preparation for board examinations, pending surgery, or general learning required one's own library or access to a hospital or university library. Now, online learning often supplements printed material, and as time progresses, print may become even less important in the education of physicians in general and orthopaedic surgeons in particular. Nevertheless, ambitious authors continue to write or edit books, publishers continue to print them, and orthopaedists buy enough of them to make it somewhat profitable. In 2004, for example, Wolters Kluwer's imprint Lippincott Williams & Wilkins and Elsevier's imprints W. B. Saunders and Churchill-Livingstone offered a total of 36 books related to orthopaedics. There are titles covering arthroscopy, bone form and function, fractures, the hip, the knee, orthopaedic nursing, and posture disorders—multivolume productions costing hundreds of dollars. In addition, the AAOS publishing program produces 10 to 15 texts each year, ranging from specialty surgical texts to monographs.

Louis Bauer and Lewis A. Sayre probably published the first American books in orthopaedics in 1868 and 1876, respectively.[10,11] They had compiled their lectures given at the Brooklyn Medical and Surgical Institute and the Bellevue Medical College in New York to create 300-page texts with multiple chapters. They covered the subjects of deformities, talipes (foot deformities such as bunions), knee diseases and deformities, morbus coxarius (hip disease, usually tuberculous), the spine, ankylosis, and miscellaneous topics such as deformities resulting from nerve injury or disease.

Other texts slowly followed in the 19th century, especially those by British orthopaedists, and in the early 20th century American orthopaedists began publishing their own books in larger numbers. Willis Campbell's *Operative Orthopaedics* in the early 1930s became the model for other texts to follow.

Research in Orthopaedics

In the mid-1950s, orthopaedic surgeons realized that the future of their specialty held great promise. Individuals from diverse places and backgrounds developed new biomaterials, operations, and paradigms for treating musculoskeletal disorders. It was a time of considerable ferment in orthopaedic surgery, and it was not clear where the specialty was headed. Investigators needed financial support, and a few senior members of the specialty looked for ways to fund them to encourage research in orthopaedics. Preeminent among these was Alfred Shands, Jr. (Figure 54). His presidential address at the AOA in 1954 sparked interest in research funding and inspired the formation of the Orthopaedic Research Society (ORS) and the Orthopaedic Research and Education Foundation (OREF).[12] Joseph Barr, Jr. James Dickson, Francis McKeever, Harold Sofield, and Philip Wilson joined Shands in forming the OREF. The ORS had been established the previous year, in 1955; the OREF combined the efforts of the AOA, the AAOS, and the ORS in raising money for orthopaedic research. Shands was the son of Alfred Shands, Sr., who had been an orthopaedic surgeon and president of the AOA many years before. Shands, Jr. graduated with a medical degree from the University of Virginia in 1922 and received his residency training at Johns Hopkins. In 1930, he founded the Department of Orthopaedics at Duke University, but left Duke seven years later when he was recruited by Albert I. DuPont to head the newly established DuPont Institute in Wilmington, Delaware. Shands served in that capacity until 1962. The OREF has since provided over $52 million through 1,700 grants for research in musculoskeletal disease. The foundation employs all the techniques of modern fund-raising very effectively.

The ORS, founded in 1954 and with a current membership of 2,230, is not the fund-raising arm of orthopaedic research, but does confer grants and awards for excellence. It has an annual meeting and participates in educational activities at the Annual Meeting of the AAOS. It seeks mentors for young investigators, publishes its transactions and a newsletter, and supports the *Journal of Orthopaedic Research*. The journal presents new information on basic science, bioengineering, and clinical aspects of orthopaedic research, as well as composition, structure, and material properties of tissues important to orthopaedic surgeons.

The National Institutes of Health (NIH) also funds and conducts research in musculoskeletal diseases. The NIH began as part of the U.S. Public Health Service, the agency that provided care to the Coast Guard and Merchant Seamen.[13] During the second half of the 19th century, when European-backed bacteriologists made discoveries that helped rein in the epidemics, the Public Health Service developed "laboratories of hygiene" in an effort to bring American public health up to European standards. In 1930, the name of the Hygiene Laboratories was changed to the National Institute of Health, and several years later Congress appropriated funds to establish a National Cancer Institute. After World War II, the NIH began to fund grants for research in various medical disciplines, with a budget that went from $8 million in 1947 to $1 billion in 1966.

Orthopaedics did not fare well in the NIH grant sweepstakes, because applications for funding orthopaedic research were reviewed by the National Institute of Arthritis and Metabolic Diseases. Diabetologists seemed to dominate that institute and musculoskeletal research funding lagged. In April 1986, however, the NIH opened a new institute, the National Institute of Arthritis and Musculoskeletal and Skin Diseases (NIAMS) in response to the burgeoning significance of orthopaedic research. AAOS officers, including several former presidents of the Academy, lobbied congressional committees aggressively to achieve this. NIAMS has funded research into such musculoskeletal topics as hyaluronic acid as a biomarker for osteoarthritis, the genetic basis for bone diseases, antibody treatment of muscular dystrophy, and the relationship between the surgeon's experience and the procedure outcome for patients who have had total joint operations.

References

1. Flexner S, Flexner JT: *William Henry Welch and the Heroic Age of American Medicine.* New York, NY, Viking Press, 1941.

2. Fleming D: *William H. Welch and the Rise of Modern Medicine.* Boston, MA, Little, Brown, 1954.

3. Flexner A: *I Remember.* New York, NY, Simon & Schuster, 1940.

4. Flexner A: *An Autobiography: A Revision Brought Up to Date.* New York, NY, Simon & Schuster, 1960.

5. Flexner A: Medical education in the United States and Canada: A report to the Carnegie Foundation for the Advancement of Teaching; with an introduction by Henry S. Pritchett, president of the Foundation. Bulletin Number Four. New York, NY, 1910.

6. Henderson M: The American Board of Orthopaedic Surgery. *J Bone Joint Surg Am* 1935;17:240-242.

7. Cooper DY: The evolution of orthopaedic surgeons from bone and joint surgery at the University of Pennsylvania. *Clin Orthop Relat Res* 2000;374:17-35.

8. Derkash RS: History of the Association of Bone and Joint Surgeons. *Clin Orthop Relat Res* 1997;337:306-309.

9. Cameron BM (ed): Orthopedics mercy ship. *Orthopedics* 1959;1:293.

10. Bauer L: Lectures on orthopaedic surgery delivered at the Brooklyn Medical and Surgical Institute. New York, NY, William Wood, 1868.

11. Sayre LA: Lectures on Orthopaedic Surgery and Diseases of the Joints; delivered at Bellevue Hospital Medical College during the winter session of 1874-1875. New York, NY, D. Appleton, 1876, pp 549-551.

12. Shands AR Jr: Responsibility and research in orthopaedic surgery. *J Bone Joint Surg Am* 1954;36:695-703.

13. http://www.nih.gov/about/history.htm. (Accessed April 10, 2007)

CHAPTER 11
THE AMERICAN ACADEMY OF ORTHOPAEDIC SURGEONS

Introduction

The American Academy of Orthopaedic Surgeons (AAOS, or the Academy) was formed in 1933 by a group of orthopaedic surgeons who recognized the need for a national organization (Figure 55). (See chapter two for a more detailed accounting of the Academy's founding.) Without it, orthopaedics surely would have remained a small subset of general surgery and the revolution in musculoskeletal surgery in the last half of the 20th century would have occurred in a much different fashion. The Academy's inclusive fellowship of musculoskeletal surgeons facilitated this revolution, providing a forum for its participants to exchange new methods and advance the interests of orthopaedics. Like any large organization, however, it has had to balance the interests of the membership as a whole against the subspecialty interests of some members within it. The orthopaedic specialty societies have provided a powerful magnet to attract members seeking the fellowship of orthopaedic surgeons interested in narrower segments of orthopaedics. Thus, the Academy has worked to communicate the importance of membership in broad-based regional and national organizations. The Academy has encouraged the growth of state and regional orthopaedic societies. Also, in 1973, it formed the Board of Councilors that now consists of delegates from all 50 states in numbers proportional to the numbers of orthopaedic surgeons in each state, in the territories, and the military. In 1984, it formed the Council of Musculoskeletal Specialty Societies (COMSS) with representatives from the various subspecialty groups. In 2006, COMSS was renamed the Board of Orthopaedic Specialty Societies (BOS). Both the Board of Councilors and the Board of Orthopaedic Specialty Societies appoint members to the Board of Directors of the Academy. The AAOS also offers support services to other health care professional groups such as orthopaedic nurses, administrators, physician assistants, and special identity societies such as the Society of Military Orthopaedic Surgeons, the Ruth Jackson Orthopaedic Society, most of whose members are women, and the J. Robert Gladden Society, most of whose members are from racial and cultural minority groups.

Regional and State Orthopaedic Societies

The reputed first regional orthopaedic society, the Interurban Orthopaedic Club, held its first meeting in Boston in November 1907. A note in *The*

Tech, a student newspaper at the Massachusetts Institute of Technology (MIT), reported: "This club is an association of the younger orthopaedists of Boston, New York, Philadelphia, Baltimore, and other cities." Herman Marshall, a professor at MIT, gave a presentation on the "causation of chronic arthritis." The Interurban Orthopaedic Club still exists. It has one officer, a managingdirector, a position currently held by Edward Hanley of Charlotte, North Carolina.

The Clinical Orthopaedic Society (COS), founded in 1912 as the Central States Orthopaedic Club, offered "observations in different cities of matters related to orthopaedic surgery and the free discussion amongst its members of orthopaedic methods and teaching." COS originally drew orthopaedists from Illinois, Indiana, Iowa, Kansas, Louisiana, Michigan, Minnesota, Missouri, Nebraska, Ohio, Tennessee, and Wisconsin, and the club featured case presentations at its meetings. Seven members of the COS had a lasting effect on orthopaedic surgery, having promulgated the idea of a national organization, then actually founding the Academy. In fact, the AAOS held its first meeting in conjunction with the COS in 1933. The COS still holds annual meetings but has become a national organization and limits its membership to 750. It still requires its members to present papers accompanied by a demonstration with patients in person (by video if the patients cannot attend the meeting). The role of a regional orthopaedic society for the Midwest has been assumed by the Mid-America Orthopaedic Association.

The Western Orthopaedic Association was founded in 1932 as a result of several joint meetings of the Los Angeles and San Francisco Orthopaedic Clubs. The Los Angeles club was organized in 1922 as the first orthopaedic club west of the Mississippi River by Charles Leroy Lowman, Ellis Jones, Halbert Chancel, Alfred Gallant, Steele Stuart, John Dunlap, and John Wilson, Sr. The San Francisco group (Walter Baldwin, Howard Markel, Leonard Ely, Arthur Fisher, James Watkins, Thomas Stoddard, Edward Bull, Jack Haas, and James McChesney) organized their society a year later. The two clubs held joint meetings for several years but decided to merge in the early 1930s. The original constitution of the Western Orthopaedic Association established three chapters that subdivided the membership among three districts: northern (Washington, Oregon, British Columbia), central (northern California, Nevada, Utah), and southern (southern California, Arizona, New Mexico, Hawaii). The districts have since increased from 3 to 19.

The Eastern Orthopaedic Association began in 1970 at a Quad City Orthopaedic Club meeting in Washington, D.C. Orthopaedic surgeons from New York, Philadelphia, Baltimore, and Washington, D.C., had met informally but in large numbers for a few years; Howard Steel, a Philadelphian, made a stirring speech at the 1970 meeting that galvanized the membership into forming the Eastern Orthopaedic Association. It meets annually and, like its western counterpart, offers a scientific meeting and diverse social activities in a resort location.

The Mid-America Orthopaedic Association and the Southern Orthopaedic Association began in 1982 and 1983, respectively, with the same kind of mission statements that include education along with "fellow-ship and socialization among members." Although generally serving the Midwest and Southeast respectively, these associations overlap somewhat, both offering membership to orthopaedic surgeons in 28 states.

In addition to these regional societies, orthopaedic surgeons are orga-nized into 50 state societies. California's is the largest and Wyoming's is the smallest. State societies work locally on legislative and regulatory issues affecting orthopaedic surgeons unique to each state. Each state society also can send representatives to the Board of Councilors of the AAOS. Many of the state orthopaedic societies have fairly recent origins, but several have been in existence for decades.

The Academy's Board of Councilors

In the early 1970s, some members of AAOS felt that the Academy's the Board of Directors had lost touch with the rest of the Academy's fellowship. At several rancorous Annual Meetings, some members attempted a repudi-ation of the leadership, which they claimed had long ignored the rank and file. To avert further divisiveness, the directors of the Academy organized the Board of Councilors, providing the membership at large with a forum for discussing problems affecting orthopaedic surgeons and for offering advice to the Academy leadership through a resolution process. The chair, chair-elect, and secretary of the Board of Councilors by virtue of their offices became members of the Board of Directors of the Academy; in this way, among others, the members of the Academy had access to the leader-ship of the AAOS. The Board of Councilors held its first meeting in 1973, electing Eugene Nordby as president, Herbert Stark vice president, and Jerome Cotler as secretary. Generally, each year, the officers move up in the leadership line.

Since its inception, the Board of Councilors has convened three times a year, once at the Annual Meeting of the Academy, once in a resort-type location, and once in a major city. Since 1988, that city has been Washington, D.C., where the councilors are expected to visit their state's senators and congressmen to discuss national issues important to orthopaedic surgeons and their patients.

Orthopaedic Specialty Societies

In the early 1980s, the Board of Directors of the Academy, recognizing the strong tendency toward specialization within orthopaedics, launched an ini-tiative to retain specialists within the larger national framework of orthopaedic surgery. The directors invited the presidents and other repre-sentatives of orthopaedic specialty societies to discuss ways to prevent increasing fragmentation of the specialty. The directors decided that the Academy would sponsor a Council of Musculoskeletal Specialty Societies (COMSS) that, like the Board of Councilors, would have at least two seats on the Board of Directors of the Academy. Moreover, a full day at the

Academy's Annual Meeting would be devoted to the specialty societies, and each would have the opportunity to present a program during Specialty Day at the Annual Meeting. The criteria for an organization's membership in COMSS were carefully defined, and because members and guests at the Academy's Annual Meeting would have to buy tickets to attend a specialty society's presentation, Specialty Day generally became a profitable endeavor for the societies. Many of the specialty societies are housed at the AAOS headquarters building; while some are managed by AAOS staff members, others are totally independent of the Academy.

Related Societies

There are numerous non-physician orthopaedic organizations, each with its special focus and individual membership: orthopaedic physicians' assistants, orthopaedic nurses, and orthopaedic administrators, for example.

The American Society of Orthopaedic Physicians' Assistants was established and incorporated in 1976. It holds meetings annually and has developed a National Board for Orthopaedic Physicians' Assistants. It administers an examination and has eligibility requirements of five years of experience working for a board-certified orthopaedic surgeon. The examination covers anatomy, physiology, musculoskeletal conditions, history taking, physical examination, imaging studies, laboratory investigations, and office treatment procedures as well as perioperative care.

The American Academy of Physician Assistants (AAPA), established in 1968, represents physician assistants (PAs) in all medical and surgical specialties. Today there are almost 70,000 PAs with more than 5,000 certified PAs who practice in the orthopaedic field. There are 134 accredited PA educational programs nationwide that run an average of 26 months. Most students have a bachelor's degree and several years of health care experience. This background is necessary to prepare for the rigorous PA curriculum, which consists of classroom and laboratory instruction in the basic, medical, and behavioral sciences. Students take clinical rotations in a number of specialty areas. After graduation from a certified PA program, PAs are required to pass the Physician Assistant National Certifying Examination, which assesses their general medical and surgical knowledge. The AAPA has a joint national office with the Association of Physician Assistant Programs in the Washington, D.C., area.

The National Society of Orthopaedic Administrators (BONES Society) was founded in 1969 by four orthopaedic administrators. It also holds an annual meeting but does not offer certification or an examination. The program for the 2006 BONES Society meeting in Phoenix included sessions on "Orthopaedic Coding: Getting The Right Reimbursement," "Orthopaedic Management," "Joint Ventures," "Cost Management," and other business topics germane to administration of an orthopaedic practice. The Academy provides BONES with administrative services.

Founded in 1980, the National Association of Orthopaedic Nurses (NAON) holds an annual meeting at which members and guest speakers present papers on issues pertinent to the role of the orthopaedic nurse. In recent years, sample topics have included "A Nurse-Directed Osteoporosis Prevention Center: 20 Years and Running," "It's What Matters to Patients— Working a Partnership with Patients to Improve Care," "Unleashing the Leadership Within," and "Advancing Evidence-Based Practice in Orthopaedics through Informatics." Many other papers cover more directly clinical subjects such as pain management, deep vein thrombosis prevention and treatment, and the psychological aspects of caring for adolescents undergoing spinal fusions for scoliosis. NAON also presents continuing education courses during the Academy's Annual Meeting.

NAON offers a certifying examination through the Orthopaedic Nurses Certification Board. The eligibility requirements for taking the examination include a full, unrestricted RN license and a minimum of 1,000 hours of work experience in orthopaedics in the past 3 years. Members of NAON also have access to the association's official journal, *Orthopaedic Nursing*; many of its articles qualify for continuing education credits.

Special Interest Orthopaedic Societies

The AAOS also provides staff and services to groups organized around factors other than specialty, region, or services related to orthopaedic surgery. These include the Ruth Jackson Orthopaedic Society, the J. Robert Gladden Orthopaedic Society, and the Society of Military Orthopaedic Surgeons.

When the Academy was founded in 1933, Ruth Jackson was in active practice with Arthur Steindler treating polio patients at the University of Iowa. All male orthopaedic surgeons so engaged at that time were ensured membership in the Academy, but Jackson, despite her qualifications, was denied automatic entrance to the Academy. She had to pass the board examination first, and did so in 1937. She was, in fact, the first woman to pass the board examination in orthopaedics and was the first female member of the AAOS.

Jackson practiced for 57 years. She published numerous articles and earned a solid reputation as a serious spinal specialist with her book *The Cervical Syndrome*. She treated 15,000 neck injuries, which enabled her to write authoritatively on the subject of whiplash and more severe cervical spine trauma. Ruth Jackson died in 1993.

In 1983, a group of women who practiced orthopaedics founded the Ruth Jackson Orthopaedic Society "as a support and networking group for the growing number of women orthopaedic surgeons." The organization began with 42 members and has grown more than tenfold. The Ruth Jackson Orthopaedic Society meets simultaneously with the AAOS Annual Meeting and holds a separate biannual meeting as well. It features mentoring, networking, and listings of job opportunities for its members. The society also offers the Jacquelin Perry, MD Resident Research Award and the Dr. Alexandra Kirkley RJOS Traveling Fellowship Award. Jacquelin Perry began her professional career as a physical therapist at Walter Reed Hospital in Washington, DC. She served as such for 5 years before entering medical school at UCLA. After an orthopaedic residency at the University of California in San Francisco, she joined the staff at the Rancho Los Amigos, where she remained for the rest of her working years. She published prolifically on poliomyelitis, cerebral palsy, myelomeningocele, gait analysis, and other subjects, and overall produced more than 200 peer-reviewed articles. She participated in the development of the halo vest for the support of the collapsing and unstable cervical spine with her colleagues Dr. Verne Inman, Dr. Vernon Nickel, and Dr. Robert Waters. Alexandra Kirkley practiced at the University of Western Ontario as a sports medicine specialist and had a strong interest in research. She had a brilliant reputation as research scholar and investigator and won numerous grants to support her studies on shoulder injuries and their treatment. Her early death at the age of 40 in a small plane crash in 2002 deprived orthopaedics of a physician scientist who almost certainly would have made significant contributions to orthopaedics.

J. Robert Gladden in 1949 became the first African American certified by the American Board of Orthopaedic Surgery and the first elected to fellowship in the Academy. He was born in Charlotte, North Carolina, in 1911 and graduated from Long Island University in 1936 and from Meharry Medical College in the early 1940s. He obtained residency training in orthopaedics at Howard University and eventually became chief of orthopaedics there. The society named for him is a "pluralistic, multicultural organization designed to meet the needs of minority orthopaedic surgeons." Augustus White and Charles Nelson served as the program chairs for the inaugural scientific meeting of the J. Robert Gladden Orthopaedic Society in Lausanne, Switzerland, in July 2006. The meeting covered various aspects of musculoskeletal health disparities among women and minorities, such as etiology, evidence for disparity, and how to reduce or eliminate them. The program also considered how to increase diversity in orthopaedic faculties and residency programs. A forum was also held debating New Jersey Law S-144, which requires New Jersey physicians to take cultural competency training to obtain or retain a medical license from the New Jersey State Board of Medical Examiners. This law has evoked considerable controversy among physicians in general. With a membership in 2007 of 293, the J. Robert Gladden Orthopaedic Society also assists the Academy in recruiting minority medical students to consider orthopaedics as a career.

The Society of Military Orthopaedic Surgeons (SOMOS) was founded in 1958 "to provide a forum for the interchange of medical knowledge as it relates to the practice of orthopaedic surgery in the military." It holds an annual meeting, supports a newsletter (the *SOMOS Sentinel*), and offers membership to any orthopaedic surgeon who has served in the armed forces, including active duty, retired, or honorably discharged members. The programs of the meetings naturally contain a heavy emphasis on trauma-related subjects but also show that the members of SOMOS maintain an interest in oncology, basic sciences, and pediatrics.

SOMOS keeps military orthopaedists apprised of changing conditions and developments in continued deployments of American military forces in theaters of operations worldwide. At this writing, these include Afghanistan, Iraq, North Africa, and humanitarian operations for tsunami relief in Indonesia, relief after hurricanes Katrina and Rita, and earthquake relief in Pakistan. SOMOS has a unique and essential role in dissemination of information among orthopaedic surgeons serving in the military.

The AAOS Annual Meeting

The AAOS holds one of the most spectacular annual meetings of any medical or surgical organization in the world (Figure 56). In 2007, more than 30,000 people registered for the five-day event, which featured 33 symposia, 525 papers, more than 500 poster presentations, and 183 instructional courses. In addition, 19 individual orthopaedic specialty societies meet on Specialty Day. The Orthopaedic Research Society also meets on the days immediately preceding the Academy meeting. Widely recognized by medical specialty societies as innovative, the Academy's Annual Meeting has been modeled by others. Hands-on surgical skills courses have been offered from time to time, but in recent years most surgical instructional courses are done by skilled faculty and closed-circuit television. A highlight of the meeting is the series of presidential guest speakers who have included well-known politicians, writers, and commentators, and even a poet. In times less commercial than the first part of the 21st Century, the Academy's Annual Meeting included a display of homegrown inventions to be shared freely with colleagues in orthopaedic surgery; these annual displays were organized by the then Committee on Gadgets. Today the exhibit halls house colossal technical exhibits mounted by companies that compete for the orthopaedic surgeon's attention. Manufacturers' exhibit booths include sections for demonstrations, practice surgery on plastic models, and beautifully presented displays of devices and instruments. Approximately 450 companies exhibit each year.

The enthusiasm and energy at the annual meetings are almost palpable as Academy Fellows, residents, international visitors, and guests attend lectures and gravitate to the manufacturers' exhibits. The prestige of being selected to present a paper or serve as a course instructor attracts many applicants to compete for places on the program. The obvious benefits of selection eventually led to a system of blind review of papers so that those who evaluated submissions theoretically would not know the authors' identities. The Annual Meeting thus creates a democratic forum at which the work of any orthopaedic surgeon can be presented. When a discipline, technique, or method has achieved sufficient importance, the members of the program committee can organize a group of speakers to present a symposium on the subject. The instructional courses, on the other hand, provide members with the opportunity to learn about established state-of-the-art and gold-standard techniques from acknowledged experts. The symposia and instructional courses are evaluated by the attendees, and when the information is poorly presented, the selection committee seeks out new presenters and instructors. The faculties and presenters at these events are largely from the United States but, when appropriate, are drawn from centers throughout the world. This merit-based selection process has served the Academy and its fellows well in providing excellent ongoing instruction during an era of profound changes for the specialty. It is, in fact, difficult to imagine a format that could have accomplished this any better. The revolutions in total joint arthroplasty, arthroscopic surgery, fracture care, spine surgery, and other aspects of modern musculoskeletal surgery emerged from this unique educational forum. The Academy has been the focus for the multiple other clubs, societies, and associations that feed into it and rely on its services. Much of this revolves around the Annual Meeting, arguably the Academy's most important component.

The Academy meeting venues have changed over its 75-year existence. During the early years, the meeting usually took place in Chicago at the Palmer House Hotel. As meeting attendance surged, the AAOS had to find larger facilities to accommodate it. By the late 1960s, it had outgrown the Palmer House and moved on to cities such as Las Vegas, San Francisco, Atlanta, New Orleans, and Orlando, which had capacious convention centers and hotel facilities for large crowds of physicians and exhibitors. The Academy had scheduled the 2006 meeting for New Orleans, but Hurricane Katrina damaged its convention center, hotels, and services so severely that the city could not host the meeting. Ironically, this forced the Academy to move back to Chicago in 2006 for its Annual Meeting after more than a 30-year absence, but to McCormick Place, one of the world's largest convention centers, rather than to the Palmer House. Despite the date and location changes in 2006, attendance reached levels similar to previous years, a good indication of the current vitality of the organization. Successfully moving such a large meeting in less than six months is evidence of the skills of the Academy's meetings staff.

The Academy's Publishing Program

The Academy has been publishing educational books for orthopaedists and others for more than 70 years. The most popular series, or at least the most long-lived, is the *Instructional Course Lectures* volumes. Since 1942, there has been an annual volume published, based on courses given at the Academy's annual scientific meeting. First published in 1942, the series has continued in each year that there has been an Annual Meeting of the Academy. In 1986, the Academy itself began publishing these books as opposed to using an outside commercial publisher. The Academy has had a publications committee since 1947 when, according to board of directors minutes, there were so many publications being published that a group charged to organize and oversee the process had become mandatory.

The Academy's most popular publication is not aimed at orthopaedic surgeons. *Emergency Care and Transportation of the Sick and Injured* was first published in 1971 as a training text for persons desiring to become emergency medical technicians (EMTs). Based on a series of courses for "ambulance attendants" developed by the Academy's Committee on Injuries in the mid-1960s, the book, now in its ninth edition, became a best seller in vocational publishing. The first edition appeared at the same time that national training standards for ambulance drivers were being developed by the U.S. Department of Transportation; prior to that time there were no training standards for ambulance drivers, and ambulances often were converted station wagons rather than vehicles designed specifically for emergency services. Given its appearance at such a critical time, the Academy's book became the text of choice for literally hundreds of thousands of potential EMTs in its early years. With early editions sporting an orange cover, the book became known as the "Orange Book" and over the years it has had a tremendous impact on prehospital care in the United States and throughout the world, and has been translated into five languages. Orange remains the de-facto color symbolic of prehospital care, largely because of the Orange Book. Through a copublishing arrangement with Jones and Bartlett Publishers of Sudbury, Massachusetts, the Orange Book line of textbooks and ancillary publications includes more than 40 titles.

Similarly, a book based on a concept by Montana orthopaedic surgeon Robert K. Snider called *Essentials of Musculoskeletal Care*, first published in 1997, is written for primary care physicians, rather than orthopaedists. With an audience much larger than the orthopaedic community, *Essentials* has also been extraordinarily successful. It offers advice on basic musculoskeletal conditions for the nonorthopaedist.

At an educational workshop in 1979, the consensus among the participants was that the ever larger flood of orthopaedic information was exceeding the capability of orthopaedists to keep up. In response, the Academy developed a home study program entitled *Orthopaedic Knowledge Update* (*OKU*), which consists of a textbook based on three years of articles appearing in the orthopaedic literature and a general self-assessment examination. Published every three years since 1984, the highly successful *OKU* series presents a comprehensive view of new developments in the field and has spawned the publication of eight specialty *OKU*s.

Through its Committee on Evaluation, the Academy has been publishing self-assessment examinations since 1973. Its program consists of the Orthopaedic Self-Assessment Examination, 13 Orthopaedic Special Interest Examinations (OSIEs), and the Orthopaedic In-Training Examination. The orthopaedic self-assessment examination covers the entire field and consists of 250 questions. Each special interest examination on such topics as adult reconstruction, sports medicine, and spine and pediatric orthopaedics has 150 questions. The OSIEs are available on the Internet and on CD-ROM. The Academy is one of only two medical specialty societies that publishes an in-training examination for residents; in all other specialties the in-training examinations are products of the respective certifying boards.

In 1992, the Committee on Publications presented to the Council on Education a proposal to begin publishing an orthopaedic review journal, the *Journal of the American Academy of Orthopaedic Surgeons* (*JAAOS*). The proposal approved by the board of directors that year described a bimonthly publication of some 60 pages of editorial content with subjects chosen in light of an overall orthopaedic curriculum, and with invited authors. Under the leadership of John W. Frymoyer, the journal's first editor, *JAAOS* immediately became popular with Academy members. In fact, the concept of publishing articles only from invited authors soon fell by the wayside as numerous orthopaedic surgeons and others submitted articles for consideration in the new journal. A sign of its continuing popularity is that *JAAOS* moved to monthly publication in 2005.

The Academy's Continuing Medical Education (CME) Programs

Continuing medical education programs have included courses for physicians and non-physicians since 1964. Following its first course for ambulance attendants in New York City in September 1964, the Academy presented its first course for physicians: a trauma course in Atlanta in November 1964. In the early days of AAOS CME, course chairs were given great responsibility for their courses; beyond recruiting other faculty members, they usually made hotel arrangements and handled course registration within their own office, as the Academy lacked the staff to provide these functions that now seem commonplace.

One of the largest single efforts of the Academy in this area was a series of courses in the early 1970s designed to instruct orthopaedic surgeons on the proper use of chymopapain injections in the care of low back pain patients. Prohibited by the Food and Drug Administration from teaching chymopapain procedures until the drug was approved by the FDA, and given the large public demand for such treatments at the time, the Academy was challenged by tremendous demand and limited resources. Although the courses eventually met the demand, it took several years to train all those who desired this type of training. Although this type of procedure generally has fallen from favor, the training the Academy provided was a tribute to the volunteer faculty and the administrative staff.

Other courses on a wide variety of topics have been a staple of the Academy's program throughout the years. Organized by relevant CME committees, these programs generally address one specialty area in orthopaedics, as conceived by the course director and codirector and the volunteer faculty, which numbers approximately 20 orthopaedic surgeons per course.

In 1993, the AAOS joined forces with the Arthroscopy Association of North America (AANA) to construct and outfit the Orthopaedic Learning Center at a total cost of approximatly $10 million. Built at the Academy's headquarters building in Rosemont, Illinois, the OLC consists of a 5,600 sq. ft. surgical skills lab with 24 fully outfitted learning stations, along with appropriate space for instrument storage and preparation as well as separate facilities for storage and preparation of cadaveric specimens. In addition there are two lecture rooms and locker rooms, and in late 2006 the lab's audiovisual equipment was upgraded to high-definition quality. The Arthroscopy Association of North America and the Academy use the OLC for courses approximately 28 weekends per year. Other weekends and during the week, the OLC is used by industry, other medical societies, and individuals for courses and research and development requiring cadaveric specimens.

In the mid-1990s, the Academy helped its members understand the dynamics and deal with the complexities of managed care organizations through a series of seminars and conferences. These educational programs included such titles as "Managed Care, The Basics" and "Winning at Risk." AAOS also has published monographs on managed care, an audio series of conversations with practice management experts, and numerous articles and items at the Practice Management Center on its Web site.

The Academy's Electronic Media Program

Other technologies the Academy has used over the years have included sound-slide programs, 16mm movie films, and videotapes. Each of these media has been featured at the Academy's Annual Meeting, with Academy members producing the programs and submitting them to the relevant Academy committee for possible selection to be shown at the meeting. Most orthopaedists in the United States are familiar with the sight at the Academy's meeting of large numbers of orthopaedic surgeons sporting headsets and peering intently at a computer screen or video monitor, as they learn new techniques or review the work of the orthopaedists who developed the program. After the Annual Meeting, the authors of the programs donate them to the Academy, which makes copies for sale to orthopaedists who could not attend the meeting.

The Academy was the first medical specialty society to publish on CD-ROM. In 1987, the editor of *Orthopaedic Knowledge Update 3*, Dr. Robert Poss suggested that the Academy publish the full text and illustrations of all three *OKU*s on a CD-ROM as a new product to accompany *OKU 3*. He had learned about CD-ROM publishing technology by reading a story in the *Harvard Crimson* that the classics department at Harvard, had captured much of the knowledge of ancient Greek civilization and published it on a series of CD-ROMs. That storage capacity intrigued him as he thought about *OKU 3*. In addition to the text and illustrations of three full-length textbooks, the CD-ROM published in 1990 also included many of the original articles upon which the textbook was based. In embracing this new publishing technology, the Academy was challenged not only by the technical intricacies of capturing the content of three books, but with educating its potential market about what a CD-ROM was and how to access the data contained on it. Perhaps because orthopaedic surgeons often like new technology, the CD-ROM publishing program was a success from the outset with sales of the first CD-ROM exceeding 2,000 copies.

Other trendsetting electronic publishing by the Academy has included interactive multimedia education programs beginning in the mid-1990s. "Orthopaedic Grand Rounds" was a subscription series covering most specialties in orthopaedics and included patient cases selected by subject matter experts who guided the learner through the decision-making process in the care of these patients. With questions and answers relating to the individual patients, these programs included illustrations, x-rays, and videos of procedures. As CD-ROMs gave way to DVDs, storage capacity increased, which allowed for higher quality video and more complex educational programming. A series of extremely rich multimedia programs debuted in 2003 with "The Athlete's Knee," in which the learner could choose from a number of different learning experiences. Each of 10 different patients presents with a different chief complaint, mechanism of injury, patient history, and set of comorbidities. With the vast set of learning resources included on the DVD, the program includes primary research articles, surgical videos, illustrations, and imaging studies related to each patient problem.

The Academy Online

The AAOS first established its Internet presence in June 1995 with the launch of a very primitive site. Ahead of its time, AAOS was one of the first associations to do so. Over time, the site grew in size (to 30,000 static pages before a recent re-design), mission, and complexity. In 2000, the AAOS launched both Your Orthopaedic Connection (the AAOS patient education Web site) and the Personal Physician Web Sites (OrthoDoc). Using OrthoDoc and AAOS-supplied templates, any member can build a Web site for patients and the public dynamically linked to Academy resources. Later in 2000, template-driven Group Practice Web Sites were also made available to the members. The site allows the public to Find an Orthopaedist by searching the Academy's database of members by name, city and country. The AAOS member Web site was redesigned first in 2001 and subsequently in 2006.

The AAOS Web site is extensively interfaced with the internal association management system software. The software uses the Academy database to authenticate members and users of the Web site, to determine product pricing in the online catalog, for dues payments, course registrations, Find an Orthopaedist, the private membership directory, Annual Meeting registrations, committee appointment program applications, committee roster listings, address changes, and for other ancillary data. Information changed in the database is immediately reflected on the Web site. Likewise, information collected on the Web site is automatically transferred into the database. Since 2003, it has been mandatory that all poster and podium session abstracts be submitted online. The number of abstracts submitted in 2003 was 3,289. By 2007, this number had increased to 4,069.

The AAOS has used its Web site for E-commerce applications since 1996. In 2006, more than $9.3 million was garnered via the Web site, nearly 20 percent of the Academy's entire yearly revenues. This includes product sales, course registrations, dues payments, Annual Meeting registrations, and placement service fees. With online Annual Meeting registration first offered for the 1998 meeting, in 2007 almost 8,800 members and allied healthcare professionals pre-registered using the Web site (72% of the total).

The Academy has also used the Internet for educational purposes with its members. In 2001 it established *Orthopaedic Knowledge Online*, as a member-benefit service for continuing medical education. Originally conceived as a type of just-in-time education, *OKO* was intended to be a refresher for those wanting to review videos of surgical procedures. However, as *OKO* developed, it was expanded to include a template-driven online textbook or journal. Under the direction of William Grana and John Sarwark, *OKO* consists of more than 100 clinical topics, most with accompanying videos, a text-based review section, and continuing medical education activities based on clinical topics. *OKO* has forged relationships with nine specialty societies for the development and review of content. In addition, it has a virtual bookstore with selected AAOS texts available online, and a link to the Academy's Educational Resources Catalog. With more than 20,000 active users, *OKO* is updated at least monthly.

The Academy's Growing Presence Internationally

During the late 1980s international orthopaedic surgeons started attending the AAOS Annual Meeting on a regular basis. From a modest 250 attendees in 1988, today internationals comprise nearly one third of all physician attendees at the Annual Meeting, with participants coming from more than 100 nations of the world. In 1997 the Academy membership passed a bylaws amendment that allowed for a new class of membership, the International Affiliate Member. There are almost 4,000 International Affiliate Members today, many of whom attend the Annual Meeting on a regular basis. As international interest and awareness of the AAOS Annual Meeting has grown, so has demand for its educational products and services. Recognizing this trend early, and knowing international markets and customers were "the next new frontier" for AAOS, in 1994 the board of directors recommended and authorized a dedicated international function be established within the organization. A new international committee was created and international staff hired to begin the long-range strategic planning process to grow global relationships and activities. Today, AAOS is involved in global activities at many levels and continues to look for new opportunities to help meet its primary mission of orthopaedic surgeon education and improved musculoskeletal health care for patients worldwide.

As the world's third largest orthopaedic publisher, AAOS benefits from a robust and growing international rights and distribution business managed by International Department staff. AAOS works with independent book distribution agents to have its English language print and electronic education products distributed worldwide and is an active participant in the annual Frankfurt Book Fair held each October in Frankfurt, Germany, AAOS books, journals, and electronic media products are available as translated editions in eight world languages. In 2007, international product sales reached an astounding $1 million, contributing to 14 percent of total product sales revenue.

Organized through the AAOS international committee and hosting international orthopaedic societies, each year AAOS conducts seven to nine international education programs throughout the world. Participation is by invitation only; AAOS does not conduct independent education programs in any country other than the United States without the express personal invitation of the national or regional orthopaedic society in any country or region. Program proposals are presented to the International Committee for review and approval a minimum of 18–24 months in advance of the planned program. U.S. faculty size can be as small as three or four or as large as twenty. The majority of programs are incorporated into the scientific program of a society's annual scientific congress, though some are delivered as independent, free-standing programs. Cooperative agreements are reached over details of program logistics, faculty travel, and housing and so forth. As appropriate, AAOS staff may accompany faculty and assist with on-site logistics and also work at the AAOS exhibit stand provided by the program host. AAOS staff manage the daily oversight of program development and implementation, working directly with the AAOS course director and faculty and the International Committee member liaison assigned to the program.

In addition to the cooperative education program ventures noted, AAOS also undertakes humanitarian outreach programs and scholarship programs on an annual basis, and this aspect of AAOS global initiatives is expanding. In 2008 AAOS hopes to begin the first of a four-year-long program of Basic and Advanced Orthopaedic Education for the West Africa region. AAOS also remains active in other areas of the world, including Iraq and parts of Latin America.

Inaugurated in 2005, the AAOS Annual Meeting Guest Nation Program was established to foster greater awareness and recognition of the contributions made to the practice of orthopaedics from the many nations of the world, and also enhance the very real and already robust international flavor of the AAOS Annual Meeting. Further, it is intended to raise awareness of the social and cultural richness of the many countries of the world. To date, Spain, Argentina, and Thailand have been honored with Guest Nation status. A number of planned special events are built into the five-day AAOS Annual Meeting.

Communicating with Members

Like most associations, AAOS has devoted much energy and significant resources to communicating with its members. With the Academy, such communication has taken numerous forms. Largely relying on letters from the president in its early years, the Academy's communication program took a step up in 1953 when it began publishing its *Bulletin*. Over the years the *Bulletin* was published according to a number of schedules: intermittently, quarterly, and bimonthly. Subjects covered in the *Bulletin* have included Academy events, personalities, health care policy, and ethics and professionalism. In early 2007, the *Bulletin* was replaced by a tabloid style publication, *AAOS Now*, which began publishing monthly in May. This new publication has focused on major issues in orthopaedics including scientific developments, professional issues, Academy accomplishments, Academy political activities, and practice management issues. Since 1996, the AAOS has produced a daily newspaper at the Annual Meeting; originally titled *Academy News*, the publications are now the Annual Meeting daily editions of *AAOS Now*.

The AAOS has also dabbled in television. For three years beginning in April 1987, the Academy's weekly half-hour television program "Orthopaedic Surgery Update" appeared on Lifetime Medical Television. Hosted by Clement B. Sledge, the program included guest experts in two or three specialty areas discussing their approaches to musculoskeletal conditions accompanied by videos of procedures shot for this program. As part of LMT's *Physicians' Sunday*, the Academy's program drew the largest percentage of member viewers of any of the *Lifetime Sunday* programs for physicians presented by other societies. In 1993, at its own expense the Academy produced a television show broadcast on in-hotel cable channels during the Annual Meeting in New Orleans. In other years, AAOS has hired outside companies to develop and mount similar programming at the Annual Meeting.

Public and Media Relations

The AAOS has had a public relations program since the mid-1970s. It has grown in scope and complexity during the past 10 years, but prior to its major expansion in 1999 it included brochures and booklets for patients, public service announcements for radio and television, video news releases, and media training for board members and others who might be called upon to represent the Academy in the media. In 1998, a study of consumer perceptions about orthopaedic surgeons revealed the public's mixed attitudes about orthopaedic surgeons: while they respected the physicians for their knowledge and their high tech approaches to musculoskeletal conditions, in general they were less complimentary about the surgeons' abilities to communicate with patients. The study became known around the Academy as the high tech-low touch study—orthopaedic surgeons were ahead of the curve when it came to employing the latest advances in care, but fell behind in terms of relating to their patients. Additional research showed that Fellows believed that a public relations program should position orthopaedists as the best source of musculoskeletal care, differentiate orthopaedic surgeons from their competition, and raise public awareness of treatments and procedures performed by orthopaedic surgeons.

A public relations department was created in July 1999 to implement these activities under the strategic direction set by the Public Relations Task Force and later, the Council on Communications. The council was officially launched following the Academy's 2000 Annual Meeting; its first chair was Dr. Stuart Hirsch. In 2006 the Council on Communications officially became the Communications Cabinet.

The Academy's public relations goals are to enhance the image and credibility of orthopaedics, to promote the role of orthopaedic surgeons as the primary providers of musculoskeletal care, to establish the AAOS as the premier source of musculoskeletal information, and to demonstrate the difference orthopaedic surgeons make in their patients' quality of life.

The Academy's wide ranging public relations program includes the following:

- Yearly multimedia public service announcements for TV, radio, print, and advertising at airports
- A Community Orthopaedic Awareness Program consisting of PowerPoint presentations for Fellows to use in their communities
- Legacy of Heroes, a film, book, exhibit, and Web site documenting the contributions of orthopaedic surgeons in World War II
- Safe, Accessible Playgrounds. At the Annual Meeting orthopaedic surgeons and exhibitors build a playground in the host city and leave as a legacy a safe and accessible playground where children with and without disabilities can play together
- eMotionPictures: An Exhibition of Orthopaedics in Art, an art exhibition which tells the story of the impact of musculoskeletal conditions on people's lives, through artwork created by artists with orthopaedic conditions and the orthopaedic surgeons who treat them
- Humanitarian Awards, recognizing Fellows of the Academy who have distinguished themselves through outstanding musculoskeletal activities in the United States and abroad
- Patient Safety and Patient-Centered Care programs highlighting and promoting safe, effective, and timely medical care through cooperation among the physician, informed and respected patient, and a coordinated health care team
- Nationwide media relations programs promoting diversity and culturally competent care

In 2003, at the urging of John Tongue and the AAOS Council on Education, the Academy earmarked about $180,000 to train selected orthopedists in a week-long patient-physician communications education program. This cadre became the nucleus of the Communications Skills Mentoring Program (CSMP), in which these fully trained mentors provide communication skills training to residents in training as well as practicing orthopaedic surgeons. In this program, mentors have given standardized training in proven techniques to more than 4,000 orthopaedic surgeons and residents. In addition, there have been numerous articles in the *Bulletin*, *AAOS Now*, and *JAAOS* on the importance and key skills in communicating effectively with patients. It is expected that the 1998 study will be repeated to help measure the impact of the CSMP training program.

The Academy's Research Activities

The AAOS has never engaged in primary bench research, although it has lobbied for establishing and funding the intramural program in musculoskeletal diseases at the National Institutes of Health. The Academy's research activities have revolved instead around the incidence, prevalence, and economic impact of musculoskeletal conditions in the United States. Beginning in 1978, the Academy has funded and published a series of monographs that examine the overall impact of musculoskeletal conditions in terms of such measures as economic costs for treatment, loss of productivity by injured workers, days lost from school or work, and other quantifiable benchmarks. The most recent edition of this work, published in 2000, estimated the total economic impact from musculoskeletal diseases and conditions at $254 billion per year. This work, *Musculoskeletal Conditions in the United States*, was the basis and model of research activities conducted worldwide during the international Bone and Joint Decade, 2000-2010. The latest edition of this work is scheduled for publication in 2008. The Academy also has collected and published statistics on orthopaedic surgeons and orthopaedic procedures, which can be found at its Web site.

The AAOS and Medical Liability Reform

Through a multidisciplinary organization called Doctors for Medical Liability Reform, recent initiatives by the AAOS and other medical specialty societies have attempted to address these issues nationally, but the state societies potentially have a more important role because laws and regulations vary from state to state. In early 2004, the AAOS board of directors adopted tort reform as a major policy initiative, becoming a founding member of Doctors for Medical Liability Reform. In addition, the Academy used much stronger statements in its own official pronouncements on the subject of medical liability reform, for instance: "The AAOS is deeply concerned about skyrocketing medical liability costs and its effect on patient access to care" and claimed that orthopaedists are "moving away, retiring earlier, and limiting services because of the continuous threat of litigation and high insurance premiums." At the federal level, orthopaedic surgeons under the aegis of the AAOS have testified before congressional committees, such as the House Small Business Committee and the Energy and Commerce Committee, regarding the effect of excessive litigation and high insurance rates, citing loss of patient access, the beneficial effect on insurance premiums of reasonable caps on awards for pain and suffering, a General Accounting Office report that confirmed instances of reduction in services, and increased cost for orthopaedic care due to the practice of defensive medicine. The Academy has also issued strong statements on the measures necessary for tort reform such as caps, limitations on attorney fees, and restrictions on the statutes of limitations.

In 2006, these initiatives seemed to have met with some success because the United States House of Representatives voted for responsible tort reform legislation and the president, George W. Bush, said he would sign the bill. The United States Senate, however, failed to pass these measures.

The Academy offers its financial and other support to state societies dealing with the medical liability crisis at the state level but primarily focuses on legislation on the national level and providing a mechanism to curtail abuses connected with expert witness testimony.

The AAOS Professional Compliance Program

Fellows of the Academy have also complained about unqualified, untruthful, or fraudulent expert witness testimony. The high fees associated with providing expert witness testimony and the chance that an even higher fee might be contingent on the outcome of the case have led some Academy members to engage almost exclusively in this practice, to the consternation of their Academy colleagues.

The leadership of the Academy has dealt aggressively with this issue in response to continuing complaints from the membership. In 2004, it established a Professional Compliance Program that at this writing consists of the following Standards of Professionalism:

- Providing Musculoskeletal Services to Patients
- Orthopaedic Expert Witness Testimony
- Professional Relationships
- Orthopaedists–Industry Conflicts of Interest
- Research and Academic Responsibilities
- Advertising by Orthopaedic Surgeons

In the instance of expert witness testimony, or any of the Standards of Professionalism, a Fellow may file a grievance against another Fellow who is thought to have violated one of the standards, for example, testified fraudulently or inappropriately. After administrative review, the complaint is heard by the Committee on Professionalism. After reviewing the case, the committee can reject the grievant's complaint, or if it decides the complaint has merit, can recommend to the Board of Directors censure, suspension, or expulsion for the Fellow believed to have delivered the fraudulent testimony. The respondent may appeal this decision to a higher level authority, the Judicial Committee, before it goes to the board of directors, which makes the final decision.

The AAOS and Health Policy

The AAOS did not enter health politics in a meaningful way until January 1980. During the presidency of John Gartland of Philadelphia, the board of directors appropriated $100,000 to establish an office in Washington, D.C. and hired Nicholas Cavarocchi as its official lobbyist. Prior to opening that office, various officers and members (most notably Charles Heck, Phillip Wilson, and William Donaldson) had occasionally traveled to Washington, D.C., to call on members of Congress and other regulators in an effort to influence legislation and the welter of rules and regulations that Congress was enacting.

Three main issues occupied the Washington, D.C., office in its early years. The first was the development in 1986 of a National Institute of Arthritis and Musculoskeletal and Skin Diseases (NIAMS). Gartland,

Heck, and William MacAusland, Jr. testified multiple times before House and Senate committees; eventually, Congressman Claude Pepper and Senators Orrin Hatch and Barry Goldwater introduced legislation that created the national institute directly related to orthopaedics. The Academy, in fact, lobbied three Congresses for an institute to help orthopaedic surgeons obtain research grants before legislation to establish it was passed.

The Academy also worked with multiple issues related to reimbursement for orthopaedic procedures under Medicare and Medicaid. For example, orthopaedic surgeons no longer had any incentive to perform bilateral or other multiple procedures because the Health Care Financing Administration (HCFA), now called Centers for Medicare and Medicaid Services (CMS), refused payment for the second operation. Hospitals could bill successfully under the DRG system (Diagnostic-Related Groups), but physicians often could not. The Academy conducted an analysis of the ways these decisions affected patients and presented it to HCFA to adjust the payments provided for these services, and payments for bilateral or multiple procedures were approved, albeit at a reduced rate.

The Academy also worked to place orthopaedic surgeons on panels of the U.S. Food and Drug Administration (FDA) for the evaluation of new devices and procedures. The success of this effort led the FDA to create an exhibit for the annual meeting of the Academy. The FDA has been continuously involved with the Academy's Annual Meeting. As guests of the AAOS Exhibits Committee, FDA representatives take part in a walk-through of the technical exhibit hall each year on the first morning the exhibits are open. The FDA representatives assist the committee by checking for appropriate signage on the display of devices not approved for use in the United States.

The Academy also lobbied against the practice of health maintenance organizations (HMOs) of limiting patients' access to orthopaedic surgeons. Some HMOs made it difficult for patients to see an orthopaedist by creating incentives that caused primary care physicians to withhold necessary referrals. In 1993, the Academy helped organize the Access to Specialty Care Coalition, which took on the HMO industry and achieved significant concessions in terms of access to specialists. The Academy increased its efforts and expenditures on advocacy programs throughout the mid-1990s, and some members advocated doing significantly more. Constrained by its 501(c)(3) tax status, in terms of what percentage of its revenues could be spent on advocacy, the Academy formed a 501(c)(6) organization in 1997. The American Association of Orthopaedic Surgeons, as a professional trade association, rather than a not-for-profit educational institution, was not limited in what it could spend on advocacy for its members and their patients. The Academy serves the educational and research needs of its members, whereas the Association addresses economic and regulatory components of their practices. The Academy and Association boards of directors comprise the same people, and meetings of the boards are separate but held consecutively; one meeting adjourns and the other is convened.

At the time President Lyndon Johnson pushed the legislation that created Medicare through Congress in 1964, many physicians, including orthopaedic surgeons, had a fee-for-service arrangement with their patients and insurers. Physicians had the power to set prices for their services at this time, and some feared that the creation of Medicare heralded the beginning of socialized medicine. However, many physicians saw their incomes rise with the advent of Medicare because initially the federal bureaucracy allowed them to establish their own fees, which some critics said was intended to lull physicians into accepting Medicare and the new paradigm. The government's gradualism succeeded in gaining physician acceptance, but regulators soon began to change the fees physicians could expect to receive by citing runaway inflation in health care prices. The federal Medicare program established the Resource-Based Relative Value Scale (RBRVS) approximately 15 years after the enactment of Medicare. William Hsaio, PhD, and others at the Harvard School of Public Health were retained to measure resource inputs for physician services and to establish a relative value for them to begin correcting the perceived shortcomings of the existing system of customary prevailing and reasonable charges. Hsaio and his associates[1,2] suggested that application of the RBRVS system for paying physicians would eliminate imbalances between payments for physicians performing "invasive procedures" and those providing evaluation and management services. The overall game plan was set: Once the policy makers scaled down what were thought to be excessive payments to providers of invasive procedures, they could focus their attention on measuring quality and cost effectiveness in health services.

The RBRVS study, funded by HCFA, measured the time and intensity of the service, cost to the physicians who provided it, and the costs of specialty training (actual expense and income lost by the physician during training). Using this information, it devised a monetary conversion factor (dollars per unit) to determine the "reasonableness" of charges for services in all medical specialties. The Hsaio study also compared the American physicians' fees to those of Canadian physicians; as expected, it was found that Americans charged a lot more for their services. This finding, however, bolstered the main point of the Hsaio study—that American surgeons got more money for their operations than they were worth, and that many of the procedures were "overvalued." HCFA used this study to establish rates of remuneration for services, and established tight, almost draconian controls over how physicians could behave in relationship to these payments. It adopted a take-it-or-leave-it stance with regard to physician participation. Physicians, including orthopaedic surgeons, could refuse to accept the lower rates, but if they did HCFA excluded them completely from participation in the Medicare program. Because HCFA covered all individuals over 65 years of age, for most physicians, nonparticipation would have meant a severe cut in income.[3-5] Medicaid programs operated by the various states and private insurers have taken their cue from the Medicare rate schedules and generally have modified their fees downward for all physicians, including orthopaedic surgeons.

The Academy and the Future of Orthopaedics: Getting It Straight

American orthopaedics has reached maturity as a medical-surgical specialty and the AAOS is the organization that best represents it (Figure 57). Nevertheless, several issues now confront orthopaedists and the Academy and could cloud the future of the discipline. Orthopaedics could fragment irreversibly into its multiple subspecialties if its practitioners decide that their focused interests take precedence over the broader specialty of musculoskeletal health care.

Orthopaedic surgeons have more control over fragmentation than they do over the decline in Medicare payments. The mandated annual cuts in Medicare payments combined with rising expenses (particularly medical liability insurance and legal fees) are having a negative financial impact on many orthopaedists. Physicians in general and orthopaedic surgeons in particular increasingly find themselves in the position of making less for working more. On the other hand, orthopaedic surgery has provided its practitioners with incomparable career satisfaction. The hands-on experience of curing patients of musculoskeletal disorders, relieving debilitating pain with joint arthroplasty, or reconstructing trauma victims is unique to orthopaedic surgery. The keen sense of fulfillment orthopaedic surgery provides can come only to physicians who have disciplined themselves to learn its many detailed and difficult techniques. It is a true calling, one which inspires many orthopaedic surgeons to immerse themselves in lifelong learning despite all the obstacles and setbacks. Furthermore, as the science of orthopaedics advances, more reliable ways to achieve relief of suffering will be discovered by tenacious researchers. Basic scientists, and not orthopaedic surgeons, may well provide the necessary breakthroughs, but an alert clinician and a practicing orthopaedic surgeon will have to make the necessary connections, much the same way Joseph Lister saw the utility in Louis Pasteur's research.

Finally, the need for orthopaedic surgery is perpetual. The malaligned human frame will always need to be straightened, the lame will want to walk, and the broken will need to be mended. Doctors with skill and determination to take on the treatment of tumors, infections, traumatic injuries, and deformities must be available to the people who need them. The community of orthopaedic surgeons in America and the members of the AAOS comprise a fellowship of men and women who collectively are a unique national resource that must be nurtured and preserved. They have the obligation to educate their fellow citizens and representatives regarding the importance of orthopaedic surgeons' accomplishments and how much more they could achieve. Every day, all over the United States, thousands of orthopaedists provide life-enhancing and even life-saving care. The preservation and continuation of this essential service will require orthopaedic surgeons to maintain their optimism and confidence in themselves and in their profession. Their history demands it of them.

References

1. Hsiao WC, Braun P, Dunn D, Becker ER, DeNicola M, Ketcham TR: Results and policy implications of the resource-based relative value study. *N Engl J Med* 1988;319:881-888.

2. Hsiao WC, Braun P, Dunn D, Becker ER: Resource-based relative values: An overview. *JAMA* 1988;260:2347-2353.

3. Shi L, Singh DA: Cost, Access, and Quality. Delivering Heath Care in America: A Systems Approach. Sudbury, MA, Jones & Bartlett, 2004, p 483.

4. Hunt KA, Knickman JR: Financing for health care, in Kovner AR, Knickman JR (eds): Jonas and Kovner's Health Care Delivery in the United States, ed 8. New York, NY, Springer, 2005, p 75.

5. Jacobs P, Rapoport S: Public health insurance, in Jacobs P, Rapoport S (eds): The Economics of Health and Medical Care, ed 5. Gaithersburg, MD, Aspen, 2002, p 307.

Index

Page numbers with F refer to the page number in the figure section on which the figure can be found.

A

M